Psychology and the Classics

Psychology and the Classics

A Dialogue of Disciplines

Edited by
Jeroen Lauwers, Hedwig Schwall and Jan Opsomer

DE GRUYTER

ISBN 978-3-11-071009-0
e-ISBN (PDF) 978-3-11-048220-1
e-ISBN (EPUB) 978-3-11-048062-7

Library of Congress Control Number: 2018938923

Bibliographic information published by the Deutsche Nationalbibliothek
The Deutsche Nationalbibliothek lists this publication in the Deutsche Nationalbibliografie; detailed bibliographic data are available on the Internet at http://dnb.dnb.de.

© 2020 Walter de Gruyter GmbH, Berlin/Boston
This volume is text- and page-identical with the hardback published in 2018.
Typesetting: Integra Software Services Pvt. Ltd.
Printing and binding: CPI books GmbH, Leck
Cover image: Max Ernst, Oedipus Rex © VG Bild-Kunst, Bonn 2018

www.degruyter.com

Contents

Jeroen Lauwers, Hedwig Schwall and Jan Opsomer
Introduction: Psychology and the Classics —— 1

1 Embodied Cognition and the Ancient Mind

William Michael Short
1 Fundamentals for a Cognitive Semantics of Latin: Image Schemas and Metaphor in the Meaning of the Roman *Animus*-concept —— 13

Siobhan Privitera
2 *Odyssey* 20 and Cognitive Science: A Case Study —— 32

Jennifer J. Devereaux
3 Bodies of Knowledge: Metaphor and Mnemonic Practice in Ancient Historiography —— 46

Afroditi Angelopoulou
4 Feeling Words: Embodied Metaphors in *Seven Against Thebes* —— 62

Peter Meineck
5 The Affective Ancient Theatre, a Bio-cultural Cognitive Approach —— 77

Gabriel Herman
6 The Sensed Presence as an Analytical Tool in Historical Research —— 94

Alex Wardrop, Georgie Huntley and Silvie Kilgallon
7 Transforming Knowledge: Using Arts-based Activity to Explore Classics and Therapeutic Practice —— 109

2 The Hermeneutics of Psychology

Joel Christensen
1 Learned Helplessness, the Structure of the *Telemachy* and Odysseus' Return —— 129

        Lilah Grace Canevaro
2   **Anticipating Audiences: Hesiod's *Works and Days* and Cognitive Psychology —— 142**

        Marcia Dobson
3   **Why Does Orestes Stay Mad? —— 158**

        Kyle Khellaf
4   **The Elegiac Revolution: Deleuze, Desire, and Propertius' *Monobiblos* —— 171**

        Katerina Ladianou
5   **Staging Female Selves in Sapphic Poetry —— 189**

3 Reviving Classical Ideas through the Centuries

        Luca Grillo
1   **Irony in Cicero's *post reditum* Speeches —— 207**

        Paul Earlie
2   **Psychoanalysis and the Rhetorical Tradition: Theory and Technique —— 223**

        Aaron Turner
3   **Thucydides, Groupthink, and the Sicilian Expedition Fiasco —— 239**

        Richard Seaford
4   **Mystic Initiation and the Near-Death Experience —— 255**

        Jennifer Radden
5   **Burton's *Anatomy* as Classical, and Present-Day, Mind Science —— 262**

        Christopher Gill
6   **The Psychology of Psychotherapy: Ancient and Modern Perspectives —— 278**

        Bibliography —— 293

        Index —— 323

Jeroen Lauwers, Hedwig Schwall and Jan Opsomer
Introduction: Psychology and the Classics

The present volume is a direct result of a conference devoted to this topic, which was held in March 2015 at the University of Leuven, Belgium. The title of the conference, which was the same as the title of this volume, programmatically aimed to encourage a dialogue between the disciplines of classics and psychology. The links between the two disciplines are numerous, and pertain to other fields as diverse as culture, history, hermeneutics, philosophy, rhetoric, linguistics, religion and literature.

Given the rich interrelations between these fields and the defining role of classical heritage in the establishment of the discipline of psychology (stemming from Freud's great interest in the classics, which was adopted by many of his later followers), the topic immediately seems to touch upon some of the fundamental issues of contemporary scholarship in these domains. Yet, a quick look at the synergies between both fields reveals that there are indeed some topics that have lent themselves to fairly extensive collaborations over the past few decades (especially in the field of psychoanalysis), but that there are also vast areas of scholarship that have largely remained unexplored territory.

The disciplines, once fruitfully married in Freud's discourse about the human psyche, have ever since been developed into many different directions. While an individual scholar in either one of these fields may be intimidated by the sheer variety of possibilities, this volume aims to focus on the rich *opportunities* that both research traditions have to offer to each other. It is our hope that the dialogue of disciplines will offer inspiration, not only to follow the new research models introduced in this volume, but also more generally to further explore the fruitful potential of the many possible synergies between psychology and classics.

Before introducing the potential gateways through which the contributors of this volume aim to reinvigorate the dialogue of disciplines, we would like to elaborate, for a brief moment, on the paradigmatic differences within and between both fields. If we see a dialogue as a process that is built on empathy and the urge to understand each other, a good way to start is to identify the assumptions that may prevent us from truly coming to grasp with the aims and viewpoints of the 'other' discipline.

Jeroen Lauwers, Hedwig Schwall and Jan Opsomer, University of Leuven

The Universal and the Particular

A quick look at the main purpose of the disciplines of psychology and classics may already highlight a notably different approach to human nature and human production. Bluntly generalizing, we can say that classical philology and ancient history, the original hallmarks of interpretive scholarship, have emphasized the need to regard each object from antiquity as a unique source that should be studied in its own particular sociocultural context. Such a focus on the historical context quite naturally provokes a sceptical attitude towards discourses that found their premises on the supposition that modern theories of human conduct and cognition offer a direct access to the psyche of the ancients.

Psychology, for its part, is generally inspired by the scientific tradition, and aims to discover universal laws of human thinking, feeling, and behaviour. While not being blind to the potential influence of culture on individual thinking and feeling, psychology's ultimate goal is to come to an adequate understanding of how the human psyche works in general. Both traditions have good reasons for such an approach to their respective object: while it is evident that concurrent contexts influence the meaning of a particular historical object, it is equally obvious that the common biological basis of human nature and the inevitable similarity of basic social structures inspire recurring patterns in human behaviour that allow themselves to be captured in encapsulating theories.

The methodological assumptions of both fields and their influence on mutual (mis)understanding is illustrated in a lucid article by Glenn Most about the history of Narcissus from Greek mythology on to Freud and Lacan. The article, which has been published in both German[1] and Italian[2], was delivered by Most at the end of the 'Psychology and the Classics' conference, and thus became – maybe not fully intentionally, but poignantly nonetheless – a provocative statement in the face of the general optimism about the synergies between classics and psychology that were advocated by many of the contributors to the conference.

Most demonstrated the appropriations through which the Narcissus myth was transformed in order to function in the general framework of the emerging paradigm of psychoanalysis. Most's argument boils down to the interesting yet uncomfortable question: was Narcissus a narcissist? After all, as classicists would say on the basis of the ancient sources, Narcissus did not know that the young man in the water was he himself, so this rather seems to point to an object-desire than an auto-erotic subject-desire. However, psychologists may argue that

---

1 See Most (2002).
2 See Most (2007).

the level of the text and the behaviour of Narcissus may conceal deeper desires which, in the end, still can be interpreted as narcissistic. The problem of the controversy is that Freud (and the intellectual predecessors of his who introduced the term 'narcissism' in the field of psychology) clearly read more into the myth than the text itself, from a hermeneutic point of view, may allow. Yet, such a critical focus on drives that lurk beneath the level of plain behaviour and utterances is one of the very cornerstones of the psychological paradigm. Even if we were to ask Narcissus 'are you a narcissist?' and the latter would respond 'no, I'm not', there are, from a psychologist's point of view, reasons to be sceptical about this answer, if only because of the phenomenon of the 'observer's paradox' and the unreliability of self-reports.

As Most goes on to argue, the question becomes even more provocative when applied to Oedipus: did Oedipus suffer from an Oedipus complex? Again, the Sophoclean tragedy does not really seem to allow for such an interpretation, as Oedipus did not know he killed his father and slept with his mother. Still, psychologists may argue, at some more profound level of his psyche, Oedipus may have felt an unconscious drive to act the way he does, and it is only logical that the tragedy cannot make such unconscious motives explicit. Psychologists, and especially psychoanalysts, see no reason to treat Oedipus any differently from all other human beings, who, according to some psychoanalysts, are driven by the unconscious desire to have sex with their own mother and to kill their own father.

In light of the controversy between the two fields as to what counts as a legitimate interpretation, it may not come as a surprise that the relationship between classics and psychology has been somewhat problematic. Classicists, and especially those who have not really taken notice of psychoanalysis' basic theoretical framework, may well feel that Freud and his disciples consciously and wilfully abused the original mythological material in order to lend their theories some cheap credibility. And indeed, according to the traditional standards of hermeneutics, their criticisms seem quite justified. Yet it is not that hard either to imagine psychologists feeling frustrated at being misunderstood by the majority of classical scholarship, which allegedly claims an omnipotent entitlement to (their version of) the reception of the classics.

Moreover, on the basis of Most's thesis about narcissism, another fundamental question can be asked. To what extent do the origins of psychology testify to a thoroughly self-occupied stance from our modern era, which cannot simply be transposed to the ancient world? In other words, is the focus on the psyche, as Christopher Lasch argues in his controversial book *The Culture of Narcissism* (1979), in and of itself a product (or a symptom) of modern culture's narcissistic preoccupation with the self and its well-being? Is Narcissus a modern Prometheus? And, if so, what would this tell us about the mindset of the ancient philosophers whose theories form the underpinning of many psychological assumptions and therapeutic approaches?

These dodgy issues may convince (and have convinced) many to avoid this Gordian knot altogether and turn their backs on the 'other' discipline. The contributors to this volume, however, chose to tackle the tough questions about the relation between classics and psychology head on. It is not the goal to forget about the paradigmatic confines of both disciplines, but to work within these confines, discover the interpretive frictions and possibilities, and restore a dialogue to express and maybe stretch what is thus far accepted as valid research within these two fields.

A Renewed Dialogue

After all, there are indications in our current academic climate that the dialogue of disciplines may be reinvigorated by some tendencies in both domains. On the one hand, the paradigm of classical reception studies has opened a theoretical window to look at psychological findings with a fresh pair of eyes. Notably inspired by the hermeneutic models of Gadamer, classical reception studies programmatically aim to address and theorize the inevitable process of appropriation that an interpreting subject goes through in order to make sense of a text.

By refraining from an *a priori* condemnation of the dynamics of appropriation, classical reception studies have facilitated the speculative exploration of postclassical hermeneutic models as a helpful background to understand the classics in words to which contemporary scholars and audiences can relate. Applied to psychology, the reasoning would amount to the following: while we will never be able to have an exact experience of what it was like to write or read a particular text in classical antiquity, our historical knowledge about the classical text, combined with a self-aware use of contemporary psychological insights that are part of the interpretive horizon of the scholar, brings about a self-conscious dialogue between the ancient text and the modern reader, and thus produces a form of knowledge that may not coincide with the original intention of the text, but does capture something relevant about the text's reception that can be described by the scholar. The question remains, however, whether the discourse of classical reception studies, with its Foucauldian acceptance of the discursive relativity of truth, is prepared to accept the absolute scientific truth claims at which psychology aims to arrive through its experimental methods.

Indeed – and this is the second development that reinvigorates the dialogue of disciplines – the clear advancements in cognitive science have shaped new and exciting possibilities to measure all sorts of data about the human brain and its thinking processes. The results of the experiments conducted with new devices have provided evidence for a couple of theories in the fields of philosophy and psychology that were long assumed but never proven. A notable example is the philosophical argument about the theory of embodied cognition, which is now a predominant model to frame the way in which the body thinks. While it was previously a point of contestation to start from the theory of embodied mind to interpret classical texts, the present scientific evidence removes at least part of the easy criticisms that used to be made against this application. Here again, though, there is still room for debate as to what extent we can simply assume that the mind of an ancient Greek or Roman functioned in the same manner as a modern mind (see, e.g., Meineck's discussion in this volume). Despite these reservations, it is hard to deny that the current scientific advancements in psychology have a great potential to impact discussions within other branches of the humanities, including classics.

While it is tempting to focus exclusively on these 'new' developments in both disciplines, we do not wish to discard previous traditions within classics and psychology/psychoanalysis, as they form the historical backbone of the dialogue. We do not see a necessity to make a choice between the new approaches to classics and psychology on the one hand, and the more established ones on the other, and neither do the contributors to this volume.

There are at least three good reasons to keep the scope of the dialogue as broad as possible. First, we simply have not reached the point where we can say that we know enough about the classical tradition and the psyche to dismiss all the previous traditions. Our lack of absolute knowledge necessitates a cautious approach. Second, from a social-constructivist point of view, it is important to pay homage to the historical pedigree that led up to the evolutions in classics and psychology, both for reasons of historical interests and because there is a large body of critical thinking in previous traditions that allows us to address current trends with a healthy critical attitude. Third, in order to reinvigorate the dialogue in a broad fashion, it is crucial to work within the variety of traditions that are currently active in both fields, so that there is room for numerous scholars with different profiles to take part in the mapping of the shared interests and possibilities that the intersection of both fields has to offer. The reader of this volume will find a wealth of research traditions represented, both in psychology and in classics, and will receive a concrete demonstration of the possibilities that are created by combining several paradigms within these broad fields.

The Volume

The contributions in this volume could be grouped in many different ways. One could focus on notions such as the literary genre of the classical texts, the psychological theories that are discussed, the traditional scholarly field(s) in which the contribution ought to be situated, the chronology of the texts under discussion, and so on.

In order to reaffirm the dialogical aspect of this volume, however, we have taken the interaction itself as the main criterion. In other words, in assembling the chapters of this volume, we focused on how exactly the fields of classics and psychology interact and how they mutually inform each other's findings. This brings us to a division in three main parts.

In Part One, "Embodied Cognition and the Ancient Mind", contributors look at classical texts and culture from the embodiment paradigm in cognitive psychology and cognitive linguistics. In doing so, they affirm the productivity of the theories of embodied cognition to grasp aspects of ancient thought and cultural production. William Short reads Latin texts via image schemas, dynamic patterns which are formed by reiterated recognition by the human body's sensory and motor capacities. These images do not only give coherence and structure to our experience but also to a language, such as up/down schemas, center/periphery schemas and movement schemas. This experientialist account reveals supralexical patterns in a text, which can be further broken down in oppositional pairs of values. So courage and fight is described in images which consistently reflect what is full, sharp, high and near, while cowardice and flight uses metaphors connoting empty, dull, low and far. Siobhan Privitera applies the theories of embodied cognition to a very dense passage in Homer's *Odyssey* 20. She argues that the multitude of ways to talk about Odysseus' shifting emotional state is an invaluable source to grasp how the ancients felt and thought. The richness of concepts and description in Homer's folk psychology vividly involves even modern readers in this key moment in the story, and invites them to critically assess their own narrow frameworks through which they conceptualize their feelings and thought patterns. Jennifer Devereaux, too, focuses on embodied knowledge, but applies it to ancient historiography. She convincingly illustrates how narrative verbs tie in with the metaphors used in the story, creating a semantic consistency which intensifies and enlivens the narrative movement, thus highlighting the *enargeia*, a kind of implicit rhetoric which is mnemonically dense. So Quintilian's point that unfolding a story in sensorimotor terms creates emotional processes and thereby impacts on the audience's reasoning is a rhetorical technique which is further underscored by cognitive psychology. Afroditi Angelopoulou's use of the embodied cognition perspective focuses on ancient drama's potential to create emotionality, which is, of course, essential for tragedy. More specifically, in *Seven Against Thebes* she shows how embodied metaphor works as a principal cognitive tool, influencing the audience's moral reasoning process. Again the container metaphor is central: sometimes the body overflows with energy, sometimes it ejects matter as in the gustatory metaphors of disgust. Peter Meineck's focus is on drama as well, more specifically on the perception of dramatic masks by people whose image schemas have been formed by different cultures. How universal are image schemas? Can one globalize Western notions of trauma therapy? Meineck notices that though different names are given in different contexts, types can be recognized in the series PTSD, battle fatigue, shell shock, debility syndrome or the phenomenon called "Soldier's Heart". Yet he observes that each distinctive culture has "its own scopic regime", which he illustrates with a discussion of the different neural networks operating between East Asian and Western Caucasians when perceiving human faces and theatre masks. Gabriel Herman, for his part, makes a compelling argument for the universality of "the Sensed Presence", a situation in which healthy people on the verge of death are helped by supernatural powers which actually save them. His four examples cover a wide range of instances, going from the battle of Marathon in 490 B.C., the Crusades, the First World War and an operation by the Israeli army in 2009. Healing is also central to the contribution by Alex Wardrop, Georgie Huntley and Silvie Kilgallon, whose workshop "Transforming Knowledge" explored possible relevance of the classics for therapeutic practice. As in all contributions to this chapter, links between material and mental matters are surprisingly strong: the metal of baking containers which participants of the workshop could easily emboss turned out to be material evidence of an emotive process which draws on the hopes, fears, and feelings of the participant/petitioner.

Whether focusing on literary or votive objects, all contributions in this section analyzed the tight connections between kinesthetic and sensory sensations or between mental, gestural and verbal techniques of representation. Apart from the closeness of the literal and the metaphorical, contributions showed how, on the one hand, certain metaphors respond to the same kind of embodied knowledge in many different cultures, reflecting universal moral matrices; while on the other hand metaphors ground our identification in a more specific way (as rooted in a language's idiom) and make us part of a certain emotional community.

Part Two, "The Hermeneutics of Psychology" contains contributions in which psychological theories or practices fulfill a so-called "search-light function", in that psychology provides a framework to focus on particular aspects of ancient texts and phenomena which may otherwise go unnoticed, but which can form the very basis for an original dialogue between the ancient worldview and that of modern interpreters. Joel Christensen takes the psychological category of Learned Helplessness as a hermeneutic hypothesis to bring out some intuitive folk psychology that must have informed the protagonists' (lack of) agency in Homer's *Odyssey*. Lilah Grace Canevaro analyses Hesiod's *Works and Days* as a sophisticated authorial construction designed so as to mentally and cognitively engage its audience. Using Berkenkotter's categories to measure a writer's audience awareness, Canevaro manages to show us a new self-conscious Hesiod, who deploys a number of discursive techniques to convince his reader/listener of the value of the work in front of him. Marcia Dobson revisits Aeschylus' famous trilogy. Focusing on ritualist and psychoanalytical theories, she discusses Orestes' persistent incapability to operate within the confines of normality, which she interprets against the backdrop of the transitional state of fifth-century Athens, where the trilogy came into being and was first performed. Kyle Khellaf takes us to the Roman elegy. His reading of Propertius and his reception is programmatically informed by Deleuze's and Guattari's *Anti-Oedipus*. The schizoanalytic framework that was proposed by these critics works well, Khellaf argues, for the interpretation of the multifaceted *personae* who give a voice to Propertius' multiple desires, and the Propertian reception seems to correspond more closely with rhizomatic structures – testifying to an on-going process of desire – than with the branches of the Lachmannian stemmas that are mostly used in classical philology. Katerina Ladianou also reflects on multiple voices in poetry, in this case in the lyric poetry of Sappho. Inspired by Irigaray and Cixous' feminist criticisms she argues that Sappho finds her feminine voice in a vivid feminine dialogue that expels male dominance. On the basis of a close reading of two Sapphic poems, she highlights the peculiar tone of the Sapphic voice(s).

It is hard to see these interpretations of classical texts apart from their conscious application of modern theories, yet they all claim, in some way or another, to 'bring out' something true about these texts. The contributors can thus not simply be pigeonholed as adepts of some 'post-truth hermeneutics'. The sum of their interpretative efforts amounts to the following nagging question: can modern discourses about literature, the psyche or developmental psychology reveal a truth that is nevertheless inevitably anchored in a unique and distant sociocultural climate? In a determined attempt to make sense of the narrative or other patterns in ancient descriptions, the contributors advocate a vivid interaction between psychology and the classics, an interaction that sometimes seems to violate basic assumptions from the fields by which their interpretations are inspired, but may well provoke critical discussions among psychologists and classical scholars for many years to follow.

Part Three, "Reviving Classical Ideas through the Centuries", discusses various receptions of classical ideas. The classics are here regarded as a powerful source of inspiration for the critical apparatus and the very discourse of modern psychology and philosophy. Many instances in this part illustrate that modern appropriations of ancient concepts can fruitfully be reused to revisit the ancient world. Luca Grillo offers a poignant example of this, as he categorizes various sorts of irony used by Cicero. Through a close reading of numerous Ciceronian passages, he shows that the ancients practised broader types of irony than can be found in their own theorizations. Remaining in the rhetorical sphere, Paul Earlie engages in a long overdue exercise of drawing parallels between the psychoanalytic communication of the Freudian-Lacanian kind and the Western tradition of rhetoric, which distinguishes between *logos*, *ethos*, and *pathos*. He sees similarities between Socrates' maieutic method and Lacan's use of scanding, as both are supposed to lead the interlocutor to face what he ignored; Aristotle's dialectic as a method of negative critique which is always in some sense incomplete is likened to the analyst's cautious conjectures which may eventually be replaced by the patient's 'conviction'. Aaron Turner, for his part, interprets Thucydides' narrative of Athens' disastrous Sicilian campaign as an elaborate example of Groupthink. Apart from the interesting question whether the ancients were as prone as we are to the social-psychological processes that were only described in the 1970s, Turner's provocative thesis also invites some reflection about the degree to which Thucydides' narrative itself betrays its author's intuition that the presence of others has a profound impact on the thoughts and emotions of an individual. In a dense paper, Richard Seaford makes a powerful case for the ancients' knowledge and reproduction of the Near-Death Experience (NDE) in mystic rituals. Examining a number of ancient sources, Seaford shows a remarkable discursive consistency between the ancient sources themselves, *and* between ancient descriptions of the ancient rituals and modern narrations of NDE. In a thought-provoking conclusion, he strikingly opposes the communal experience of NDE in ancient Greece to the individual-physiological discourse about NDE of our modern era. The opposition may put the self-evidence of our own individualized conception of consciousness under pressure. Jennifer Radden takes on the work *Anatomy* of the sixteenth-/seventeenth-century scholar Robert Burton. Through a careful analysis of Burton's reliance on Aristotelian, Galenic and Stoic theories, she shows how his medical theorizations of the mind were decisively informed by a selection of ancient philosophies. While some of his assumptions about the human mind seem quite naïve when confronted with the current state of the art in the mind sciences, his therapeutic insights may still be very valuable to a twenty-first century public. Building further on the notion of therapy, Christopher Gill's final chapter of this volume combines ancient and modern perspectives on psychotherapy. Comparing ancient (primarily Stoic) theories with modern cognitive and behavioral therapy, Gill's paper carefully examines which elements have been handed down from the ancients to the modern mainstream, and which have been lost in the process. The Stoicism Today project which he set up with an interdisciplinary team in Exeter appears to prove the power of ancient ideas and exercises to affect people's mental health and well-being even in our modern age.

These contributions thus form a worthy provisional end to the dialogue of disciplines in this volume, as they emphasize the continuous process of appropriation through which classics and psychology have remained relevant to each other. As ancient ideas evolve, so do the researchers, and so do their theories. The process of reception thus constitutes an infinite loop of hermeneutic circles that keep the dialogue alive.

The Dialogue Continues

Looking back on the organization of the conference, on the large response it generated from the scholarly world, and on the composition of this volume, our combined efforts seem to come at a very timely moment. In order to advance as a self-conscious scientific discipline, psychology should keep in touch with its foundations, which have notably been shaped by countless (receptions of) classical ideas. Classicists, for their part, are discovering new and exciting theories to interpret ancient ideas, texts and artefacts, and this synergy may well offer a powerful plea for the persistent relevance of the classics in the future. Both disciplines have a great potential to remind each other to look both back *and* forward. Despite the potential paradigmatic frictions discussed above, there are many rewards for those who wish to tackle the big questions head on.

We are happy to see some great initiatives that keep the dialogue alive after the convention in Leuven in March 2015. Leslie Gardner organized a conference on ancient ecstatic thought and its relation to analytical psychology in London in July 2016. Peter Meineck assembled the classical scholars working with cognitive theories in New York during the Fall of 2016. And Kyle Khellaf continues his search for a Deleuzian approach to classical philology with a panel to be held at the annual SCS meeting in Boston in 2018.

No doubt this is only the tip of the iceberg. We are indeed looking forward to the evolutions in both fields, and to the new and renewed opportunities they will offer to each other for interdisciplinary research. We kindly invite our readers to learn about the remarkable potential in this volume, to feel inspired and to partake in this on-going dialogue of disciplines.

Finally we want to thank the people who helped create this book. In the first place, there are the people from the Departments of Classics, Literature, and Philosophy of KU Leuven. We also want to thank the members of the conference's scientific committee and especially Luc Van der Stockt, who has always supported this project from the very start. Next we want to express our gratitude to Vera Gonskaya, who is responsible for much of the detailed editing work. Last but not least a big thank you to all the contributors for their smooth cooperation in the publishing process.

1 Embodied Cognition and the Ancient Mind

William Michael Short
1 Fundamentals for a Cognitive Semantics of Latin: Image Schemas and Metaphor in the Meaning of the Roman *Animus*-concept

Theories developed in the so-called "second-generation" cognitive sciences have permitted significant advances in our understanding of how human beings find linguistic and other forms of symbolic representation to be meaningful.[1] In particular, since about 1980, research coming from the "embodiment paradigm" in cognitive psychology and cognitive linguistics has demonstrated just how much people's ability to make sense of their experience is underwritten by conceptual structures and cognitive processes that emerge from interactions among brain, body, and world. Rejecting any view of cognition as abstract symbol manipulation, embodiment theorists claim that thought – and hence the structure and use of language – is in fact directly grounded in the human body's sensory and motor capacities. To the extent that Classics considers itself a broadly hermeneutic discipline that aims to shed light on the meanings elaborated by members of Greek and Roman society, it therefore seems crucial for classical scholars not only to have an awareness of the findings of this "embodied" cognitive science, but also to incorporate its insights into their interpretive strategies. For this reason, in this paper I introduce certain theoretical constructs from the cognitive interdiscipline – specifically, image schemas and conceptual metaphor – that I consider key to any psychologically realistic, humanly plausible account of meaning in ancient language and literature (and indeed in ancient culture more generally) and then go on to illustrate their analytic potential through a study of Latin's metaphorical expressions of courage and cowardice.[2]

---

[1] Differing from traditional "first generation" cognitive science which viewed cognition largely in information-processing terms – a view that has been dubbed the "mind-as-computer" metaphor – the "second-generation" cognitive sciences emphasize mental processes as embodied, embedded, enacted, and extended (generally grouped as "4E theory"): see esp. Rowlands (2010); Boden (2008); Gallagher (2005).
[2] Sansò (2014) 310 states that, "Overall, there has not been much work so far on Ancient Greek within the framework of CL". This judgment may already be somewhat out of date, since one

---

Note: I wish to thank this volume's editors as well as Douglas Cairns and the press's anonymous referees for providing excellent feedback on earlier versions of this paper. The usual disclaimers apply about any remaining omissions or errors.

William Michael Short, University of Exeter

https://doi.org/10.1515/9783110482201-002

An "Experientalist" Account of Meaning

What, more precisely, does a psychologically realistic, humanly plausible account of meaning look like? In my view, it is one that adopts an explicitly "experientialist" theory of cognition, committed to the idea that, for human beings, our thinking depends fundamentally on the kind of brain we possess functioning in the kind of body we have in the kinds of physical, social, and cultural environments we typically inhabit (or have historically inhabited).[3] In other words, it is one that views concepts as embodied mental representations deriving their meaning not through their correspondence to objects in external reality, but through their link to human conceptualizing capacities and psychological functions, which are grounded in and deeply constrained by our bodily nature, as well as by the local and global socio-cultural context.[4] It is therefore one that takes a middle ground between the representationalism and functionalism of the "classical" computational theory of mind in philosophy and "good old-fashioned artificial intelligence" (Haugeland

---

can point to the studies by Douglas Cairns of Greek emotion concepts such as aidós, phriké, and érōs in the light of conceptual metaphor theory, or to the analyses that Cristóbal Pagán Cánovas and Georgis Giannakis have given of the Greek poetic images of the "arrows of love" and of the Fates as "weavers", respectively, in terms of conceptual integration theory. Kiki Nikiforidou and Silvia Luraghi have also explained the meanings of the cases and prepositions in Greek in terms of image schemas of spatial relation (and their figurative interpretations), while Rafael Martínez Vázquez and José Miguel Jiménez Delgado have shown that metaphors such as 'EXPERIENCES ARE OBJECTS' motivate the polysemy of many Greek verbs (cf., e.g., phérō in its literal and figurative senses). Meanwhile, Bruce Louden and Drew Griffiths have examined the systems of metaphor that underpin certain Homeric formulae.

By comparison, studies of the Latin language and Latin literature in the perspective of cognitive linguistics remain relatively few. Early work by Francisco García Jurado found that the sorts of orientational metaphors cognitive linguists have identified in English ('GOOD IS UP', 'BAD IS DOWN', and so forth) are also present in Plautine Latin. More recently, Luisa Brucale and Egle Mocciaro have described how the senses of Latin *per* develop from a "prototypical nucleus" in the spatial domain to cover abstract domains including causation, instrumentality, and purpose. Chiara Fedriani has produced several studies (including a monograph) of the metaphors underlying Latin's eventive and stative expression (e.g., 'EXPERIENCES ARE OBJECTS', as evidenced by *in dubio sum, sto, maneo, iaceo, haereo*). My own research has focused on how Latin speakers' preferential conceptualization of, for example, the mind, communication, and mistakenness in terms of certain image-schematic metaphors contribute to a distinctively Roman worldview: with organizing effects across different aspects of language, thought, and behavior, metaphorically structured "folk models" actually appear to function as part of the "hidden metaphysics" that defines what it means be a member of Roman society. Important first steps towards what I call a Roman "cultural semantics"; see my concluding remarks in sect. 4.

3 See esp. Lakoff/Johnson (1980 and 1999); Johnson (1987); Gibbs (1994); Grady (1997).
4 See Wilson (2002).

1985, 112) – that is, any notion that human thought consists in the syntactical manipulation of implementation-independent abstract symbol systems that mentally "re-present" the structures of an objectively existing physical world to the mind – and the "radical embodiment" of enaction theorists like Humberto Maturana and Francesco Varela, which proposes a view of cognition as the effect of flat brain-body-action-world systems and which in its strongest forms sees no need for mental representations whatsoever for implementing intelligent behavior.[5]

Such a moderately embodied theory of cognition (cf. Prinz 2008) implies a very different account of meaning than that found in traditional (formal) philosophical and linguistic semantics. Generally speaking, experientialist approaches reject "truth-conditional" theories of linguistic meaning, which posit that an utterance's meaning corresponds to the set of conditions in the world (or in any possible world) for which the utterance can said to be true. Moving beyond the view of defining categories by lists of "necessary and sufficient" features, they adopt a theory of categorization that recognizes classes characterized by nonobjective human perceptual, interactional, or purposive properties.[6] In many cases, cognitive linguists claim that word meaning may not be reducible at all to symbols expressed in amodal, propositional format and arbitrarily linked to their referents. Rather than being represented in the mind as language-like symbols, the meanings of words very often are said to actually correspond (directly or indirectly through figurative interpretation) to gestalt structures of experience or "image schemas". In cognitive psychology, an image schema is a highly abstract pre-conceptual structure of cognition that emerges through human perceptual and sensorimotor interaction with the world – as Mark Johnson (1987, xiv) writes, "a recurring dynamic pattern of our perceptual interactions and motor programs that gives coherence and structure to our experience". Image schemas may therefore be visual in nature, e.g., "long, thin shapes, or containers" (Lakoff 1987, 113–14), or more abstract representations deriving from the character of human spatial experience, such as UP/DOWN schemas, CENTER/PERIPHERY schemas and MOVEMENT schemas. As cognitive structures that are analogues of (because dependent on the same neural architecture as) sensorimotor experience and thus open to visual and kinesthetic "transformations" in mental space, image schemas provide the inferential patterns that motivate the range of senses typically characterizing the meanings of words.[7]

---

5 Maturana/Varela (1987) and (1980).
6 Cf. Rosch (1973) and (1978); Barsalou (1983); Fillmore (1985); Lakoff (1987); Johnson (1987); Taylor (1989); Atran (1993); Vallée-Tourangeau *et al.* (1998).
7 See esp. Gibbs/Colston (1995).

Image schemas may also be metaphorically interpreted, as a way of extending meaning further into abstract domains. According to the theory of conceptual metaphor, it is through the regular metaphorical mapping of bodily-based image schematic structure onto concepts not directly grounded in experience that human abstract thought is in fact possible. Recognizing the all-pervasive character of certain metaphorical patterns in language, George Lakoff and Mark Johnson argued (1980, 1999) that the clustering of metaphorical linguistic expressions around many (mostly abstract) concepts in fact reflects inherently metaphorical understandings that speakers of a language possess of those concepts.[8] Speakers of a language talk about abstract domains of experience metaphorically, that is, because they actually conceive of them metaphorically in terms of other (mostly concrete) experiences. In this embodied view of cognition, literal concepts are those formed through bodily interaction with the world, and metaphors are regular projections or mappings of conceptual content – concepts or whole structured domains of knowledge – that occur as a way of mentally representing and reasoning about abstract concepts not directly grounded in physical experience. An important claim of this theory is that metaphorical mappings are not arbitrary and unconstrained, but experientially motivated, typically by their grounding in systematic correlations in phenomenal experience. Image schemas and their metaphorical projections therefore provide a solution to the problem of how linguistic expressions and other symbols acquire their meanings, since in this view all *abstracta* are grounded, at some level, in structures of cognition that emerge from bodily experiences that are directly meaningful to human beings.

It is in this sense, then, that I take cognition and language to be embodied: namely, that human conceptualization, and thus the inferential processes guiding semantic extension, depends in large part on cognitive structures – i.e., images schemas – and construal operations that arise naturalistically from (indeed are analogues of) recurring perceptual and kinesthetic experiences. Through unidirectional mappings of image schematic structure to domains not directly grounded in experience, literal (physicospatial) understanding comes to be extended to abstract reasoning. Because they emerge from, or are grounded in, repeated human bodily movements through space, perceptual interactions, and ways of manipulating objects, image schemas – unlike Fodorian representations (amodal abstract symbols) – are thus directly meaningful representational structures. At the same time, because they are gestalt patterns of experience which capture the structural contours of our bodily interactions with the world (only secondarily imageable "in the mind's eye"), image schemas – unlike enactivist couplings, which do away

---

8 Lakoff/Johnson (1980); Lakoff (1987); Johnson (1987); Kövecses (2005) and (2006).

with mental representations altogether – are inherently multimodal structures that operate beneath consciousness. Cognitive and linguistic embodiment therefore pertains to the fact that figurative *as well as* literal understanding is based on at least partial activations of the same sensorimotor areas of the brain.[9]

Consider, for example, that in many languages what we call *anger* is conceptualized as heated fluid in a container. In English, this conceptualization is captured in idiomatic phrases such as *blow one's stack, flip one's lid,* and *let off steam,* where the notion of emotional intensity is mapped to that of the liquid's temperature, and anger's effects on the body to the pressurization of the liquid.[10] A version of this metaphor also appears in Latin, as indicated by expressions like *Quinctius quidem adeo exarsit ira* ("Quinctius so 'blazed forth' in anger", Liv. *AUC.* 35.31.13), *mortis fraternae feruidus ira* ("'Seething' with anger at his brother's death", Verg. *Aen.* 9.736), or *ardet et iram / non capit … / … exaestuat ira* (She (sc. Procne) 'burns' and cannot 'contain' her anger … she 'boils over' with anger", Ov. *Met.* 6.610–11, 623)[11]. It is the fact that such mappings involve the transfer of an organized system of knowledge from concrete physical experience (namely, how fluids behave in heated, pressurized conditions) to abstract emotional experience (namely, anger) that allows English and Latin speakers to think, and thus talk, coherently about an aspect of human life that may be difficult to comprehend in and of itself. Moreover, talking about anger in terms of hot fluid is immediately meaningful to speakers of these languages, since the metaphor is grounded in the apparently universal human experience of feeling hot and pressurized when angry. Experimental studies have shown that the occurrence of anger coincides with objectively measurable increases in skin temperature and blood pressure.[12] In this way, (part of) the physiology of anger itself affords a ready image for conceptualizing such experiences in the abstract.[13]

---

9 For the representation of metaphorical mappings in the brain, see above all Feldman (2006). Some early brain imaging studies found no evidence of neuronal co-activation during metaphor processing: see esp. Aziz-Zadeh *et al.* (2006) and Aziz-Zadeh/Damasio (2008). More recent studies, however, point to at least partial recruitment of domain-specific sensory cortex during figurative language processing: cf., e.g., Desai *et al.* (2011); Lacey *et al.* (2012); Desai *et al.* (2013).
10 See esp. Kövecses (1986).
11 Riggsby (2015)
12 E.g., Ekman *et al.* (1983); Levenson *et al.* (1990); Levenson *et al.* (1991).
13 See Kövecses (1995). Of course, an increase of blood pressure and skin temperature also characterizes the physiological response associated with other emotions, which is why we find HEAT (and conversely COLD) used metaphorically of a range of such experiences (for instance, affection or lust): cf., e.g., Williams/Bargh (2008); Wilkowski *et al.* (2009); in an ancient context, Cairns (2013) 86–87.

Latin's Metaphors of Courage and Cowardice

Cognitive linguists take as given that complex, culturally situated concepts may in fact acquire their structure and content via whole networks of metaphors. Where a concept is characterized by several distinct metaphors, cognitive linguists argue that these metaphors normally work together to produce a working understanding of the concept's various aspects.[14] While the metaphors may recruit different conceptual materials and so fail to provide a consistent overall image to conceptualization, nevertheless they fit together coherently as a system, each metaphor delivering an understanding of some dimension of the metaphorically defined concept. In this respect, consider Latin speakers' conceptualization of courage and cowardice in terms of *animus*, which is delivered by the system of metaphors illustrated by Figure 1.

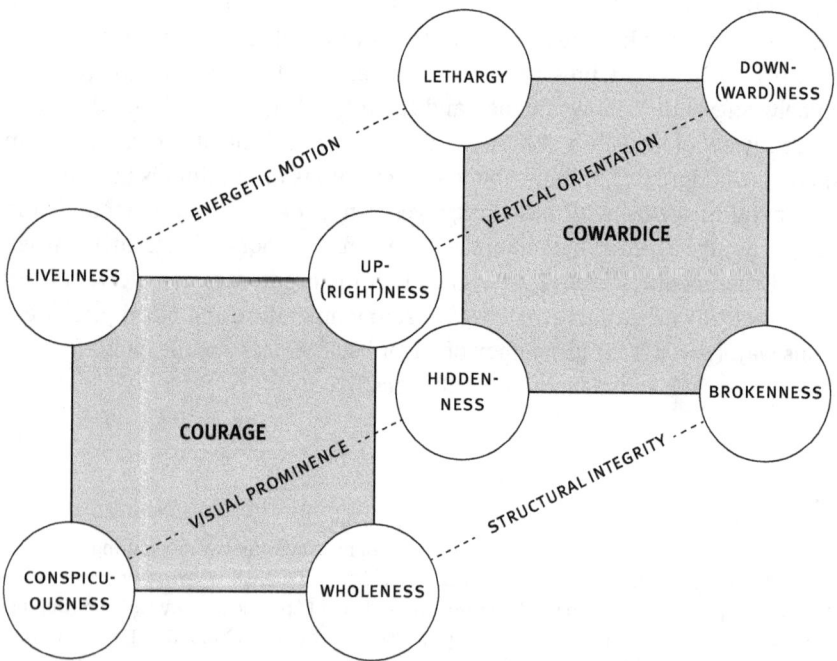

Figure 1: Metaphorical source domains contributing to Latin speakers' conceptualization of courage and cowardice.

---

14 On the character and function of such metaphor systems, see Danesi/Perron (1999) and Kövecses (2006).

What this figure shows is the set of images converging on *animus* as a way of expressing the concepts *both* of courage *and* of cowardice: that is, the images that metaphorically capture Latin speakers' understanding of courage and cowardice as distinct but inextricably related aspects of experience. As the figure shows, this understanding is delivered by highly schematic (rather than richly elaborated) images drawn from a limited number of concrete bodily source domains. It also shows that each of these domains provides a pair of contrasting image schemas to conceptualization, mapping reciprocally correlated physical concepts to those of courage and cowardice (as well as their relation).

Let us see in somewhat greater detail what each of these conceptual mappings entails.[15] Take the VERTICAL ORIENTATION metaphor. In this metaphor, *animus*

---

[15] Discovering large-scale metaphorical mappings of this sort begins from dictionary and corpus work. Because the linear alphabetical ordering of traditional lexicons tends to obscure figurative associations that structure the semantic system at a higher order than the individual lexeme, reference works like Meissner's *Latin Phrase Book* or the Langenscheidt *Grundwortschatz Latein*, which organize single-word expressions as well as phrasal lexical items under broad subject headings, can often provide preliminary evidence of conceptual metaphors. Alternatively, *n*-gram searches can be conducted for occurrences of target-domain vocabulary items. Careful examination of contextual usages will produce a tabulation of source-domain words used metaphorically of the target in question. Once initial metaphorical relations have been identified in this way, searches must be performed for occurrences of the whole range of vocabulary items belonging to each identified source domain with those of the target domain, in order to establish their degree of conventionalization in the language, as well as their internal mapping structure. (Synonym and antonym dictionaries like Ramshorn's or any of the *gradus ad Parnassum* type are useful here). Metaphors recruiting a highly circumscribed set of source-domain words, or that are restricted to a particular author or time period, or that occur only in fixed phrases, will be of limited relevance in this respect.

Given the overall set of source-to-target correspondences, generalizations can then be made about the conceptual mapping(s) underpinning the linguistic expressions (A search that yields expressions such as *bellum exstinguere* and *cuncta bello ardent* might lead us to posit a conceptual mapping of FIRE to WAR, for instance). In some (less interesting) cases, the mappings may involve only a single source-domain concept and target-domain concept; in others, it will involve whole systems of concepts. For the latter, it will be necessary to determine (possibly relying on statistical frequencies) which of the conceptual mappings is the more central (the metaphor's "main meaning focus": Kövecses 2003), and which are logical entailments of this central mapping based on Latin speakers' conventional knowledge of the source domain. Of course, classification of linguistic expressions as manifestations of any given conceptual metaphor is not always straightforward. Sometimes, an expression may appear to reflect multiple mappings simultaneously. Though this may complicate the analyst's neat categorization, it should hardly be surprising, since experience itself, which provides the grounding of and motivation for metaphors, is not easily segmentable. For an example, see n. 14.

is imagined as a kind of physical object or structure and courageousness corresponds to *animus* being in a state of vertical up(right)ness. Thus, Latin speakers employ verbs referring literally to "lifting up" (*tollere*) or "setting up(right)" (*erigere*) with *animum* or *animos* to convey the meaning we might express in English as "taking" or "gathering" or "plucking up" one's courage or, equally, "giving" or "instilling" or "inspiring" courage. For example, Livy describes Marcellus rallying his men at Nola as literally "'setting up(right)' the spirits of his own men" (*suorum militum animos erigeret*, AUC. 23.45.5), while Livy's epitomizer conveys the notion that the Parthians took courage from Crassus' death by saying that they "'stood up' their spirits" (*animos erexerant*, Ann. Flor. Ep. 4.9). Similarly, to express that the Trojans became very emboldened, Vergil writes that they literally "'lift up' their spirits to the stars" (*animos ad sidera tollunt*, Aen. 9.637) – *ad sidera* representing, according to the logic of the metaphor, the maximum of bravery. This is why the author of the *Bellum Africanum* can also describe Caesar as "carrying before himself a 'tall spirit'" (*animum enim altum ... prae se ferebat*, 10.3) to mean that he was brave, or why the author of the Latin *Iliad* can say that the Greeks and Trojans "'set up straight' their spirits" (*instaurant ... animos*) to capture the idea that they fight with renewed courage: what is tall and straight is by nature "up" and thus metaphorically "courageous".[16]

Correspondingly, cowardice is construed as a condition of down(ward)ness of *animus*; that is, to behave like a coward is to have one's *animus* oriented in some way "down". Latin speakers therefore use words referring literally to "falling"

---

[16] It is possible that figurative usages of *excitare* with *animus* in the sense of "embolden" (cf. Cic. Man. 6.4, *quod maxime vestros animos excitare ... debeat*; Resp. 41.9, *ad animos imperitorum excitandos ... perfectus*; Anon. Bell. Afr. 81.2, *animos eorum excitabat*; Sen. Contr. 10.2.17, *non est utile rei publicae excitari hostium animos*) can be accounted for in terms of this metaphor, as well – if we consider the literal meaning of the verb to be something like "build, erect, construct" (cf. Cic. Leg. 2.68, *sepulcrum altius ... excitari*; Caes. BG. 5.40.2, *turres*; Suet. Claud. 1, *tumulum*; Sen. Ep. 52, *aedificium*; etc.). Alternatively, it may emerge from an ontological metaphor in which *animus* is construed in terms of a human or even animal agent (i.e., "move, stir, shake, set in motion (a person or animal)" > "set the spirit in motion" > "embolden"); this kind of "personification" of *animus* would certainly not have been unusual in Latin (cf., e.g., Sen. Phaed. 112, *quo tendis, anime? quid furens saltus amas?*; 163, *animusque culpa plenus et semet timens*, 255–56, *moderare, alumna, mentis effrenae impetus, / animos coerce*). If the latter, it might be better to analyze this image as part of the ENERGETIC MOTION metaphor or even the VISUAL PROMINENCE metaphor of courage, as "causing to move out" (*ex-citare*) implies a change from a state of hiddenness to one of conspicuousness. But I am inclined to take *excitare animum* as reflecting a sort of structural metaphor because of expressions like Plaut. Trin. 132, *exaedificaret suam incohatam ignaviam*, where "emboldening" is clearly construed metaphorically as "building (up)" *animus* (as if something akin to *oppidum, domum, templum, navem ...*).

(*cadere*) or "sending down" (*demittere*) in conjunction with *animus* to convey what we might express again in English as "losing" or "giving up" courage. For instance, to express that the Crustumini lost the conviction to go through with the war they had begun against the Romans, again Livy writes that their "spirits had 'fallen'" (*ceciderant animi*, AUC. 1.11.3). Likewise, Caesar uses the construction *animo deficere* (literally, "to break down from courage") to express the idea of losing courage in the face of some difficult circumstance, as in "Marcius Rufus ... entreated his men not to give up courage" (*ne animo deficient*, BC. 2.43.1).[17] Elsewhere, the image of *animus* as "thrown down" (*perculsus*) or simply "low" (*humilis*) or "lying flat" (*iacens*) is used to convey notions of cowardliness – as, for instance, when Cicero asks of the Gauls, "Do you think, judges, that with their military cloaks and breeches they are behaving at all like cowards", literally, "with their courage sunk down and near-to-the-ground?" (*animo demisso atque humili*, Font. 33), or when Propertius exhorts himself to turn from elegiac cowardliness to epic courage: *surge, anime, ex humili; iam, carmina, sumite vires* (2.10.11).

In the images of the STRUCTURAL INTEGRITY metaphor, on the other hand, courage is construed as the wholeness and cowardice as the brokenness of *animus*. Thus, to give courage to a person is, literally, to "make fast" (*firmare* and its compounds) or "tie together" (*colligere*) or "harden" (*indurare*) or "make whole" (*integrare*) the *animus*. In Plautus' *Amphitruo*, for example, Alcmena declares her resolve to endure her husband's absence "with a strong and 'bolted-on' spirit" (*animo forti atque offirmato*, 656). When Caesar assures the Gauls that he will prevent further settlement of their territory by the Germans, this "'made fast' their spirits" (*animos verbis confirmavit*, BG. 1.33.1). And Livy recounts that the Volsci and Aequi, under attack by the consul Valerius, "when they had 'tied together' their courage (*animos collegissent*) ... rallied and held their own" (AUC. 3.60.11).[18] At the same time, to deprive someone of courage is to "break" (*frangere*, but also *corrumpere* or *adflictare*) the *animus* – as when once more Livy writes that Postumius, "after depriving (literally, 'breaking') the Aequi of their courage in skirmishing (*cum leuibus proeliis Aequorum animos fregisset*), forced an entrance into the town" (AUC. 4.49.9), or when Valerius Maximus tells us that "Hannibal beat down the strength of the Romans more than he 'broke' their courage" (*magis vires*

---

17 Cf. also Verg. Aen. 3.259–60, *cecidere animi*; Ov. Fast. 3.225, *tela viris animique cadunt*, Luc. Sat. fr. 27.9 = Non. 286M, *re in secunda tollere animos, in mala demittere*; Caes. BG. 7.29.1, *ne se admodum animo demitterent*; Sall. Jug. 98, *demisso animo fuit*; Caes. BC. 3.112.12, *ne negotio desisteret neve animo deficeret*.
18 Cf. also Verg. Georg. 4.386, *firmans animum sic incipit ipsa*; Sall. Cat. 46.3, *confirmato animo*; Liv. AUC. 42.60.3, *dum perculsi milites animos colligerent*; Sen. EM. 104.22, *hi iubebunt ... animum indurare*,; Hom. Lat. Il. 614–15, *Apollo / integratque animum*.

Romanorum contudit quam animos fregit, Mem. 3.2.11).¹⁹ The same image likely underwrites, as well, the meaning of the word *murcus* mentioned by Ammianus Marcellinus as soldiers' jargon for a coward: *Res Gestae* 15.12.3, *aliquando quisquam in Italia munus Martium pertimescens pollicem sibi praecidit, quos iocaliter murcos appellant,* "Once in a while someone in Italy fearing military service cuts off his own thumb – and they call these men, derisively, *murci*". If, as Edwin Fay has suggested (1905: 398), *murcus* can be derived from *mulcare* ("strike, maul, mutilate"), this word directly figures the coward as someone who is "mutilated".²⁰

In the VISUAL PROMINENCE metaphor, courage and cowardice are expressed instead in metaphorical terms of the conspicuousness or hiddenness of *animus*.²¹ Hence expressions like *magno animo esse* (literally, "be with a big spirit") or *ingenti animo* ("with a huge spirit") or *praestanti animo* ("with a standing-forth spirit") or *excellenti animo* ("with a towering spirit") that signify courage.²² This metaphor probably also accounts for formulations in which courage is construed as the "increasing" or "growing" of *animus*: e.g., *praesidio legionum addito nostris animus augetur* ("The spirit 'increases' for our men from the additional support of the legions", Caes. *BG*. 7.70.3) and *veritus ne vanis tot conatibus suorum et hostibus cresceret animus* ("He (sc. Scipio) feared the enemy's spirits would 'grow' by his men's so many futile attempts", Liv. *AUC*. 28.19.16).²³ Conversely, the coward is typically portrayed as "hiding" or "lying concealed" by Latin authors: cf., e.g., *quid ergo ille ignavissimus / mihi latitabat?* ("Why is that utter coward hiding from me?" Plaut. *Trin*. 926–27) and *utrum inclusum atque abditum latere in occulto atque ignaviam suam tenebrarum ac parietum custodiis tegere?* ("Was he to lurk about in the dark, shut in and hidden, concealing his own cowardice with the safeguards of shadows and walls?" Cic. *Rab*. 21). The archaic word *cussiliris* given by Festus as

---

19 Cf. Liv. *AUC*. 26.13.1, *fregit animos*; 32.31.2, *animos fregisset*; 38.16.14, *infregit animos*; Val. Flacc. *Arg*. 6.283–84, *corripuit fregitque animos*; Prop. *Carm*. 5.6.51, *frangit et attollit vires in milite causa*; Sall. *Jug*. 31, *piget dicere ... ut vobis animus ... conruptus sit.*
20 The etymology is not treated by De Vaan (2008), nor does *murcus* appear in this sense in the *OLD*, although a possible by-form *murcidus* attested by St. Augustine (*Civ*. 4.16) for the comedies of Pomponius is given with the meaning "lazy, inactive".
21 Perhaps no principled distinction can actually be made between the mappings of the VISUAL PROMINENCE and VERTICAL ORIENTATION metaphors, since in human experience what is up is typically easier to see and what is down is typically more difficult to see. Here, however, I treat the two metaphors as discrete, to better highlight the systematicity of each mapping.
22 Cf. Cic. *Deiot*. 36, *magno animo et erecto est*; Caes. *BG*. 7.10, *hostium impetum magno animo sustineant*; Sall. *Ep. ad Caes*. 7.10, *ingentem eorum animum subegit*; Cic. *Phil*. 14.36, *fortissimo praestantissimoque animo exercitum castris eduxerit*; Caes. *BC*. 3.4.4, *Rhascypolis praeerat, excellenti virtute*.
23 *Crescere animum*, "embolden" may again suggest a metaphorical view of *animus* as a kind of human, animal, or even vegetal entity: see above, n. 12.

a synonym for *ignavus* also appears to metaphorize the coward directly as "covering up" or "hiding".²⁴ Though several etymologies have been proposed, the most plausible derivation is from *cossim in lira*, literally, "cowering (on the thighs) in a furrow", its figurative sense of "coward" thus apparently developing by reference to the threat avoidance behaviors characteristic of some animals.²⁵

Finally, in the images of the ENERGETIC MOTION metaphor, courage corresponds to liveliness (of *animus*) and cowardice to lethargy. This can be seen in formulations like *animus alacer* or *strenuus*, literally a "quick" or "lively spirit", as in, for instance, *tuumque simul promptum animum et alacrem perspexi ad defendendam rem publicam* ("I perceived at the same time your 'ready and quick spirit' for defending the Republic", Cic. *Fam.* 3.11.4) or *postquam omnium animos alacris videt, cohortatus, ut petitionem suam curae haberent, conventum dimisit* ("When he (sc. Catiline) sees their 'quick spirits', he charged them to attend to his interest at the election of consuls and dismissed the assembly", Sall. *Cat.* 21.5), and, likewise, in *quod si animo strenuo fecissent, futurum ut aduersarii non possent resistere* ("If they had done it 'with a quick spirit', their foes would have been unable to resist", Nep. *Dat.* 6.4).²⁶ The converse construal of cowardice as lethargy is well known from uses of *ignavus*, meaning, etymologically, "not active" (*in-gnavus*): e.g., '*conpertum ego habeo, milites ... neque ex ignavo strenuum neque fortem ex timido exercitum oratione imperatoris fieri*' ("'I am well aware, soldiers ... that a brave army cannot be made of a cowardly one, nor a strong one from a weak one, simply by a speech of its commander'", Sall. *Cat.* 58.2).²⁷ But the metaphor extends to uses of *segnis* and *iners* as well: cf., e.g., *nec Turnum segnis retinet mora* ("Nor does any cowardly delay hold Turnus back", Verg. *Aen.* 10.308) and *tam sis hostis iners, quam malus hospes eras* ("Be as cowardly an enemy as you were evil a guest!" Ov. *Ep.* 13.44).

---

24 I.e., Paul. Fest. p. 50, 13 Müller, *cussilirem pro ignavo dicebant antiqui*.

25 Walde-Hofmann (1954) I, 162. Cf. Rheden (1907) 699, "die Bezeichnung ist sehr anschaulich, offenbar hergenommen von Vögeln und anderen Tieren, die sich, um sich der Beobachtung und Bedrohung zu entziehen, in eine Furche ducken".

26 Cf. Col. RR. 11.1.17, *cum uigore et alacritate animi praecedentem eum tamquam ducem strenue sequatur*; Caes. *BG.* 1.46.4, *multo maior alacritas studiumque pugnandi maius exercitui iniectum est*; Sen. *Cons. Helv.* 12.8.5, *alacres itaque et erecti quocumque res tulerit intrepido gradu properemus*; Val. Max. *Mem.* 3.2.3, *alacri animo suos ad id proelium ... cohortatus est*; Caes. *BC.* 3.92.4, *est quaedam animi incitatio atque alacritas naturaliter innata omnibus, quae studio pugnae incenditur*; Tac. *Hist.* 2.14, *strenui ignavique in victoria idem audent*.

27 Cf. also Cic. *Inv.* 1.92, *indignum esse ab homine ignavissimo virum fortissimum Aiacem necatum*; Liv. *AUC.* 2.46.5, '*adeo ignauissimos hostes magis timetis quam Iouem Martemque per quos iurastis?*' and 5.28.8, *Postumius suis in tutum receptis cum contione aduocata terrorem increparet ac fugam, fusos esse ab ignauissimo ac fugacissimo hoste*.

As may be seen from these (and numerous other) examples, certain conventional, everyday ways of expressing the concepts of courage and cowardice in Latin are conveyed by metaphors drawing on images of concrete human bodily and physical experience. In these metaphors, images of bodily experience are predicated of *animus* in a regular and consistent fashion as a means of expressing the fact of someone's "having" courage or not. The metaphors are regular in the sense that they organize the figurative meanings of whole semantic fields. Each metaphor, that is, operates at a level of sense making that is supralexical, rather than belonging to the semantic structure of any individual word (e.g., the LIVELINESS metaphor structures the meanings not only of *ignavus* but of the range of terms designating laziness). They are consistent in the sense that they recruit pairs of contrastively related image schemas toward the expression both of courage and of cowardice, each metaphor thereby projecting the relational structure of the literal domain onto the figurative domain. Let me emphasize, then, that from the perspective of the cognitive linguistic theory of metaphor, it is these metaphors *per se* that make sense of Latin speakers' talk of courage and cowardice and in fact constitute their conceptualization of these categories vis-à-vis *animus*. Without these metaphors, Latin speakers would have an understanding of these categories that was very impoverished.

Alternative Metaphors

This is not to imply that Latin speakers did not also possess other (and other metaphorical) ways of conceptualizing courage. Evidence indicates that a much wider set of images actually converged on this conceptualization. For instance, courage may be conceived as a sort of substance that "fills" the body, as when Turnus "'fills' the Rutulians with daring courage" (*Rutulos animis audacibus implet*, Verg. Aen. 7.475). Or courage may be imagined as a kind of physical object "given" to someone (by the hands), as when again Turnus taunts the Trojans as "the sort of soldiers to whom trust in an intervening moat and the delays of trenches ... 'give' courage" (*quibus haec medii fiducia valli / fossarumque morae ... / dant animos*, Verg. Aen. 9.142–44) or Athena literally "'hands over' courage to the young man" (*animos iuveni ... ministrat*, Hom. Lat. *Il.* 396).[28] Courage may also be conceived in metaphorical terms of spatial proximity: Cicero, for example, reporting that his arrival in Cilicia

---

[28] However, Valpy (1828) 263 derives *ministro* from *minus* by analogy with *magister* < *magis*, the vocalization of the first syllable paralleling *comminus* and *eminus*.

emboldened Cassius, writes that courage literally "came near to" Cassius (*Cassio ... animus accessit, Att.* 5.20.3). In another frequent metaphor, courage is a kind of fire. Giving courage is therefore setting *animus* aflame (*inflammare* or *accendere* or *incendere animum*), as when Allecto promises to, literally, "'set their spirits on fire' by lust for senseless war" (*accendamque animos insani Martis amorem*, Verg. *Aen.* 7.550).[29] Courage is also sharpness: for instance, Livy recounts that after the capture of New Carthage, Scipio instituted a new training regimen for his soldiers and thus "'sharpened' their bodies and spirits for war" (*corpora simul animosque ad bellum acuebant, AUC.* 25.51.7).[30] The overall set of metaphors delivering Latin's concept of courage can thus be represented as in Figure 2.

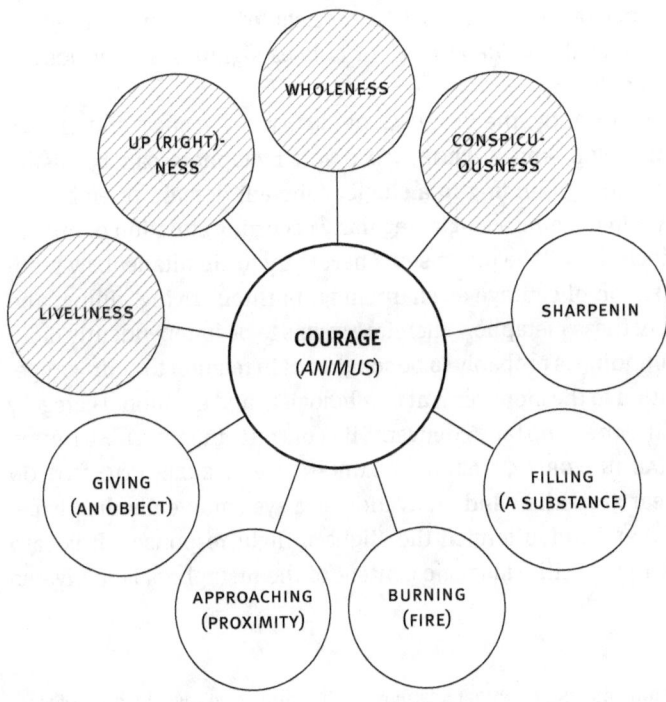

Figure 2: Overall set of metaphors delivering Latin speakers' concept of courage in terms of *animus*.

---

29 Cf. Verg. *Aen.* 12.426, *primusque animos accendit in hostem*; Cic. *Man.* 6, *vestros animos ... inflammare ... debeat*; Liv. *AUC.* 2.46.7, *accendamus militum animos*; 3.61.8, *accendit animos*; 6.14.10, *accendunt militum animos*; 26.44.8, *ad accendendos militum animos*; etc.

30 Almost exactly the same expression occurs at *AUC.* 35.35.9, *non sineret sub tectis marcescere otio sed educeret et in armis decurrere cogeret, simul animos acueret et corpora exerceret*. SHARPNESS of *animus* may also signify anger, as apparently in Verg. *Aen.* 1.57, *mollitque animos et temperat iras*.

Nevertheless, I believe the VERTICAL ORIENTATION, STRUCTURAL INTEGRITY, VISUAL PROMINENCE, and ENERGETIC MOTION metaphors can be distinguished from these others in several important respects. To begin with, they are regular and consistent in a way the others are not: that is, as already noted, they structure meaning pervasively across Latin's semantic system, over periods of the language and at different levels of the linguistic code, whereas the others tend to be (usually generically) more restricted. And they recruit images always in pairwise fashion toward the conceptualization of both courage and cowardice, whereas the other metaphors are univocal, tending to focus on the metaphorical characterization of courage alone. For example, while a "sharp" *animus* signifies courage, images of "dullness" typically denote stupidity in Latin (Bettini 2011, 50–51). And while "giving" *animus* to a person or for *animus* to "come near to" a person means being emboldened, the "removal" or "departure" of *animus* signifies instead loss of consciousness or even death.

Perhaps most importantly, the VERTICAL ORIENTATION, STRUCTURAL INTEGRITY, VISUAL PROMINENCE, and ENERGETIC MOTION metaphors can be distinguished in terms of their grounding in a single, coherent domain of embodied experience. It is hard to imagine a single, regularly occurring situation of human embodiment that includes *all* the dimensions necessary to simultaneously motivate a conceptualization of courage as sharpening, burning, giving, filling, and approaching. Each of these metaphors therefore seems to be independently motivated, and their grounding is probably to be sought not in relation to courage specifically, but in relation to the more general psychological and emotional category whose understanding they appear to deliver.[31] By contrast, the VERTICAL ORIENTATION, STRUCTURAL INTEGRITY, VISUAL PROMINENCE and ENERGETIC MOTION metaphors have clear grounding and motivation as a system in embodied experiences of what Walter Cannon termed the "fight-or-flight response". It is easy enough to see how the specific imagistic content of the metaphors is motivated

---

31 The BURNING, FILLING, and SHARPENING metaphors each characterize a whole range of emotion concepts. One immediately thinks of Latin elegists' use of "burning" as a metaphor especially for erotic love. It is equally common, though, to find hope and joy – as well as grief and anger – construed metaphorically as fire. And even as "filling" the *animus* means giving courage, it is also possible to "fill" someone or someone's *animus* with other emotion-substances: with love (as, for instance, in Naev. fr. 136, *animum amore capitali compleuerint*) or with superstition (as in Liv. AUC. 29.14.2, *impleuerat ea res superstitionum animos*), or hope, or happiness, or longing. "Sharpening" metaphorically captures emotional arousal in general, which is why *acer* and *acutus* often have the sense of "impassioned". The PROXIMITY metaphor has perhaps the widest scope: "coming near to" or "approaching" can express the occurrence of all sorts of mental states, above all "agreement" (as in expressions like *ipse quoque huic sententiae accedo*, Iust. Dig. 36.2.12.6).

by the set of autonomic physiological reactions and stereotyped bodily behaviors associated with these scenarios.[32] The images of the ENERGETIC MOTION metaphor, for instance, appear to be grounded in felt sensations related to the release of adrenal catecholamines (especially epinephrine and norepinephrine), which prepare the body for quick action by accelerating the heart rate, increasing blood pressure and muscle tensity, and providing additional glucose to the bloodstream as a boost of available energy for rigorous exertion.[33] Because this mechanism actually becomes mobilized in scenarios where an individual has determined that "fight" is the more adaptive course of action – in other words, in "courage" scenarios – liveliness thus affords a ready metaphorical image for understanding this category. On the other hand, the lethargy image is likely motivated by the fact that in "flight" conditions, digestive functioning, muscle contraction, heart rate, and breathing are slowed to preserve metabolic resources, proprioceptively and perhaps objectively perceived as a kind of physical sluggishness taken to be characteristic of – and so a salient metaphorical image for – cowardice. The image may also be grounded in the tendency of human beings to resort to "tonic immobility" or "freezing" in situations of extreme danger, where "fight" is not favorable and escape by feigning death represents the better option.

At the same time, UP(RIGHT)NESS and CONSPICUOUSNESS are apt images for courage because the "fight" scenario entails an increase in apparent height, size, and stability, due to protrusion of the chest and raising of the head and neck brought about by involuntary contraction of the back muscles, along with bracing of the legs. Pupil dilation and horripilation, while enhancing vision and environmental sensitivity, also tend to give an impression of increased size. Images of cowardice as down(ward)ness and hiddenness are instead likely grounded in the typical "flight" behaviors of lying prone on the ground (collapse) and concealment, not to mention the body's attempt to appear smaller (and so less threatening to a predator) by contracting the muscles of the front of the body, pulling the shoulders, head, and spine inward and down. The STRUCTURAL INTEGRITY metaphor may also depend on effects of the release of epinephrine and norepinephrine during "fight" or "flight". These neurotransmitters are known to be related to so-called "phantom limb" perception: their availability to the nervous system has in fact been shown to correlate positively with the onset and maintenance of phantom sensations.[34] One of their effects, in other words, appears to be

---

[32] The classic treatment is Cannon (1953). See now esp. LeDoux (1996); Panksepp (1998); Porges (2011); Everly/Lating (2012).
[33] For details, see Usdin *et al.* (1976) and Makara *et al.* (1983).
[34] Cf. Allen (1990); and esp. Sherman *et al.* (1989).

to induce a perception of the body as an integrated whole (even in cases where the body is not physically whole). If "fight" involves sustained release of these chemicals, this would account for the WHOLENESS image of courage, whereas their diminishment from the bloodstream and nerve fibers in the "flight" scenario could produce a (consciously or unconsciously) perceived disruption of the "body schema" coming to be interpreted of cowardice in metaphorical terms of brokenness.[35]

Concluding remarks

I have dwelt on the metaphorical structuring of Latin's conceptualization of courage and cowardice via embodied image schemas, and on the likely experiential grounding of these conceptual metaphors, to be able to suggest what I believe an experientialist account of meaning can bring to classical studies. In positing that sense-making emerges from embodied experience, such an approach offers, minimally, a model of linguistic meaning capable of explaining lexical polysemy in a systematic fashion. More than this, though, it offers a model of cultural meaning. In treating figurative associations pervasive and highly conventionalized in the linguistic system as reflecting conceptual (not only semantic) structures, such an approach can help identify the sorts of meanings that Latin speakers will tend to rely on in constructing and in interpreting "texts" of all kinds – including those inscribed through the aesthetic codes of visual representation – and that thus link together Roman society's various imaginative activities into a cohesive signifying order. As one immediate example, consider Trajan's Column. Though it is probably impossible to reduce the meaning of the column and its relief to a single overarching message, Per Gustaf Hamberg's claim (1945, 116–19) that it is meant above all to advertise the emperor's "manly courage" (*virtus*) seems undeniable. In this light, the placement of Trajan's statue at its top seems motivated by the metaphorical understanding of what is courageous as being "up". In effect, the column itself, with what Salvatore Settis (1988) called the constant vertical directional "impulse" of its decoration, literalizes in its physical form the metaphor of courage as up(right)ness. In this sense, the

---

[35] The same effect could be attributed to the release of cortisol by the parasympathetic nervous system, following "fight-or-flight". High levels of cortisol are known to severally disrupt hippocampal functioning, and the hippocampus has often been seen as a crucial brain area in the maintenance of the body schema. See MacLachlan (2004).

metaphor provides a principle of topographical organization for the construction and decoration of the column, as well as the mechanism of its interpretation.

More broadly, such an approach provides the sort of "experience-near" perspective that has recently been advocated in the study of ancient cultures. An "experience-near" perspective, as we know, privileges "native" ways of knowing and of representing the world, rather than concepts belonging to the observer's own cultural framework (concepts that Geertz 1973, 481–82 calls "experience-distant"). By illustrating how human-universal structures and processes of conceptualization give rise to the idiosyncratic meanings subtending a particular society's symbolic activities, image schema theory provides exactly the sort of language-independent, "etic" framework of analysis that can enable an "emic" accounting of Latin speakers' conceptual system. Especially when combined with a culturally-comparative perspective – since this helps highlight how speakers of different languages may elaborate different metaphorical models on the basis of the same images schemas, or how different languages and cultures capture the "same" concept through sometimes very different metaphorical images. Indeed, comparing Latin's metaphors of courage and cowardice with those from other languages reveals that cultural understandings of these categories are highly variable. In Greek, for example, courage may be conceived as a sort of smoke or vapor in the body (θυμός being connected with Latin *fumus* already by Onians 1954, 44–58).[36] Greek speakers also appear to favor animal imagery, especially of the lion, wild boar, wolf, or leopard for courage and of the deer or cattle for cowardice.[37] Many modern European languages conceptualize courage and cowardice instead through "heart" images, often in conjunction with an OBJECT metaphor: cf., e.g., Italian *prendere* and *perdere corraggio*, French *prendre* and *perdre courage*, and German *den Mut finden* and *verlieren*.[38] In Mandarin Chinese, courage is imagined in relation to the gallbladder, however: "gall-capacity (*dan-liang*)" means "courage" and the brave person is said to have a "big gall (*dan-da*)", whereas a coward has a "small gall (*dan-xiao*)".[39] Thus, while Latin speakers' metaphors may be based on experiences shared by presumably all

---

36 Cf., e.g., Hom. *Od.* 10.461, θυμὸν ἐνὶ στήθεσσι λάβητε; *Il.* 6.256, 7.152, θυμὸς ἀνῆκεν; *Od.* 2.315, ἀέξεται ἔνδοθι θυμός. See now Caswell (1990) 6–8.
37 See esp. Schnapp-Gourbeillon (1981) and Lonsdale (1990). The HIDDENNESS metaphor of cowardice in Latin – where the coward is directly likened to the cowering animal – suggests these images are not entirely foreign to Roman culture, either.
38 Gutiérrez Pérez (2008).
39 Yu (2003).

human beings, their privileging of such experiences in metaphorical conceptualization appears to constitute a distinctive feature of their signifying order.[40]

In providing an "experience-near" perspective, such an experientialist approach thus addresses a significant deficit of classical studies: namely, that while the ostensible objective of most research is to reconstruct the meaning(s) of some cultural artefact in a way that conforms as much as possible to historical context, scholars nevertheless tend to analyze the repertory of Roman culture's meanings in terms of categories that belong to their own intellectual and cultural framework. The danger, of course, is not beginning our reflections from such "etic" categories – this is inevitable and in fact necessary – but remaining exclusively within them, viewing them as natural categories that are true in an ahistorical sense and never even minimally questioning whether or how Latin speakers elaborated similar conceptualizations. At the same time, it is obviously undesirable to aim exclusively at the "emic", since this poses the risk of losing any sense of how any particular symbolic configuration is distinctive and meaningful within a larger cultural or linguistic context. As Clifford Geertz wrote (1983, 58), "THE TRICK IS *NOT* to get yourself into some inner correspondence of spirit with your informants", the result of which would be something like the proverbial "ethnography of witchcraft written by a witch". The trick is instead to involve the etic and the emic in a productive dialectic that highlights where conceptualizations diverge and so avoids predetermining the meaning of cultural forms by subsuming them to presumably analogous conceptual categories.[41]

To be clear. In advocating that Classical Studies incorporate cognitively-informed methodologies, I am not suggesting that scholars of Greek and Latin need to suddenly start talking about post-synaptic depolarization, dendrodendritic inhibition, and backpropagating action potentials (we already have our own opaque technical jargon). There is the danger of losing sight in the neuroscientific weeds of how human beings (and not just cognitive systems) go about making sense of their world. Nor am I implying we should view the classical languages as simply a resource for supporting the universalizing claims of some cognitive linguists. In showing that Latin speakers' meanings depend to some extent on cognitive structures and processes shared by all humans, there is the danger

---

[40] What accounts for Latin speakers' privileged conceptualization of courage and cowardice in such markedly embodied terms is, I would suggest, the particular symbolic affordances that the human body seems to have presented to them for representing and understanding psychological and emotional phenomena of all sorts. I have shown elsewhere the Latin speakers' understanding of most aspects of mental activity: Short (2012) and (2013).
[41] Cf. Bettini (2009).

of downplaying their sociocultural situatedness. What I am suggesting we need is an approach that does not hesitate to describe Latin speakers' mental contents in scientifically validated ways and in terms of recognized brain-based mechanisms of meaning construction, but that does so at a level of abstraction functional to characterizing what is different about those "contents"[42] – while recognizing, at the same time, that human embodiment can and does impose certain constraints on the proliferation of meaning cross-culturally. This is because the image schemas and image-schematic scenarios that underpin even highly abstract, culturally situated concepts – along with the construal operations of which image schemas are susceptible – are specified by the nature of the human body and by our bodily interactions with the natural and social environment. Opportunities for metaphorical projection are also subject to limitation, since mappings of image-schematic structure must preserve the cognitive topology of the concrete source domain in the metaphorical target domain and thus possible figurative relations are constrained by the internal structuring of concepts.[43] Probably even the most imaginative metaphorical images of literary production can be shown to derive from conventionalized patterns of figurative associations (by way of the elaboration, extension, combination or questioning of established mappings: cf. Kövecses 2005). Indeed, to be meaningful in the first place, what is imaginative and creative must relate at a certain order to that which is conventionalized and ordinary.[44]

---

42 Cf. Detienne (2002) and (2005); Bettini (2009).
43 For the "Invariance Hypothesis", see Lakoff (1993) and Turner (1990). Brugmann (1990) offers a critical view.
44 See esp. Lakoff/Turner (1989) 67–72.

Siobhan Privitera
2 *Odyssey* 20 and Cognitive Science: A Case Study

The *Odyssey* is a poem about physical and psychological journeys. It documents Odysseus' voyage home from Troy, all the while being intensely concerned with his psychological transition from helpless victim and ceaseless wanderer to self-determining hero and lord of Ithaca. Both journeys hinge primarily on Odysseus' exceptional mental aptitude: on his ability to undergo and overcome arduous trials with cunning and intellect, to adopt and maintain convincing disguises, and to endure circumstances that other Homeric heroes would find intolerable with fortitude and patience. Odysseus' thoughts and emotions are thus the subject of particular narrative interest and attention through the epic: he is furnished with a full mental life to which the poet frequently refers in explaining his intentions, motivations, and actions. As is common in Homer, the poet conveys these psychological processes using metaphor, metonymies, and similes that draw their source material from the physical world, as well as nonverbal behaviour as a means of delineating cognitive activity. In using techniques such as these, the narrator consistently advocates an interpretation of mind that consists of brain, body, and world, and presents his cast of characters as individuals whose psychological experiences are structured by interactions between them.

In this sense, the picture of mind given by Homer is fully consistent with the embodied theory of cognition developed in second generation cognitive science, which advocates a view of cognition as structured and conceptualized by phenomenological experience. "A culture's emotional categories are experiential", Cairns argues, "based on the interaction of embodied human beings with their environments *via* metonymies and metaphors that derive from such experience".[1] But if Homer can be seen as an advocate of embodiment *ante litteram*, in using

---

[1] Cairns (2016) 1. The valuable findings provided by these studies concern not only scientific but literary analysis. Early work on conceptual metaphor and poetic representation, for example, demonstrates that despite an historic tendency to view the construction and understanding of poetry as an elevated and isolated process, poetic expression and imagination are inextricably embedded in everyday language and experience. These studies are too numerous to delineate in full here; but recent and significant contributors to the field include Lakoff/Johnson (1980), Lakoff/Turner (1989), Kövesces (2000), and Zunshine (2006) and (2015).

Siobhan Privitera, Australian National University

https://doi.org/10.1515/9783110482201-003

such techniques, the narrator also capitalizes on a culturally embedded set of metaphorical images of mind the allows his audience to engage their own experience in interpreting the narrative. This study aims to show how methodologies from cognitive science—but especially regarding conceptual metaphor—can be constructively applied to accounts of complex psychologies in the Homeric poems. It thus participates in a growing discussion of how recognizing the co-dependency of mind, body, and world can bring us to a more precise understanding of how thought and emotion is presented by the Homeric narrator.[2] Homeric representations of mind constitute a "phenomenology of experience" that the narrator develops throughout his poems; that is, a reconstruction of the psychological workings of his characters that draws on the physical, material, perceptual, interactional, and evolutionary via conceptual metaphor. He facilitates audience interpretation and understanding in appealing to these universal, everyday aspects of experience. Furthermore, the poet reveals the extent to which sense-making and meaning are shaped and constrained by our bodies, cultures, interactions with others, and evolutionary development.[3]

To begin to see the way in which Homer conceptualizes his characters' internal experiences, consider the beginning of *Odyssey* 20, in which a disguised Odysseus, unable to sleep, deliberates his impending revenge against Penelope's suitors (5-30). More broadly, this internal debate is a recurring narrative device that occurs elsewhere in moments of crisis, where a Homeric hero, struggling with over-whelming, unfavourable odds, chooses between self-preservation and

---

[2] The application of these theoretical models to Homeric psychology is recent, but not new. Cairns, Scodel, and Minchin incorporate insights from cognitive linguistics in their own work on Homeric psychology and social interaction, and demonstrate, to great effect, how understanding the co-dependency of mind and body in structuring abstract experience enriches our approach to the Homeric material. See, for example, Minchin (2001a), (2001b), (2007), and (2008), Scodel (2008), and Cairns (2005), (2012), (2013), and (2016).

[3] More traditional studies in classical philology interpret the process by which audiences understand the psychologies of literary characters using concepts of Einfühlung ("empathy") and Verstehen ("understanding"); see Dilthey (1976) and Schleimacher, whom the former cites extensively; for a history of the scholarship on both concepts, see Harrington (2001) and Nowak (2011). My own perspective is somewhat different; unlike these studies, I argue that we interpret the psychology of Homer's characters because of our own first-person familiarity with similar experiences. In doing so, my approach is similar to that of Cairns', who argues of φρίκη, for example (2014) 86: "To be sure, φρίκη is a subjective experience, but it is a subjective experience with an external, visible aspect, and it is this external, visible aspect that allows us to relate *that person's* visible shudder, *via* the implicit theory of mind that we develop from infancy, to our own subjective experience of shuddering and of the emotions of which shuddering is a symptom".

perseverance.[4] In a more specific sense, internal monologues provide compelling insight to the psychological workings of Homer's characters; but the *Od.* 20 passage has attracted special attention because of its dense psychological imagery and interplay: within twenty-five lines, there are two similes, eight metaphors, three monologues, didactic uses of memory, nonverbal behavior, and multiple references to psychological terminology.[5] This passage thus demonstrates the full range of ways in which the Homeric poet conceptualizes his characters' internal experiences, and provides an accessible means for making sense of complicated thought processes. "The passage prefigures later Greek ways of conceptualizing psychological interplay", Gill explains, "but it also exemplifies the scope for presenting cohesive internal relationships within Homeric terminology".[6]

Accordingly, the *Odyssey* 20 passage opens with metaphors of physical space, containers, and boundaries (5–13):

ἔνθ' Ὀδυσεὺς μνηστῆρσι κακὰ φρονέων ἐνὶ θυμῷ

κεῖτ' ἐγρηγορόων· ταὶ δ' ἐκ μεγάροιο γυναῖκες

ἤϊσαν, αἳ μνηστῆρσιν ἐμισγέσκοντο πάρος περ,

ἀλλήλῃσι γέλω τε καὶ εὐφροσύνην παρέχουσαι.

τοῦ δ' ὠρίνετο θυμὸς ἐνὶ στήθεσσι φίλοισι·

πολλὰ δὲ μερμήριζε κατὰ φρένα καὶ κατὰ θυμόν,

ἠὲ μεταΐξας θάνατον τεύξειεν ἑκάστῃ,

ἦ ἔτ' ἐῷ μνηστῆρσιν ὑπερφιάλοισι μιγῆναι

ὕστατα καὶ πύματα·

---

4 Scully (1984) 14 articulates the most dominant view of these monologues in arguing that, "[t]he private thoughts of a hero question the values of heroic activity as he could never do publicly. Thus, it is the privileged domain of the soliloquy to convey the anxiety of the hero as he moves from indecision to resolution, from fear to courage, from thought to re-affirmation of heroic action". For other examples of Homeric internal monologues, but especially battlefield soliloquys, see *Il.* 11.403ff. [Odysseus], 17.90ff. [Menelaus], 18.5ff. [Achilles], 20.343ff. [Achilles], 550ff. [Agenor], 22.98ff. [Hector]; *Od.* 5.298ff. [Odysseus]. See Pelliccia (1995), Richardson (1993), and Gill (1996) for scholarly discussions of Homeric internal monologues.

5 Gill (1996) in particular discusses this passage in detail as an example of psychological conflict; Pelliccia (1995) 177 states that, "the importance of the passage cannot be exaggerated" and continues at 122f that, "[i]ts singularity, however, can: in relation to "ordinary" Homeric psychology what is depicted in the scene differs in degree rather than in kind". See also Jahn (1987), Caswell (1990), and Halliwell (1990) for further discussion.

6 Gill (2001) 786.

Odysseus lay there awake, devising evils in his *thumos* for the suitors as those women were coming from the hall, the ones who had mixed with them before this, providing happiness and laughter for each other. His *thumos* swelled in his own *stēthos*, and he debated anxiously in his *phrēn* and *thumos*, whether to rush upon and make a death for each of them, or to let them mix with the arrogant suitors one last and final time.[7]

Odysseus plans the events of the follow day inwardly (μνηστῆρσι κακὰ φρονέων ἐνὶ θυμῷ, 5), and his second internal debate is introduced by the formulaic, "he debated anxiously in his *phrēn* and *thumos*" (μερμήριζε κατὰ φρένα καὶ κατὰ θυμόν, 10). In both these examples, the θυμός and φρήν are deliberative spaces that, in terms of cognitive semantics, correspond to the "mind as a container" image schema: to a figurative conceptualisation of our psychological capacities as having definable boundaries and in-out orientations.[8] These metaphors are common elsewhere in Homer, where gods place ideas and motivations in the heads of mortals, and people hide their thoughts from others within their minds. Thetis, for example, beseeches Achilles to reveal his thoughts to her in *Iliad* 1 (μὴ κεῦθε νόῳ, ἵνα εἴδομεν ἄμφω, 363), while Iris incites in Helen a desire for her past life in Book 3 (Ὣς εἰποῦσα θεὰ γλυκὺν ἵμερον ἔμβαλε θυμῷ| ἀνδρός τε προτέρου καὶ ἄστεος ἠδὲ τοκήων, 139–140).[9] We have similar expressions in the English language: consider, for example, "I need to clear my mind", "my brain is full of interesting ideas", and "he's empty-headed".[10] Odysseus' *deliberative* content, furthermore, corresponds to the "ideas as objects" schema, in which his possible choices (his plans for the following day and his more immediate intentions with the maidservants) are stored, examined, and processed within the container-mind. On a conceptual level, these metaphors depend on the kinds of bodies we have, the way we define and move through space, and the way we manipulate objects in our environment. As Lakoff and Johnson explain:

> We are physical beings, bounded and set off from the rest of the world by the surface of our skins, and we experience the rest of the world as outside us. Each of us is a container, with a bounding surface and an in-out orientation. We project our own in-out orientation onto

---

7 All translations are my own.
8 The fullest explanation of container metaphors is in Lakoff/Johnson (1980) 29–32.
9 The same formula occurs at 16.19 [Achilles to Patroclus], and similar wording at 18.74 [Thetis to Achilles]. In these two further cases, thoughts are likewise represented metaphorically as physical objects that can be hidden from others. For further examples of gods putting thoughts or motivations in the minds of mortals, see *Il.* 2.451–452 [Athene and the Achaians], 5.512–513 [Apollo and Aeneas], 13.82 [the two Ajaxes]; *Od.* 19.485–486 [Eurycleia]; 23.260 [Odysseus and Penelope].
10 See Lakoff/Johnson (1980) 198; Kövecses (2000).

other objects that are bounded by surfaces. Thus we also view them as containers with an inside and an outside.[11]

More specifically, we manipulate our environment from a very early age with our hands – throughout their first year of life, a child learns the boundaries and capabilities of their bodies by physical testing their surroundings – and objects within it – through play.[12] Had we evolved without them, Wilson and Gibbs argue, we might not have developed metaphors like "grasping a concept" or "throwing out an idea".[13] That we have hands, therefore, that we use in interacting with our world from an early age, informs how we understand these cognitive structures; the fact that we also have bodies which move through space and orientate themselves based on the objects around them and, indeed, think of our bodies as objects themselves, help us to conceive of abstract concepts metaphorically as their own definable containers with bounded surfaces. This bodily basis for these metaphors not only inform the way we, in the every day, structure our mind and thoughts as containers and objects, but also the narrator's presentation of Odysseus' psychological functioning in *Odyssey* 20.

In the opening lines, therefore, the *mechanics* of Odysseus' thought processes are embodied using container metaphors. The majority of this passage is, however, dedicated to describing his *emotional* response – it is, primarily, a representation of an individual who struggles in controlling his anger, frustration, anxiety, and indecision at a time of extreme emotional pressure. The broader context of this passage is important: it is the night before Odysseus and Telemachus take revenge on the suitors, cleanse their household, and re-establish proper order in Ithaca. This is the culmination of Odysseus' journey home from Troy; it is therefore essential that he not reveal his identity until the proper moment, though he still struggles with his reaction to the things he sees and experiences in his home. In order to convey this struggle metaphorically, the narrator employs concepts of heat, fire, and motion in the "hungry man" simile. Odysseus has just exhorted himself to calm down, citing his imprisonment in Polyphemus' cave as evidence that he is capable of maintaining self-discipline and control in

---

11 Lakoff/Johnson (1980a) 29.
12 Gallagher (2005) 1.
13 Wilson/Gibbs (2007). See also Gibbs' (2006a) 441–442 discussion of metaphors that describe abstract concepts in terms of grasping and throwing; in this study, he argues that these metaphors entail a kind of "embodied simulation", in which "conceiving of abstract entities as physical objects enables people to perform mental actions on these objects as if they possessed the properties of real-world, concrete, physical entities" (442).

even worse situations (18–21). Though this rationale works for his κραδίη, which remains "unceasingly enduring", Odysseus himself is unable to rest (25–30):

> ὣς ἔφατ', ἐν στήθεσσι καθαπτόμενος φίλον ἦτορ·
>
> τῷ δὲ μάλ' ἐν πείσῃ κραδίη μένε τετληυῖα
>
> νωλεμέως· ἀτὰρ αὐτὸς ἑλίσσετο ἔνθα καὶ ἔνθα.
>
> ὡς δ' ὅτε γαστέρ' ἀνὴρ πολέος πυρὸς αἰθομένοιο,
>
> ἐμπλείην κνίσης τε καὶ αἵματος, ἔνθα καὶ ἔνθα
>
> αἰόλλῃ, μάλα δ' ὦκα λιλαίεται ὀπτηθῆναι,
>
> ὣς ἄρ' ὅ γ' ἔνθα καὶ ἔνθα ἑλίσσετο μερμηρίζων,
>
> ὅππως δὴ μνηστῆρσιν ἀναιδέσι χεῖρας ἐφήσει.
>
> μοῦνος ἐὼν πολέσι.

> So he spoke, accosting his own *ētor* in his chest, and, in great obedience, his *kardia* remained unceasingly enduring. But he himself tossed back and forth. As when a man at a fire turns a stomach back and forth, full of fat and blood, and is eager to roast it very quickly, so Odysseus tossed back and forth, debating anxiously how to lay his hands on the shameless suitors, being alone among many.

On the one level, this simile describes Odysseus' body language, in which the dense and repeated use of terms corresponding to quick, back-forth movements such as ἑλίσσω, ἔνθα καὶ ἔνθα, and αἰόλλω describe the manner in which he tosses and turns in his bed. But on the same hand, they also reflect his indecision as he struggles in settling on a plan for the following day – all these terms give us more information about Odysseus' conflicted thoughts, appearing in line 28 as μερμηρίζω (to debate anxiously). The narrator's repeated use of ἔνθα καὶ ἔνθα, which appears three times in five lines, and especially with ἑλίσσω (to roll), best encapsulates this process, in which separate choices are concretised in terms of physical distance, and emotional toil is described as rapid, whirring movements.[14] To draw is more closely back to the simile, Odysseus both physically and mentally shifts between one choice and another – like a sausage over a fire – as he struggles internally. In drawing heavily on ideas of rapid movement and physical distance, this simile corresponds to the sorts of things we might do when

---

[14] This particular metaphor was later used as source material by Apollonius, in which Medea, after waking from a dream about Jason, debates whether or not to go to her sister's bedchamber (*Argonautica* 3.651–655). The same terminology is used of Medea as for Odysseus in the *Od.* 20 passage, where ἔνθα καὶ ἔνθα and ἑλίσσω describe both her inner mental turmoil and her very literal back-forth movement over her bedrooms threshold.

processing difficult information or making hard decisions: we might toss and turn, pace back and forth, or rock our heads from side to side. It is not only that the physical component of Odysseus' emotional experience is, therefore, very familiar to us, but also that these nonverbal behaviours contribute to a conceptualisation of indecision as being, in concrete terms, frenetic movement or disparate locations.[15] In line with this, Colombetti, citing Gibbs' and Sheets-Johnstone's phenomenological accounts of emotion experience, describes how linguistic expressions and metaphors can "reveal the *dynamical* and *kinetic* character of emotional experience".[16] This is precisely what we have here: it is not just that the narrator renders Odysseus' psychological turmoil as a two-part, physical and mental account of emotion; instead, the physiological experience of emotion (tossing and turning in his bed) actually *structures* and *frames* the psychological one (internal decision-making and formulating plans). To be specific, the audiences is given access to Odysseus' psychological conflict and restlessness *via* their familiarity with and experiences of physical nonverbal behaviour and somatic experiences of anxiety and anger; the narrator, in presenting the relationship between the mind and the body in this way, demonstrates his understanding of the extent to which they mutually structure and influence each other.

This internal debate is made difficult by the psychological pressure under which Odysseus operate at this point in the narrative. In this sense, the simile also encapsulates the *intensity* of his emotional experience, in which his anger roasts him like a blazing fire, and his eagerness is likened to the hunger and desire of the starving man. The characteristically cunning Odysseus struggles to

---

15 Conflict, whether in the sense of different decisions or disagreement, is sometimes metaphorised as physical distance in Homer. In *Iliad* 1.6–8, for example, the narrator describes Agamemnon's and Achilles' psychological dissonance using concepts of physical separation: ἐξ οὗ δὴ τὰ πρῶτα διαστήτην ἐρίσαντε| Ἀτρεΐδης τε ἄναξ ἀνδρῶν καὶ δῖος Ἀχιλλεύς.| τίς τάρ σφωε θεῶν ἔριδι ξυνέηκε μάχεσθαι (From the time when first they were set apart having quarrelled, the son of Atreus, leader of men, and god-like Achilles. Who of the gods brought them to fight in bitter strife?); and Diomedes' heart is described as being 'divided' two ways in *Il*. 13.455–457. A more modern example of a similar idea is in Frost's *The Road Not Taken* (1916), which begins with, "Two roads diverged in a yellow wood, and sorry I could not travel both and be one traveller". One interpretation of this poem is that Frost employs the concept of a journey as a metaphor for life; this kind of metaphor is used in everyday speech, in which important decisions are forks in the road, different choices are diverging pathways, and difficulties are rough terrain. Like Homer, then, Frost describes psychological processes using concepts of physical distance. Within this context, as Lakoff/Turner (1989), audiences have an automatic, inbuilt apparatus for understanding these connections that is directly sourced from their experiences in and interactions with the outside world.
16 Colombetti (2014) 119.

formulate a plan because of the rage he feels towards the maidservants, his frustration at his inability to act, his anxiety for the day ahead, and his eagerness to kill the suitors. Words like μάλα (exceedingly), ὦκα (swiftly), and πολύς (mighty) express this in a literally sense; but αἴθω (to burn) and ὀπτάω (to roast) do so in a metaphorical one. So it is not just that Odysseus is angry – he is intensely so and, if we follow the simile, it inhibits his inability to think clearly, even despite his rapidly churning mind.

Accordingly, neurobiological and psychophysiological studies show that extreme emotion is physiologically felt as heat and pressure – as an increase in temperature and blood pressure in the body.[17] These studies demonstrate that anger can trigger "flight or fight" responses in individuals, in which humans and animals respond to threats or challenges with a general discharge of the sympathetic nervous system – one of the two parts of our autonomic system that regulates unconscious action. More specifically, the adrenal medulla (a part of the adrenal gland) produces hormones that discharge catecholamines (but especially norepinephrine and epinephrine/adrenaline) into the body. With respect to nonverbal behaviour, catecholamines can cause physiological changes that prepare an organism for quick action and strenuous physical activity; some of these effects include increases in heart rate blood pressure, muscle tensity, and glucose levels.[18] But these same symptoms are also consistent with modern studies of fear and anxiety, which suggest that both emotions have strong bases in evolutionary development. In a recent article, Öhman argues that fear and anxiety are "closely related emotional phenomena originating in evolved mammalian defense systems".[19] He continues:

---

[17] Ax (1953); Innes/Millar/Valentine (1959).

[18] One of the first major studies of "fight or flight" responses was Cannon (1929), but for a more recent discussion of the neurobiological underpinnings of this process, see Jansen et al. (1995). Boyd (2008) 92–93, additionally, argues that these impulses might be the reason that humans develop games specifically aimed at refining their skills and abilities in these areas (i.e. "flight" games might include chase, tag, running, "fight" games include wrestling and throwing, and recovery of balance includes skiing, surfing, and skateboarding). In line with this, Boyd (92) argues that, "The more often and the more exuberantly animals play, the more they hone skills, widen repertoires, and sharpen sensitivities. Play therefore has evolved to be highly self-rewarding. Through the compulsiveness of play, animals incrementally alter muscle tone and neural wiring, strengthen and increase the processing speed of synaptic pathways, and improve their capacity and potential for performance in later, less forgiving circumstances." On this point, see also Bekoff (2007) 100.

[19] The distinction between fear and anxiety as two emotional experiences is still a topic of debate in the sciences. The American Psychiatric Association identifies anxiety as a 'pre-stimulus' (anticipatory or propositional) response to perceived future threats. Fear, on the other hand, is

> Fear is a functional emotion with a deep evolutionary origin, reflecting the fact that earth has always been a hazardous environment to inhabit. Staying alive is a prerequisite for the basic goal of biological evolution ... even the most primitive of organisms have developed defense responses to deal with life threats in their environment.[20]

In line with this, a study by Arrindell and his colleagues identify four basic motivating factors in experiences of fear: (first) interpersonal events or situations (i.e. criticism, rejection, and conflict), (second) death, injury, blood, and illness, (third) animals, and (fourth) agoraphobia.[21] Each of these factors, Öhman argues at p. 711, has its basis in evolutionary pressures, where urges to survive and propagate, establish safe kin groups and secure environments, and avoid social humiliation and status threats drive the development of certain fears and shape our most commonly occurring fears.[22] Put more simply, at p. 712:

> Evolution has equipped humans with a propensity to associate fear with situations that threatened the survival of their ancestors ... thus the development of phobias is jointly determined by genetic predispositions and specific environmental exposures.

While Odysseus is angry, we also know that fear and anxiety are motivating factors for his internal conflict: Odysseus is "alone among many" (μοῦνος ἐὼν πολέσι, 30), and these unfavourable odds prevent him from acting sooner; he has just come from his emotional night-time interview with Penelope; and he has reunited

---

'post-stimulus' in that it has a current, identifiable target. Öhman (2005) 710, following Lader/Marks (1973), explains the distinction between the two: "Fear denotes dread of impending disaster and an intense urge to defend oneself, primarily by getting out of the situation. Clinical anxiety, on the other hand, has been described as an ineffable and unpleasant feeling of foreboding." In contrast to both these arguments, however, Epstein (1972) 311 concludes that fear and anxiety are defined by different coping behaviour: "*Fear* is an avoidance motive. If there were no restraints, internal or external, fear would support the action of flight. *Anxiety* can be defined as unresolved fear, or, alternatively, as a state of undirected arousal following the perception of threat."

20 Öhman (2008) 709–710.
21 Arrindell *et al.* (1997) 79.
22 Homeric examples of experiences of fear include *Iliad* 7.214–218 [Hector and the Trojans], 10.91–95 [Agamemnon], and 13.280–284 [Idomeneus' "cowardly man"]. Accordingly, each these groups exhibit different kinds of physical behaviour consistent with "flight-or-fight" impulses, as well as experiences of fear and anxiety: the coward's, Hector's, and Agamemnon's heart-rates accelerate (μεγάλα πατάσσει), the coward's skin changes colour (ἄλλυδις ἄλλη); the coward (οὐδέ οἱ ἀτρέμας ἧσθαι ... θυμός), the Trojans (τρόμος ... γυῖα ἕκαστον), and Agamemnon (τρομέει δ' ὑπὸ φαίδιμα γυῖα) are unable to control the shudder of their muscles; and the coward's teeth chatter (πάταγος δέ τε γίγνετ' ὀδόντων).

with his nursemaid, Eurycleia, to whom he has expressed, indirectly, his anxiety at the prospect of being discovered prematurely, even by his wife (19.479–481):

> αὐτὰρ Ὀδυσσεὺς
> χείρ' ἐπιμασσάμενος φάρυγος λάβε δεξιτερῆφι,
> τῇ δ' ἑτέρῃ ἕθεν ἆσσον ἐρύσσατο φώνησέν τε·
> "μαῖα, τίη μ' ἐθέλεις ὀλέσαι; σὺ δέ μ' ἔτρεφες αὐτὴ
> τῷ σῷ ἐπὶ μαζῷ· νῦν δ' ἄλγεα πολλὰ μογήσας
> ἤλυθον εἰκοστῷ ἔτεϊ ἐς πατρίδα γαῖαν".

> Then Odysseus reached for Eurycleia, grabbed her throat with his right hand, pulled her closer with the other, and said: "Good Mother, why do you want to destroy me? You yourself reared me at this breast of yours, but now, after suffering great sorrows, I have come, in the twentieth year, to my homeland".

That Odysseus' fear, anxiety, and anger are partially conceptualized using concepts of intense heat, pressure, and motion is, within this context, compelling; it suggests not only that the simile introduced by the narrator has its roots in everyday physical processes, but also that he expects his audience to have an implicit understanding of the phenomenological aspects of emotion experience. To put it more simply, the process by which we understand this simile is a comfortable and natural one because the metaphorical correspondence between heat and anger is based in physiological and evolutionary pressures: as Darwin observed early on, and as stated above, anger exhibits itself in human and non-human primates as an acceleration of the heart and circulatory system, reddened skin and increased body temperature, and distended veins in the face and neck (2009[1872], 235).[23] Conversely, rationality and calm are often physiologically felt and metaphorically understood as a decrease in body temperature: Shakespeare's Theseus in *A Midsummer Night's Dream*, for example, juxtaposes irrationality and anger with rationality and calm when he states that, "Lovers and madmen have such seething brains, such shaping fantasies, that apprehend more than cool reason ever comprehends" (5.1.4–6). The image schemata on which these metaphors are based – "anger is a boiling liquid", "love is a flame", "passion is heat", "dispassion is cold" – all have their deepest roots in the physiological effect of these experiences on the body.[24] In presenting Odysseus' anger in this way, the narrator taps into physical, perceptual, and evolutionary dimensions of our experience;

---

23 Darwin (2009 [1872]) 235.
24 Kövecses (2000) 39 and 147–148.

our understanding of this internal process, furthermore, is made possible by our implicit and subconscious theory of mind – the process by which we intuit thoughts, beliefs, intentions, and emotions to others – which enables us to make inferences about Odysseus' psychological state based on our own historical, first-person experience with extreme emotion[25] and, in a more mundane sense, of the affect of fire and heat on bodies.

The narrator also makes extensive use of canine imagery in describing Odysseus' emotional response, in a cluster of metaphors and a simile that borrows from the instinctual behaviour of animals in threatening situations. The first example of this is at line nine, where Odysseus' θυμός is roused to anger by the maidservants' behaviour. The main verb in this clause, ὀρίνω (to rouse or stir) is elsewhere commonly used in Homer of men and animals;[26] here, it introduces the more obvious link between Odysseus and the instinct-driven, protective dog in the successive verses (13–17):

> κραδίη δέ οἱ ἔνδον ὑλάκτει.
>
> ὡς δὲ κύων ἀμαλῇσι περὶ σκυλάκεσσι βεβῶσα
>
> ἄνδρ' ἀγνοιήσασ' ὑλάει μέμονέν τε μάχεσθαι,
>
> ὥς ῥα τοῦ ἔνδον ὑλάκτει ἀγαιομένου κακὰ ἔργα.
>
> στῆθος δὲ πλήξας κραδίην ἠνίπαπε μύθῳ·

> And his *kardia* growled inside him. As a dog steps around her weak puppies and growls at a man she does not recognise, eager to fight, so Odysseus growled inside him, indignant at their evil actions, and pounded at his chest and reproached his *kardia* with words.

The simile, in providing more information about what Odysseus can only do inwardly and covertly, closely couples his instinctual response, territoriality, and rage with that of the dog who, circling her puppies (the much-depleted Ithacan household), growls at a strange man (the suitors and maidservants). Modern scholarship on the evolutionary roots of nonverbal behaviour has found that human and non-human primates engage in threat displays in similar ways. Darwin's early comments on this point are apt:

---

[25] See Cairns (2013) 86, who argues a similar point of φρίκη: "φρίκη is an experience of an animal, but what the application of the term pinpoints is the visible aspect of that experience in the eyes of others. When this term is applied to an emotional experience, what we are dealing with is (in the strict sense) the phenomenology of emotion, i.e. the shared, third person perspective that we all have ... of what it is like to experience the emotion in the first person".

[26] Of human emotions, see *Il.* 2.142 [Achaians], 3.395 [Helen], 13.418 [Antilochus]. ὀρίνω is also commonly used of natural phenomena; for example, of the wind and sea: *Il.* 2.294, 9.4, 11.297–298.

> The uncovering of the canine tooth is the result of a double movement ... the action is the same as that of a snarling dog; and a dog when pretending to fight often draws up the lip on one side alone, namely that facing his protagonist.[27]

Homer also draws close connection between aggressive behaviour in humans and animals, but especially when individual threat displays involve the baring of teeth in a mirthless smile from beneath the brow (*Il.* 7.211–213, 15.607–609). In these cases, the bristled brow, described using the verb βλοσυρός, is used elsewhere in early hexameter poetry to denote an animal's 'shaggy' or 'bristling' coat (*Sh* 175, 191). The *Odyssey* 20 example is especially important, however, for two main reasons. First, in drawing close connections between the behaviour of Odysseus and the dog, it more explicitly delineates the evolutionary basis for Homeric metaphors and simile.[28] In describing Odysseus in this way, the narrator provides his audience with an accessible means for understanding his emotional state that is based in our deepest, most subconscious evolutionary roots. Second, this passage is especially interesting because these particular lines have been used for evidence that the Homeric narrator had an understanding of conceptual metaphor. To be specific, we might see how the simile of the snarling dog is used in concretizing the abstract thought processes in the metaphors of the surrounding lines (13, κραδίη δέ οἱ ἔνδον ὑλάκτει; 16, ὥς ῥα τοῦ ἔνδον ὑλάκτει ἀγαιομένου κακὰ ἔργα). In doing so, the narrator borrows from the physiological in order to conceptualise the psychological, in which the repeated use of ὑλακτέω characterizes both the dog's actual physical behaviour and Odysseus' emotional response.

---

27 Darwin (2009 [1872]) 247. See Redican (1982) for a more modern study on deimetic behaviour; based on studies of humans and animals, at pp. 226–227, he argues that: "In its complete form, as often seen in most taxa of Old World monkeys and apes, the display is characterized by a slightly to full open mouth with upper lip tensed over the teeth and corners of the mouth brought forward, and the upper and often lower teeth are not usually visible; especially in profile; the ears are usually flattened against the head; the gaze is fixed upon the percipient; the eyebrow may be furrowed; and the nostrils may be flared." For other examples of the application of this idea to aggressive smiling in Homer, see Clarke (2005) 38–39. See also Goffman (1967) 24–26 on the aggressive use of "face-work".

28 As Rose (1979) points out, additionally, the narrator often describes Odysseus using canine elements in the *Odyssey*; in addition to the *Od.* 20 passage, he cites 14.21–22, 29–32, and 17.291–327. Another good example of this is in *Od.* 20, where Odysseus smiles inwardly in anticipation of his revenge against the Suitors (301–302): ὁ δ' ἀλεύατ' Ὀδυσσεύς| ἧκα παρακλίνας κεφαλήν, μείδησε δὲ θυμῷ| σαρδάνιον μάλα τοῖον. This is the only use of the noun σαρδάνιος in archaic hexameter poetry; Levine (1984) 5, Rutherford (1992) 229, and Clarke (2005) 38 argue that it is likely related to σαίρω, "to grin, grimace", the underlying image being of a dog baring its teeth threateningly. See also Fenik (1974) 180–186; Lateiner (1995) 194.

There is one further use of canine imagery in this passage, in which Odysseus recollects his time in Polyphemus' cave (18–21):

"τέτλαθι δή, κραδίη· καὶ κύντερον ἄλλο ποτ' ἔτλης,

ἤματι τῷ, ὅτε μοι μένος ἄσχετος ἤσθιε Κύκλωψ

ἰφθίμους ἑτάρους· σὺ δ' ἐτόλμας, ὄφρα σε μῆτις

ἐξάγαγ' ἐξ ἄντροιο ὀϊόμενον θανέεσθαι."

"Endure this, *kardia*. You once endured an even worse ["more dog-like"] thing, on that day when the Cyclops, uncontrollable in strength, ate my strong companions: you endured it, until *metis* led you from the cave, though expecting to die."

In comparing his prior and current circumstances, Odysseus attempts to control himself; in this sense, his reference to Polyphemus' cave might be understood as a didactic use of memory, in which the past provides a framework by which Odysseus can psychologically resolve his present challenge.[29] This connection hinges primarily on the double meaning of κῆδος, which denotes both one's possessions and extended family. More specifically, the Suitors deplete Odysseus' household (and literally consume his possessions) as Polyphemus devoured his companions; the Ithacan Palace, as a site that poses an immediate threat to Odysseus, might be likened to the cave itself; and the Suitors' failure to adhere to the obligations of the host-guest relationship, which threatens to strip Odysseus of both his belongings and his return, is similar to that of Polyphemus' in *Odyssey* 9. It is perhaps interesting, additionally, to consider the simile used in *Od.* 9, in which Odysseus' companions are likened to puppies as Polyphemus kills them (288–290):

"ἀλλ' ὅ γ' ἀναΐξας ἑτάροισ' ἐπὶ χεῖρας ἴαλλε,

σὺν δὲ δύω μάρψας ὥς τε σκύλακας ποτὶ γαίῃ

κόπτ'·"

"But he jumped up and put his hands on my companions, grabbed two at once and smashed them, like killing puppies, against the earth".

---

29 Memory serves this function elsewhere in Homer. Hector, for example, recollects a prior encounter with Poulydamos (*Il.* 22.99–103), in which, in not following his advice, several of Hector's men had died. As in the *Odyssey* 20 passage, there is a link between Hector's past experiences and current circumstances, in which the former acts as instruction for the latter, and a framework by which he can structure his thoughts.

In this sense, the past becomes a framework by which he can manage the present and the future. It is in recognizing the similarities between these two experiences that Odysseus reaches the conclusion that, as with Polyphemus, dealing with the suitors and the maidservants with forethought and endurance are best; on an extra-narrative level, the use of canine elements in both passages may reinforce the significance of this past experience for Odysseus' present psychological processes.

This study consists of a three-way dialogue. First, it reaffirms the enormous potential of cognitive science to expand our knowledge and understanding of psychological functioning in Homer. Second, it establishes the Homeric poems as a valuable corpus of material that, as an artefact of mind, lends weight to the the findings of scientific survey and analysis. Finally, this study positions Homer's narrative within a wider scholarly movement—cognitive poetics—which contends that literary minds are as complex and multi-modal as our own. Accordingly, the narrator expresses Odysseus' unstable and tempestuous psychological state primarily using embodied metaphors that have, notably, both universally determined and culturally specific components. As we have seen, metaphors of fire, heat, and motion are universal phenomena that are, in part, based in physiological components of emotion experience, such as rises in body temperature, higher levels of adrenaline, and physical restlessness; but the wider use of terms such as ἔνθα καὶ ἔνθα and ἑλίσσω elsewhere in the Homeric corpus also informs the narrator's use of spatial imagery. The narrator's deployment of canine imagery likewise combines familiar and universal evolutionary elements with (1) culturally-specific understandings of aggressive behavior and (2) connections with earlier narrative action that impact upon Odysseus' current psychological state. Cognitive science therefore not only enables us to recognize how pervasively the narrator employs embodied metaphor in his poetry, but also aids us in navigating a complex set of physiological, psychological, cultural, interactional, and evolutionary pressures that inform his representation of psychological functioning. In examining these connections in greater depth, and with respect to modern studies of cognition, we reach a more precise understanding of how narrators and audiences conceive of individuals as cohesive wholes. For Homer, in other words, as in the everyday, "there is no such thing as a naked brain".[30]

---

[30] Barrett (2011) 135.

Jennifer J. Devereaux
3 Bodies of Knowledge: Metaphor and Mnemonic Practice in Ancient Historiography

"If we, with our superior knowledge, were to say to them that a given core element was false, I imagine they would be glad for the information. ... If, on the other hand, we were to say to an ancient historian that a given example of *exaedificatio* was untrue, he would no doubt reply, with some indignation, 'It *must* have been like that'".

– Anthony J. Woodman[1]

History is described by Antonius in the second book of Cicero's *De oratore* as the witness of time (*testis temporum*), the light of truth (*lux veritatis*), the life of memory (*vita memoriae*), the teacher of life (*magistra vitae*), and the messenger of antiquity (*nuntia vetustatis*).[2] This raises the question: What does it mean to be a truthful witness of *time*? I would suggest that since "truth" in ancient historiography is often *that which is plausible*,[3] and what is most plausible is that which is most commonly understood – namely bodily sensation and emotional states[4] – truthfulness entails a qualitative approach towards time. What I mean by a qualitative approach towards time will become clear, but, in general, it refers to the fact that narrative time is largely created through action, and verbs of narration often seem to exhibit a unique relationship to metaphor in ancient historiography, which accounts for their qualitative property. Even verbs we don't automatically expect to carry metaphorical or emotional weight, do, and metaphors extended through verbal elements demonstrate that the elaboration of truth can

---

1 Woodman (1988) citing Wiseman (1981).
2 Orat.2.36.
3 Woodman (1988) identifies this through Thuc. 1.22.4 (καὶ ἐς μὲν ἀκρόασιν ἴσως τὸ μὴ μυθῶδες αὐτῶν ἀτερπέστερον φανεῖται: ὅσοι δὲ βουλήσονται τῶν τε γενομένων τὸ σαφὲς σκοπεῖν καὶ τῶν μελλόντων ποτὲ αὖθις κατὰ τὸ ἀνθρώπινον τοιούτων καὶ παραπλησίων ἔσεσθαι, ὠφέλιμα κρίνειν αὐτὰ ἀρκούντως ἕξει) and Cic.*Inv.* 1.9 (*inventio est excogitatio rerum verarum aut veri similium, quae causam probabilem reddant*).
4 Cf. Schubert et al. (2008) 177; Yu (2008); Gibbs (2005) 67.

Note: My heartfelt gratitude to Thomas Habinek for his support and guidance throughout this ongoing project. Special thanks to William Short for organizing our panel and to Douglas Cairns for his response. Thanks also to Michael Carroll for his helpful comments.

Jennifer Devereaux, University of Southern California

https://doi.org/10.1515/9783110482201-004

be done by means of content elaborating content, that is, by action elaborating action. The movement of the narrative – literally and figuratively – develops the stuff of *vita memoriae* through a form of teaching that involves storytelling, otherwise known as *inventio*. This fictional element of ancient historiography has been well discussed by Anthony Woodman and Timothy Wiseman, among others,[5] with the former drawing a neat distinction between *monumenta* – the kernels of truth, or 'hard core' – at the center of historical narrative, and their artistic elaboration (*ornamenta*), the crafting of which was informed by the rhetorical practice of *inventio*. Obviously there are many ways to artistically elaborate and render a narration vivid. This paper will explore what seems to be a particular way of doing so that suggests an adjustment of emphasis in the opening quotation is called for:

> If, on the other hand, we were to say to an ancient historian that a given example of *exaedificatio* was untrue, he would no doubt reply, with some indignation, 'It must have been *like* that'

It is a seemingly minor but arguably significant change of emphasis that rests on reframing the term *plausible* in such a way as to draw attention to the fact that although scholars have long recognized the use of rhetorical devices in history-writing, they overlook a deeper connection that has the potential to enrich our understanding of the historian's art and of their potential impact on their audiences. That said, I will obviously not be able to provide the depth and breadth of analysis necessary to make any broad-sweeping claims at this time, but I do hope to demonstrate that there are levels of implicit rhetoric seemingly occurring within an embodied framework that warrant further study. By "embodied framework" I refer to the theory of embodied cognition that postulates that aspects of the agent's body beyond the brain play a significant causal or physically constitutive role in cognitive processing. It is a theory of cognition that postulates language is grounded in the bodily states that comprise emotions,[6] an hypothesis that enjoys the support of mounting evidence, including that which indicates some degree of sensorimotor involvement in the processing of verbal language,[7] which in turn produces subconscious bodily states that influence emotion and impact reasoning processes,[8] suggesting that perceptual and motor

---

[5] See esp. Grant (1995); Gill/Wiseman (1993).
[6] Cf. Glenberg *et al.* (2008).
[7] Cf. Aziz-Zadeh *et al.* (2006); Kaschak *et al.* (2009); Thelen *et al.* (2001); Feldman (2006); Lakoff (2008); Zwann/Madden (2005); Desai *et al.* (2011).
[8] Cf. Damasio (2010) (esp. p.117).

representations play a role in retrieving information in memory[9] and may have something to do with bodily movement reinforcing memory.[10]

Hidden Metaphors

To begin exploring the role of sensorimotor knowledge in the composition of texts, we may consider *De orat.* 3.7 and *AUC* 21.40 in parallel. Their comparison illustrates the sort of conceptual coherence that will be of interest to us as we move forward. The first expresses Cicero's reaction to the death of Crassus, the second recounts the challenges faced by Hannibal's Carthaginians as they cross the Alps. The passages demonstrate a certain conceptual consistency with each other not strictly evident in the propositional content of the texts. This paper will suggest that this conceptual consistency is evidence of a narrative technique described and displayed in rhetorical treatises, appearing in similar forms with some regularity in ancient historiography.

> *De orat.*3.7
> *O fallacem hominum spem fragilemque fortunam, et inanes nostras contentiones, quae medio in spatio saepe franguntur et corruunt et ante in ipso cursu obruuntur, quam portum conspicere potuerunt!*
>
> Ah, how treacherous are men's hopes, how insecure their fortunes! How hollow are our endeavors, which often break down and come to grief in the middle of the race, or are shipwrecked in full sail before they have been able to sight the harbour! (Rackham)

> *AUC* 21.40
> *Effigies immo, umbrae hominum, fame frigore, inluvie squalore enecti, contusi ac debilitati inter saxa rupesque; ad hoc praeusti artus, nive rigentes nervi, membra torpida gelu, quassata fractaque arma, claudi ac debiles equi.*
>
> They are but the semblance, the shadows of men, wasted away with hunger and cold, with filth and squalor; bruised and crippled amongst the rocks and cliffs; moreover, their limbs are frost-bitten, their muscles stiffened by the snow, their bodies numb with cold; their arms shattered and broken, their horses lame and feeble. (Foster)

---

9 Zwann (2005) 3.
10 Cf. Sutton/Williamson (2014), esp. p.316: "... accumulated experiences are actively embodied in actions. I need not explicitly recollect any specific past events, or even recognize that I am remembering, unless my smooth coping is disrupted. As Edward Casey puts it, such memory is intrinsic to the body: 'because it re-enacts the past, it need not represent it' (1987: 147, 178)."

In Cicero, in the description of the death of Crassus, the abstract concept of *the human condition* is indirectly metaphorized into a ship(wreck). It is fragile and hollow, which relates to a propensity for breakage, and in particular to ship hulls, given that *frangitur* is *le mot juste* when referring to shipwrecks. The accepted reading of *obruuntur* here in Cicero is indeed *shipwrecked*, and this meaning was later utilized by Livy (*AUC* 30.10). The metaphor in Cicero is poetic, a style of writing generally frowned upon in historiography from the time of Thucydides.[11] However, the structure of the metaphor – its emotionological framework[12] – is iterated through a mixture of metaphor and plain language by Livy. Through conceptual iteration, not unlike that which exists between *franguntur*, *corruunt*, and *obruuntur*, the Carthaginians are disintegrated and lost to obscurity. Made stiff like statues (*effigies: rigentes, torpida*) and cold like the dead (*umbrae: frigore, praeusti, gelu*), they are then suggested through metonymy to be fragile with *quassata fractaque*, the net result of *enecti ac debilitati*. Together with the breaking metaphors referring to frustrated ends in both passages, *obruuntur* and *enecti* seem conceptually related and thus strengthen the connection between the passages at a deeper cognitive level. *Obruo* has the core meaning of *to cover, flood, submerge, or bury beneath weight or force*, and extends to the figurative sense of *to obscure by superior effectiveness* or *importance*. *Eneco*, meaning *kill, stifle, destroy, exhaust* and *torment*, has *to execute* as one of its earliest and best attested meanings, that is, *to put to death in pursuance of a sentence*, so it is perhaps most accurate to say of *eneco* that it indicates the putting to death of someone by a person in a position of authority, a conceptual parallel to the figurative meaning of *obruo*.

Heightening the interest of this particular parallel is the biological metaphor that is intertwined with Livy's use of *eneco*. Just after Livy, Columella (2.11.1) uses the verb in reference to plants (*enecentur*) dying from cold (*frigora*; *gelu*) due to their roots having been exposed and severed by a hoe, with cold likely metonymically referring to physical manifestations of cold, such as snow and ice. With this in mind, consider the conceptual metaphor for *effigies* in Livy against the simple causal description by Columella:

---

11 Cf. Woodman (1988) 7.
12 Cf. "the *living* handbook of narratology" (http://wikis.sub.uni-hamburg.de/lhn/index.php/ Cognitive_Narratology#Emotion.2C_Emotion_Discourse.2C_and_.E2.80.9CEmotionology.E2.80.9D): "Every culture and subculture has an emotionology, which is a framework for conceptualizing emotions, their causes, and how participants in discourse are likely to display them".

Livy: *effigies(umbrae)* = *frigore et gelu* + *enecti* + *rigentes* + *fracta* [13]
Columella:[14] *frumenta(radices)* + *detegantur* + *succidantur* + *frigora et gelu* = *enecentur*

Due to a high degree of conceptual overlap evident in the propositional content of these texts, one can imagine that a biological understanding of death informs Livy's conceptual metaphor, bringing it into parallel with Cicero's use of *obruo*, particularly given that frost and ice have weight and literally cover the exposed roots. Such conceptual consistency between otherwise disparate narratives of failure in turn demonstrates that a biological process gains intentional force when used by an effective speaker skilled in rhetoric, like Scipio. That is to say, both *obruo* and *eneco* have similar conceptual content, and here are used in similar conceptual milieus that situate them in a shared space wherein to fail, broadly construed, is to be disintegrated by someone or something more powerful *by nature*. In the Livy passage, that authority figure is ultimately Scipio, who speaks the words in a hortatory speech to his troops after crossing the Po, effectively using rhetoric to shatter the Carthaginian ranks in a manner analogous to shattering an effigy – an act of *damnatio memoriae*.[15] This in turn runs parallel to Cicero's shipwreck that metaphorizes life, or a goal within it, as a journey, and describes death's denial of life's highest honors to Crassus in similar terms of breakage, because the same conceptual framework about failure underlies both passages. It thus seems that not only does Cicero use the metaphor to define his view on the human condition, but he also betrays a conceptual structure for tacitly talking about defeat that can be identified in otherwise dissimilar passages, like *AUC* 21.40.

---

13 I compound *umbrae* due to Livy's pairing and the simple fact that effigies in the physical world correspond to shades in the underworld in Roman culture, much as a plant corresponds to its roots in agriculture.

14 Col.2.11.1: *Quidam negant eam quicquam proficere, quod frumenti radices sarculo detegantur, aliquae etiam succidantur ac, si frigora incesserint post sartionem, gelu frumenta enecentur;satius autem esse ea tempestive runcari et purgari.*

15 I have previously suggested (2016) "that through the embodied understanding of Scipio's words the Carthaginians are not only *phantasiai*, but also *figurae sententiae* that structure the relationship between the speaker (Scipio; Livy) and his audience (soldiers; readers): through rhetoric Scipio has already begun the process of shattering the Carthaginian ranks in a manner analogous to shattering an effigy – an act of *damnatio memoriae*".

The Body and Narrative Structure

As we move forward, we will turn towards the body and consider a form of iteration that constructs metaphorical concepts through the arrangement of the text. This may have been done for the sake of appealing to shared feeling (cf. *commiseratio Rhet.Her* 4.28). As we will see, it was a technique already employed by Herodotus, who relies on an aggregate of the embodied experience expressed by a striking metaphor to describe Cambyses' internal response to the realization that his brother's death was unnecessary (3.64, ἔτυψε ἡ ἀληθείη Καμβύσεα):

> ἐνθαῦτα ἀκούσαντα Καμβύσεα τὸ Σμέρδιος οὔνομα **ἔτυψε ἡ ἀληθείη** τῶν τε λόγων καὶ τοῦ ἐνυπνίου· ὅς ἐδόκεε ἐν τῷ ὕπνῳ ἀπαγγεῖλαι τινά οἱ ὡς Σμέρδις ἱζόμενος ἐς τὸν βασιλήιον θρόνον ψαύσειε τῇ κεφαλῇ τοῦ οὐρανοῦ. μαθὼν δὲ ὡς μάτην ἀπολωλεκὼς εἴη τὸν ἀδελφεόν, ἀπέκλαιε Σμέρδιν· ἀποκλαύσας δὲ καὶ περιημεκτήσας τῇ ἁπάσῃ συμφορῇ ἀναθρῴσκει ἐπὶ τὸν ἵππον, ἐν νόῳ ἔχων τὴν ταχίστην ἐς Σοῦσα στρατεύεσθαι ἐπὶ τὸν Μάγον. καί οἱ ἀναθρῴσκοντι ἐπὶ τὸν ἵππον τοῦ κολεοῦ τοῦ ξίφεος ὁ μύκης ἀποπίπτει, γυμνωθὲν δὲ τὸ ξίφος **παίει** τὸν μηρόν· τρωματισθεὶς δὲ κατὰ τοῦτο τῇ αὐτὸς πρότερον τὸν τῶν Αἰγυπτίων θεὸν Ἆπιν **ἔπληξε**, ὥς οἱ καιρίη ἔδοξε **τετύφθαι**, εἴρετο ὁ Καμβύσης ὅ τι τῇ πόλι οὔνομα εἴη· οἱ δὲ εἶπαν ὅτι Ἀγβάτανα. τῷ δὲ ἔτι πρότερον ἐκέχρηστο ἐκ Βουτοῦς πόλιος ἐν Ἀγβατάνοισι τελευτήσειν τὸν βίον. ὁ μὲν δὴ ἐν τοῖσι Μηδικοῖσι Ἀγβατάνοισι ἐδόκεε τελευτήσειν γηραιός, ἐν τοῖσί οἱ ἦν τὰ πάντα πρήγματα· τὸ δὲ χρηστήριον ἐν τοῖσι ἐν Συρίῃ Ἀγβατάνοισι ἔλεγε ἄρα. καὶ δὴ ὡς τότε ἐπειρόμενος ἐπύθετο τῆς πόλιος τὸ οὔνομα, ὑπὸ τῆς συμφορῆς τῆς τε ἐκ τοῦ Μάγου **ἐκπεπληγμένος καὶ τοῦ τρώματος** ἐσωφρόνησε, συλλαβὼν δὲ τὸ θεοπρόπιον εἶπε 'ἐνθαῦτα Καμβύσεα τὸν Κύρου ἐστὶ πεπρωμένον τελευτᾶν.

> *The truth of the words and of a dream struck Cambyses the moment he heard the name Smerdis; for he had dreamt that a message had come to him that Smerdis sitting on the royal throne touched heaven with his head; and perceiving that he had killed his brother without cause, he wept bitterly for Smerdis. Having wept, and grieved by all his misfortune, he sprang upon his horse, with intent to march at once to Susa against the Magus. As he sprang upon his horse, the cap fell off the sheath of his sword, and the naked blade pierced his thigh, wounding him in the same place where he had once wounded the Egyptian god Apis; and believing the wound to be mortal, Cambyses asked what was the name of the town where he was. They told him it was Ecbatana. Now a prophecy had before this come to him from Buto, that he would end his life at Ecbatana; Cambyses supposed this to signify that he would die in old age at the Median Ecbatana, his capital city; but as the event proved, the oracle prophesied his death at Ecbatana of Syria. So when he now inquired and learned the name of the town, the shock of his wound, and of the misfortune that came to him from the Magus, brought him to his senses; he understood the prophecy and said: "Here Cambyses son of Cyrus is to die."*
> (A. D. Godley)

In a scene dependent upon the memory of Cambyses, the reader encounters various violent forms of physical contact in close succession (παίει, ἔπληξε, τετύφθαι), culminating with a direct metaphorical parallel (ἐκπεπληγμένος καὶ τοῦ τρώματος), which weaves together cause (being struck by the truth) and effect (being stunned by the wound). The internal experience of Cambyses is conceptualized not only by the metaphors that frame it, but also through the intervening verbs that connect to them. The truth and the wound are united in sense through a compounding of sensory experience.[16]

In general, the so-called pity evoked by this technique might be best understood as the ability to recognize common or shared experience. For example, we find the experience of Carthaginian soldiers framed by Livy with a tactile metaphor that sharpens the picture of Hannibal, whose hortatory speech is undermined through the use of extended metaphor that runs parallel to the propositional content of the text, wherein his men struggle in desperation (*desperatio in omnium voltu emineret*) to overcome the Alps:

> ... *Hannibal (dixit) ... uno aut summum altero proelio arcem et **caput Italiae in manu ac potestate habituros** ... omnis enim ferme via praeceps angusta **lubrica** erat, ut neque sustinere se ab **lapsu** possent nec qui paulum titubassent haerere adfixi vestigio suo, aliique super alios et iumenta in homines occiderent. Ventum deinde ad multo angustiorem rupem atque ita rectis saxis ut **aegre expeditus miles temptabundus manibusque retinens** virgulta ac stirpes circa eminentes demittere sese posset. Natura locus iam ante praeceps recenti **lapsu** terrae in pedum mille admodum altitudinem abruptus erat. ... Taetra ibi luctatio erat via **lubrica non recipiente** vestigium et in prono citius pedes **fallente**, ut seu manibus in adsurgendo seu genu se adiuvissent, ipsis adminiculis **prolapsis** iterum corruerent. (AUC 21.35–36)*

> ... *Hannibal (said) ... after one, or, at the most, two battles, they would have in their hands and in their power the citadel and capital of Italy .... For practically every road was steep, narrow, and treacherous, so that neither could they keep from slipping, nor could those who had been thrown a little off their balance retain their footing, but came down, one on top of the other, and the beasts on top of the men. They then came to a much narrower cliff, and with rocks so perpendicular that it was difficult for an unencumbered soldier to manage the descent, though he felt his way and clung with his hands to the bushes and roots that projected here and there. The place had been precipitous before, and a recent landslip had carried it away to the depth of a good thousand feet. Then came a terrible struggle on the slippery surface, for it afforded them no foothold, while the downward slope made their feet more quickly slide from under them.* (Foster)

---

[16] I have previously suggested (2016) that Herodotus here relies on an embodied understanding of what it is to have one's flesh penetrated to communicate an "image" of experience and the "feelings" that accompany it, and that the internal state that the metaphor seeks to render for the reader becomes clear with the literal verbs of striking that follow and extend the experience associated with the metaphorical phrase.

Through the metaphorical structuring of the episode, the actors' sense of desperation is rendered similar to trying to hold onto something that insists on slipping away, and, by virtue of metonymy, the deceived (*fallente*) feet of the soldiers stand for the soldiers themselves, who literally fall forward and, in metaphorical terms, go to ruin (*prolapsis*). The tacit relationship between the feeling of despair, the tactile metaphor, and the literal meanings of words that extend from its emotionological framework merge embodied experience with propositional content and thereby ground memory in psychosomatic experience.

I would suggest that these passages are "mnemonically dense" due to the number of semantically stable verbal elements that surround and extend the sense of the metaphors.[17] The body and its movements provide a qualitative commentary on temporal experience, a phenomenon that seems to inform Aristotle's *Rhetoric* (3.11.1 : 1411b), in which we are told the importance of putting things before the eyes (πρὸ ὀμμάτων ποιεῖν). To demonstrate this, Aristotle provides a Euripidean example that exhibits both activity and metaphor (ἐνέργεια καὶ μεταφορά). Such a combination runs parallel to the numerous examples taken from Homer, who is praised for representing inanimate things (ἄψυχα) as being animate (ἔμψυχα). This preference for animation is echoed by Cicero through a fragment of Pacuvius (*De orat*.3.157), who metaphorizes a storm at sea by using a string of verbs that evokes bodily trembling (*inhorrescit, coruscat, contremit*). Verbs help to enact emotion, because emotion is integrated with the body, which plays a vital role in generating emotion with some degree of predictability, something that neuroscience understands in terms of emotional processes unfolding in sensorimotor terms,[18] and classical scholars can understand through Quintilian (cf. 8.3.71: *omnis eloquentia circa opera vitae est ... et id facillime accipiunt animi, quod agnoscunt*),[19] who, like Cicero before him, identifies passages thick with bodily experience as being the reliable sort for crafting emotional experience. It is a technique that might be understood as the ability to recognize common or shared experience, something that Hellenistic poetry's convention of depicting plights of emotion through physical movement confronts.[20]

---

[17] I have previously (2016) drawn on Eviatar Zerubavel's (2003) 26 "Mountains and Valleys" version of historical narrative to make this claim. He observes that the social shape of the past is formed through narratives that are comprised of various *mnemonic densities* that differentiate extraordinary social realities from ordinary ones through a pronouncedly qualitative approach towards time. Zerubavel is working on a significantly larger scale, but I argue that the macro and micro approaches are part of the same historical topography.
[18] Damasio & Damasio (2006).
[19] Webb (2009).
[20] Cf. Kubiak (1981) 16ff. for examples.

The use of semantically consistent verbs to extend metaphor is readily found in Roman rhetoric and historiography, and is a pattern likely related to iteration appealing to pity. Outside of metaphorical phrases, the verbs found in historiography generally carry their core meaning, as seen in the Herodotus example above, where the verbs that occur between the two metaphorical phrases about being "struck" mentally describe actual striking. Insight into the practice of iterating the core meaning of verbs to extend and refine the emotional content of the narrative appears early on in Cicero's *De oratore* (1.12), wherein we learn that those trained in the art of persuasion utilize the common sense of words:

> ... *dicendi autem omnis ratio in medio posita, communi quodam in usu, atque in hominum more et sermone versatur ... in dicendo [autem] vitium vel maximum sit a vulgari genere orationis atque a consuetudine communis sensus abhorrere.*
>
> ... *while the whole art of oratory lies open to the view, and is concerned in some measure with the common practice, custom and speech of mankind ... in oratory the very cardinal sin is to depart from the language of everyday life, and the usage approved by the sense of the community.* (Sutton and Rackham)

So that speech (or text) is ornamented by metaphor in a clear way (*De Orat.* 3.166–167):

> *Sumpta re simili verba eius rei propria deinceps in rem aliam, ut dixi, transferuntur. Est hoc magnum ornamentum orationis, in quo obscuritas fugienda est.*
>
> *Something resembling the real thing is taken, and the words that properly belong to it are then, as I said, applied metaphorically to the other thing. This is a valuable stylistic argument; but care must be taken to avoid obscurity.* (Rackham)

Metaphor can be extended to evoke so-called pity by virtue of the common meanings of verbs that constellate around the metaphor, which, when read within an embodied framework, convey the emotional content entailed by the metaphor.

Take for example an iterative model of emotional contagion found at *De orat.*2.190:[T][*21]

> *Neque est enim facile perficere, ut **irascatur**, cui tu velis, iudex, si tu ipse id lente ferre videare; neque ut oderit eum, quem tu velis, nisi te ipsum **flagrantem** odio ante viderit; neque ad misericordiam adducetur, nisi tu ei signa doloris tui verbis, sententiis, voce, vultu, collacri-*

[*21] Passages noted with a superscript "T" were located with USC's *Text Analysis, Crawling and Interpretation Tool* (TACIT). TACIT was developed by the University of Southern California's *Computational Social Sciences Laboratory*, headed by Dr. Morteza Dehghani. With special thanks to Niki Parmar for her work in writing the Latin stemmer.

*matione denique ostenderis; ut enim nulla materies tam facilis ad **exardescendum** est, quae nisi admoto **igni ignem** concipere possit, sic nulla mens est tam ad comprehendendam vim oratoris parata, quae possit **incendi**, nisi ipse **inflammatus** ad eam et **ardens** accesserit.*

For it is not easy to succeed in making an arbitrator angry with the right party, if you yourself seem to treat the affair with indifference; or in making him hate the right party, unless he first sees you on fire with hatred yourself; nor will he be prompted to compassion, unless you have shown him the tokens of your own grief by word, sentiment, tone of voice, look and even by loud lamentation. For just as there is no substance so ready to take fire, as to be capable of generating flame without the application of a spark, so also there is no mind so ready to absorb an orator's influence, as to be inflammable when the assailing speaker is not himself aglow with passion. (Sutton and Rackham)

In republican and imperial Latin, anger, among other so-called passionate emotions, is frequently ignited or set ablaze. Emotions, just like fire, are combustible and prone to spread. Cicero discusses this phenomenon while frequently touching upon the conceptual metaphor in a short span of text, which suggests that instruction on iteration and emotion is an aspect of the composition itself. The application of a rhetorical strategy linked to arousing emotion in a discussion about arousing anger not only points to the depth and complexity of the treatise's structure, but also suggests that the iteration of metaphorical elements in texts outside of rhetoric have a relationship to exactly this type of training.

Exemplifying the architecture supplied by cognitive metaphor to historical narrative is *AUC* 42.54,[T] wherein the inhabitants of Mylae do not wish to surrender to Perseus of Macedon. The mob, ignited by their desperation, rushes together to create a sudden eruption on account of irrational anger:

*Quae res cum infestiorem hostem ad oppugnandum fecisset, ipsos **desperatione veniae** ad tuendos sese acrius **accendit**. Itaque per triduum ingentibus utrimque animis et oppugnata est urbs et defensa. Multitudo Macedonum ad subeundum in vicem proelium haud difficulter suppetebat; oppidanos, diem noctem eosdem tuentes moenia, non vulnera modo sed etiam vigiliae et continens labor conficiebat. Quarto die cum et scalae undique ad muros erigerentur et porta vi maiore oppugnaretur, oppidani depulsa vi muris ad portam tuendam **concurrunt eruptionemque repentinam** in hostis faciunt; quae cum **irae** magis **inconsultae** quam verae fiduciae virium esset, pauci et fessi ab integris pulsi terga dederunt fugientesque per patentem portam hostes acceperunt.*

This impertinence both made the enemy more vehement in the attack and fired the citizens, through despair of obtaining pardon, to defend themselves more vigorously. Therefore for three days with great spirit on both sides the city was attacked and defended. The numbers of the Macedonians were easily sufficient to undertake the battle in relays; the townspeople, guarding the walls day and night without relief, were worn out not only by wounds but also by wakefulness and unbroken toil. When on the fourth day ladders were lifted against the walls on all sides and also the gate was attacked with greater violence, the townspeople, after thrusting back the assault on the walls, rallied to guard the gate and made a sudden sally against the enemy; this being more the result of heedless rage than

>in genuine confidence in their strength, the small number of weary men, routed by fresh opponents, turned tail and in their flight let the enemy in through the open gate. (Sage and Schlesinger)

The structure of the passage is notable for its fidelity to the elements of passionate emotion identified by Conceptual Metaphor Theory (CMT). According to CMT, cross-culturally, the loss of control over anger is similarly – though not identically – conceived of as erupting out of humans as though their bodies were pressurized containers. It is a consequence of the universality of actual physiological mechanisms, such as becoming hot when angry (cf. *accendit*). It is also generically conceptualized as being caused by internal stress (cf. *desperatione veniae*), as being unintentional (cf. *quae res accendit ipsos*), and as being sudden and violent (cf. *eruptionemque repentinam*).[22] *Accendit ... irae inconsultae* as a form of iteration works together (conceptually not grammatically) with the other constituents to develop the emotional clarity of the narrative through the structuring of the story with, in this case, a nearly universal metaphorical schema. Cicero demonstrates with his heavy use of fire imagery that anger is underwritten by the repetition of metaphorical elements associated with the emotion being evoked. We see this also in Livy, who approaches time *qualitatively*. Thus, one can see that Cicero and Livy reveal that a relationship between mind, emotion and body informs the structure of ancient narratives.

The Emotional Body and Collective Memory

Cognitive metaphors also, of course, structure the narrative environment of poetic texts, as we see, for example, in Vergil (*A*.2.304–16)[T] who internalizes the external to render the anger of Aeneas and his allies hot by transferring the flames of nearby houses (*flamma, ardet, igni*) to them (*ardent animi: furor iraque*). In rhetoric, the transference of emotion can be conceived of similarly, moving from speaker to audience.[23] Cicero demonstrates this in terms of another emotion – disgust – with the same technique demonstrated in *de Orat*.2.190 in *Phil*. 2.67. After metaphorizing Antony into a Charybdis (*quae Charybdis tam vorax*), numerous words denoting either consumption or a pouring out appear in context (*effuderit, absorbere, potabatur, consumpta, devorare*). Wealth is poured out or discharged like bodily fluid; furniture, clothing, and all manner of things are swallowed; wine

---

22 Cf. Gibbs (1992) and (1994); Kövecses (2005); Riggsby (2015).
23 Cf. *De orat*. 2.185–216.

is drunk for days on end; richly embroidered couches are consumed; cities, kingdoms, houses and gardens are devoured. Since we are told in *De oratore* (3.163) that Charybdis is explicitly a non-visual metaphor, we should consider that the audience, rather than being led to the impossible image of an unseen mythological creature, are instead led to imagine the creature by means of a purely visceral experience – one intended to connect Antony not only to the concept of danger and destruction, but also to the embodied understanding of overindulgence and vomiting.[24] In essence, a metaphorical creature stands in for the emotion associated with the physical distress that accompanies overconsumption, which is evoked through the narrative structured by the metaphor, which acts as a locus around which communities of memory and morality can coalesce.

Similar experiential structures underwrite the fear of the Samnites in *AUC* 7.36ᵀ. Here we find Decius Mus crossing through the Samnite camp.

> Iam evaserant media castra, cum superscandens uigilum strata somno corpora miles **offenso** scuto praebuit sonitum; quo **excitatus** vigil cum proximum **movisset erectique** alios **concitarent**, ignari cives an hostes essent, praesidium **erumperet** an consul castra cepisset, Decius, quoniam non fallerent, clamorem tollere iussis militibus torpidos somno insuper **pavore exanimat**, quo praepediti nec arma inpigre capere nec obsistere nec insequi poterant.

> They had already got half way through the camp, when a soldier in stepping over the bodies of some sleeping sentries struck his shield and made a sound. A sentry was awakened by this, and having shaken his neighbor, they stood up and began to rouse the rest, not knowing whether they had to do with friends or foes, whether the party on the hill were escaping, or the consul had captured the camp. Decius, seeing that they were discovered, gave the order to his men, and they set up such a shout that the Samnites, who had been stupefied with sleep, were now in addition breathless with terror, which prevented them from either arming promptly or making a stand against the Romans or pursuing them. (Foster)

The passage is structured by a ubiquitous metaphor – *metu perculsus* – which is created anew with the conceptual relationship of *offenso .... pavore* and that which intervenes, namely numerous verbs at home in expressions of fear.[25] The internal experience of consciousness involved with *excitatus* is mirrored in the external world with *erecti*, with *movisse* correlating to the former and *concitarent* to the latter – both conceptually and grammatically. In turn, the reference to rupture in terms of the possibility of the consul attacking is conceptually linked to the embodied actions which precede it. This is particularly likely, given Livy's demonstrated understanding of strong emotion as a cause of rupture in *AUC*

---

24 Devereaux (2016).
25 E.g. *metum excitatum* (*De off*.2.75); *metu moverentur* (*Ver*.2.1.81); *metu concitarentur* (*Ver*.2.5.163).

42.54 above. The presence of the word in the context of an intense emotion tacitly provides emotional clarity when met with the eventual expression of intense emotion that characterizes the passage as a whole: *pavore exanimat*. Again, a grammatical relationship between elements does not hold throughout the passage, but a low-level conceptual, embodied relationship that carries the activity of the narrative into the mental disposition of the enemy soldiers does. Similar to what we find in Herodotus, wherein emotional and sensory experiences merge, the striking of the shield merges with being terrified, or, as it were, being struck by fear. Without using the metaphor directly, and without detailing the internal experience of the soldiers in the propositional content of the text, the quality of the soldiers' internal state is nonetheless evoked, because metaphor is not just an analogy – that which is evident on the face of the text – but is something even more essential: a prompt to shared experience that entails the text. The striking of a shield ultimately results in terror, with the mental transition entailed qualitatively understood as a physical process characterized by arousal, movement, and rupture. The qualitative experience of time for the Samnites, terrified (albeit inadvertently at first) by the Romans, is effected by the narrative structure, which in turn affects the way the story is remembered. The frightening experience of the Samnites "rings true" thanks to the "kernel of truth" provided by embodied experience, which, in all of the narratives discussed herein, ultimately functions to underwrite Roman collective-identity with emotional resonance.

In the above passage we thus find iteration that is similar in form and effect to that found in rhetoric and poetry. Recognizing this particular method of eliciting emotion, we are then able to draw deeper connections to and important distinctions from parallel passages, such as the following from Sallust's *Bellum Iugurthinum* (99), wherein enemy troops react similarly when startled awake by the instruments and shouts sounded at the order of Marius:

> *Deinde ubi lux adventabat, defessis iam hostibus ac paulo ante somno captis, de inproviso vigiles, item cohortium turmarum legionum tubicines simul omnis signa canere, milites clamorem tollere atque portis **erumpere** iubet. Mauri atque Gaetuli, ignoto et horribili sonitu **repente exciti**, neque fugere neque arma capere neque omnino facere aut providere quicquam poterant: ita cunctos strepitu clamore, nullo subveniente, nostris instantibus, tumultu formidine **terror quasi vecordia** ceperat. denique omnes fusi fugatique arma et signa militaria pleraque capta, pluresque eo proelio quam omnibus superioribus interempti. nam somno et **metu** insolito impedita fuga.*

> And then, when day approached, and the enemy were fatigued and just sinking to sleep, he ordered the sentinels, with the trumpeters of the auxiliary cohorts, cavalry, and legions, to sound all their instruments at once, and the soldiers, at the same time, to raise a shout, and sally forth from the camp upon the enemy. The Moors and Getulians, suddenly roused by the strange and terrible noise, could neither flee, nor take up arms, could neither act, nor provide for their security, so completely had fear, like a stupor, from the uproar and shouting, the

absence of support, the charge of our troops, and the tumult and alarm, seized upon them all. The whole of them were consequently routed and put to flight; most of their arms, and military standards, were taken; and more were killed in this than in all former battles, their escape being impeded by sleep and the sudden alarm. (Watson)

Not only is the story similar – sleeping soldiers roused by a noise are sent into confusion as a result of being disoriented by sleep and fear and are unable to escape a bad fate – but so is the language used: *erumperet: erumpere; excitatus: exciti; pavore:formidine/terror/metu* (note also *clamorem tollere and cepisset ... capere: capere ceperat*).[26] However, the quality of the fear is described by Sallust through a simile (*terror quasi vecordia*) rather than evoked through the narrative (cf. *offenso excitatus movisset concitarent erumperet pavore exanimat*). Sallust uses a simile that likens one state of mind to another with minimal embodied action. To flee, to do, to provide, to be able: all are concepts of action that are devoid of specificity in terms of bodily movement. Livy's narrative is more cohesive in these terms. Striking, stirring, moving, moving together, bursting forth and losing breath combine to qualify and thereby historicize *pavore exanimat* in a way that differs from Sallust's *terror quasi vecordia,* although both depend upon embodied notions of arousal and rupture (*excitare* and *erumpere*) for their full meaning. At the core of the difference between these two otherwise similar passages is the relationship of words that connect fear to the notion of rupture. In Livy, the notion appears in the text after the frightened soldiers have been embodied through the conceptual content. The narrative is experiential. In Sallust, a reference to rupture is instead followed by an abstract mental state that proceeds from it, rather than recreating it. It is a subtle distinction that clarifies the nature of the emotional appeal used by Livy, who takes pains to choreograph movement to engage his readers.

Probabilities

Movement and rupture, the latter of which is an element of uncontrolled emotional response, were indeed at the core of the way in which emotion was understood and expressed by Roman authors, and it is my suggestion that attention to how these concepts are expressed is valuable to our understanding of the texts as sites of memory. To get closer to what I am suggesting, consider the expres-

---

26 It is worth noting that both authors iterate *capere*, a verb of grasping. Verbs of grasping are associated with mental states that could be at play here. Cf. Short (2012).

sion *motus animi*. *Motus animi* is a term for emotion found throughout rhetorical, historiographical, poetic and philosophical texts, seeming to betray an intuitive understanding of emotion in terms of the common experiences that arises out of the blueprint of our bodies, our senses, and our shared physical world.[27] These experiences forge common understandings that members of a shared culture use to create meaning.[28] That meaning is the product of not only a shared culture, but of a shared psychology characterized by common understandings of embodied activities that are in turn used to imaginatively structure more abstract ideas and events. By way of common bodily experiences, individuals are understood to be "truthful" users of language.[29] It is a litmus test that pleads consideration in terms of so-called "literary truth" and the Roman commitment to the construction of truth being a social enterprise.[30] That is to say, with common bodily experience and the emotions associated with narrative ringing "true", it becomes evident that the propositional content of historical narrative is transformed into the rhetoric of history through the embodied nature of linguistic processing – *pathos* is where literary truth resides.[31]

With this in mind, the fact that ancient historiographers' use of detail depended on the effect they intended, irrespective of the amount of dependable material available,[32] can be observed to reflect the principles of narrating exempla outlined by the elder Cicero in *De partitione oratoria* (71), as well as Crassus' lesson on the ornamentation of style in the third book of *De oratore* (211–12). The senior Cicero imparts that direct argumentation is not involved in the exhibiting of past actions. Instead, style is used to gently influence emotion (*ad animi motus leniter tractandos*) and amplify the certainty of the statements being made (*ea quae certa aut pro certis posita sunt augentur*). Crassus, in turn, explains that the manner in which rhetoric is used and the degree to which it is expressed is dictated by practical sagacity (*scire quid quandoque deceat prudentiae*). *Prudentia* may mean 'discretion' in Crassus' mouth, but in the writing of historiography, *prudentia* surely would retain some good part of its primary sense: *a foreseeing*. Thucydides established this for writers of history, who tell of things that took place and will take place again, given human nature (1.22.4). And yet, we have up until this point largely missed the expositions of human nature that

---

[27] Schubert *et al.* (2008) 177.
[28] Cf. Yu (2008); Gibbs (2005) 67.
[29] Devereaux (2016).
[30] Habinek (2005a) 73; see also Habinek (2005b); for literary truth and historiography, see Grant (1995) 94 and Woodman (1988).
[31] Cf. Feldherr (1998) 8 n.24.
[32] Cf. Paul (1982); Wheeldon (1989).

occur in historiography as a part of the emotionological structuring of narratives designed to be remembered precisely because they will occur again as a consequence of that very nature.

Conclusion

I have taken up valuable space to provide the ancient texts as fully as possible, together with accepted translations, so as to demonstrate what is left unseen when one does not attend to verbal structure at the level of embodied concepts. Human nature, as the ancients perceived it, emerges through the telling of events, the action of which is often suspect in its factual accuracy, but is vividly truthful in terms of embodied experience. It is my suggestion that the nature of this truth is central not only to the persistence of events in memory, but also to the form that memory takes. In our own time we are coming to understand how influential cognitive metaphors are on the way people reason about complex social problems, due to their ability to unconsciously categorize emotional experience.[33] From this perspective one can gain a new understanding of the deep connection between rhetorical devices and history-writing, and observe the impact that an embodied messenger of antiquity (*nuntia vetustatis*) can have on the memory of its audiences. This messenger is, of course, the ancient historian himself. Metaphor enables the witnessing of time (*testis temporum*) in terms of the truth of experience (*lux veritatis*) and the animation of memory (*vita memoriae*), thereby allowing emotion to inform history's lessons on human nature and its attendant probabilities (*magistra vitae*). This suggestion recognizes that it is the author, who, by the sharing of sensorimotor and perceptual images through the text, creates a collaborative relationship with readers that can be shared in across time and space. It is for this reason, were we to say to an ancient historian that a given example of *exaedificatio* were untrue, he would assuredly reply, with due exasperation: 'It must have been *like* that'.

---

[33] Cf. Thibodeau/Boroditsky (2011) and (2013); Modell (2009).

Afroditi Angelopoulou
4 Feeling Words: Embodied Metaphors in *Seven Against Thebes*

This paper evaluates, from an embodied cognition perspective, ancient drama's potential to create emotionality, one of tragedy's essential qualities. I begin with a brief consideration of the underlying cognitive mechanisms of embodiment that enable the elicitation of affective responses, thus facilitating our emotional engagement and participation. Particularly at the linguistic level, I offer a microanalysis of emotional metaphors in *Seven Against Thebes*. I focus on the role of embodied metaphor as a principal cognitive tool, aiming to show that we should reassess its active role in constructing and communicating emotional meaning, as well as influencing the audience's moral reasoning process.

Affectivity *qua* lack of indifference, τὸ μὴ ἀναίσθητον, as Plutarch would have it,[1] is an essential element for the negotiation and understanding of the theatrical and dramatic levels of performances, and also a constituent element of ritual, of which ancient drama forms part. During the theatrical experience, "emotions were orchestrated in important ways that contributed to the process of creating a community through common experience".[2] Such an approach, to which I am sympathetic, stresses the affective response, rather than an intellectual understanding of ancient performances. Watching drama was primarily an emotional, multisensory experience, the apprehension of which required visual, auditory, tactile, thermal, olfactory, gustatory and kinesthetic qualities. Such experience is made possible largely by the mind's affectivity. As Giovanna Colombetti posits, "The mind, as embodied, is intrinsically or constitutively affective; you cannot take affectivity away from it and still have a mind".[3]

The emphasis here lies on the idea that the mind/brain is shaped by the body in its interaction with the physical and cultural world. Indeed, a rapidly

---

1 *De Gloria Atheniensium* (348C-D): ἤνθησε δ' ἡ τραγῳδία καὶ διεβοήθη, θαυμαστὸν ἀκρόαμα καὶ θέαμα τῶν τότ' ἀνθρώπων γενομένη καὶ παρασχοῦσα τοῖς μύθοις καὶ τοῖς πάθεσιν ἀπάτην, ὡς Γοργίας φησίν, ἣν ὅ τ' ἀπατήσας δικαιότερος τοῦ μὴ ἀπατήσαντος, καὶ ὁ ἀπατηθεὶς σοφώτερος· τοῦ μὴ ἀπατηθέντος. ὁ μὲν γὰρ ἀπατήσας δικαιότερος, ὅτι τοῦθ' ὑποσχόμενος πεποίηκεν· ὁ δ' ἀπατηθεὶς σοφώτερος εὐάλωτον γὰρ ὑφ' ἡδονῆς λόγων τὸ μὴ ἀναίσθητον.
2 Bouvrie (2011) 144.
3 Colombetti (2014) 2.

Afroditi Angelopoulou, University of Southern California

https://doi.org/10.1515/9783110482201-005

growing body of experimental research highlights the role of bodily experiences in a variety of psychological processes, from basic attention and memory to social perception, attitude, inference, and judgment.[4]

It seems worthwhile to reassess the experiential effects of the spoken word in the context within which it operated, the Attic theater, and its role in communicating emotional meaning through the body and its sensorimotor system. Language is 'inherently multimodal,' using many modalities linked together – sight, hearing, touch, motor actions, and so on.[5] Accordingly, linguistic interpretation is grounded on the ways people perceptually and kinesthetically interact with objects and events in the world, a cognitive process that renders the communicative potency of language "not merely symbolic, but also somatic".[6]

Such a perspective explains why watching drama, listening to (or reading) a story is primarily a deeply visceral experience. Peter Meineck underscores the particularly strong connection between viewer and viewed via the empathic responses elicited during dance performances; the tragic mask facilitated such connection, drawing attention to the performer's body, in which emotion was incarnated.[7] According to the *embodiment* hypothesis, perceiving and thinking about emotion involve perceptual, somatovisceral, and motoric re-experiencing of the relevant emotion in one's self. Neuroscience tells us that, "people can readily, and mostly unconsciously, create simulations of real-world events as they communicate with others, hear stories, solve problems, and even perceive motionless displays".[8] If indeed language is closely tied to embodied imagination, the interpretation of stories involves creating a reenactment, feeling the emotions of others as if they were our own.[9]

Plato's prescient notions of the potential impact of language's sensory impressions come remarkably close to such insights. As he suggests in the *Republic*, all the "frightening and dreadful names" that "make everyone who hears shudder" (φρίττειν) must be struck out, lest the guardians "are made softer and more malleable by such shudders" (μὴ ἐκ τῆς τοιαύτης φρίκης θερμότεροι καὶ

---

4 Lee/Swartz (2014).
5 Gallese/Lakoff (2005).
6 Foroni/Semin (2009) 173.
7 Meineck (2011) 135–8 and (2012). He reports numerous studies, which show that there is an increase in neural activity when the dance is familiar to the onlookers. Such was the case with the Athenians, themselves 'expert dancers,' when watching the choruses in tragedies.
8 Gibbs/Matlock (2008) 164.
9 See Foroni/Semin (2009). Recent experiments have shown that language comprehension (e.g., understanding the verb *to smile*) leads to physical simulation of the events to be comprehended.

μαλακώτεροι τοῦ δέοντος γένωνται).[10] Plato's language captures an important aspect of ancient drama's affectivity, namely its potential to actively "shape" the listener's moral disposition and ethical makeup.

Elsewhere in the *Republic* he raises the question concerning the nature of the relationship between imitation, and the process of vicariously sharing or taking on the states of others, one of "the subcomponents of the multifaceted construct that is empathy";[11] he constructs a link between feelings of "shudders," "feeling with" (συμπάσχειν)[12] the characters on stage, and the ethical implications of such emotional attunement, conceiving of any kind of emotional "disturbance" (ταράξειεν) as a sign of vulnerability, a sort of "deformity" (ἀλλοιώσειεν).[13]

Plato's discussion, though unconsciously, points to the now widely accepted claim that the bodily changes as a response to features of the world are inextricable from emotions, which, as philosopher Jesse Prinz submits, "are perceptions of our bodily states. To recognize the moral value of an event is to perceive the perturbation that it causes".[14] The body, through the elicitation of empathic responses towards the other's distress, fear or sadness, alerts us to moral transgressions, which are often associated with such feelings.[15]

Tragic plays frequently represent emotions as embodied appraisals. The body, in its symptoms and expression, makes its presence felt through dramatic language, which gives access to these internal processes as a way of response towards the external events of the play. We, the external audience and readers, are thus able to gauge and interpret somewhat safely the significance of such events in terms of the social and cultural milieu in which they are set, guided by the degree and manner of affectivity they produce. For instance, when the

---

[10] *Republic* 387b-c. These observations bear a striking resemblance to the idea of the plasticity of our brain, subject to change due to its constant integration with the external environment, since we as human beings are embodied and physically embedded in it (Borghi et al. (2010); Clark (2003)). It is also worth comparing this idea with physical theories of the of fifth century BCE: "the so-called pluralists help foster a new understanding between people and the larger world. For they embed people in this world [...] as composite objects engaged in an ongoing process of becoming" (Holmes (2010) 101).

[11] Zaki/Ochsner (2012) 207.

[12] *Rep.*10. 605c-d: οἶσθ' ὅτι χαίρομέν τε καὶ ἐνδόντες ἡμᾶς αὐτοὺς ἑπόμεθα *συμπάσχοντες* καὶ σπουδάζοντες ἐπαινοῦμεν ὡς ἀγαθὸν ποιητήν, ὃς ἂν ἡμᾶς ὅτι μάλιστα οὕτω διαθῇ.

[13] *Rep.* 2. 381a: ψυχὴν δὲ οὐ τὴν ἀνδρειοτάτην καὶ φρονιμωτάτην ἥκιστ' ἄν τι ἔξωθεν πάθος ταράξειέν τε καὶ ἀλλοιώσειεν;

[14] Prinz (2005) 99.

[15] As preeminent neuroscientist Antonio Damasio (1994) 226 posits, "the body contributes more than life support and modulatory effects to the brain. It contributes a *content* that is part and parcel of the workings of the normal mind" [author's emphasis].

chorus in the *Agamemnon* shudders (πέφρικα) at Cassandra's allusion to Thyestes' feast on his own children, we can deduce with some certainty that Aeschylus ties the particular emotional experience with themes of a deeply moral and religious nature like kin killing, ritual pollution and intra-familial violence.[16] Such marked use illustrates how a near-universal, physical, embodied experience is also context-induced, becoming enmeshed in a network of culturally conditioned appraisals.

The conveyed psychological states reflect the emotional response of both internal and external audiences when confronted with the subversion of a sociomoral order the integrity of which is crucial for human civilization. As Syvønne des Bouvrie put it, "Members of a society do not only have to learn basic categories and values but also to learn how to feel 'correctly' about these categories and values".[17] We as audience are thus invited to participate by simulating the 'shuddering' elicited by the events in the narrative.[18]

One of our earliest extant tragedies, *Seven Against Thebes*, is concerned with the subversion of certain moral foundations of sociopolitical life that have a universal resonance because they largely reflect the world's moral matrices. Social psychologist Jonathan Haidt posits that there is a limited number of built-in psychological systems organized "in advance of experience" pertaining to violations of sanctity, authority, loyalty, which eventually get to be diversified through time and across cultures.[19] Athenian drama provides us with the particularities of the community's externalization of certain emotional and intuitive processes *qua* reactions towards such 'universal' violations. These reactions, conditioned by cultural and social influences, are constituents of a particular cultural knowledge, which has been acquired by the members of the community in a sustained, deep, cognitive, affective and motoric way.[20]

The subject of the *Seven* revolves around the problematic of Polynices' corrupt *nostos*, his homecoming with an invading army. The prospect of the city's capture frames the narrative, which, as was quite often the case with Athenian tragedy, reflects feelings of deep anxiety towards violence resulting from warfare.[21] As Chaniotis and Ducrey observe,

---

16 *Agamemnon* 1242–4: Τὴν μὲν Θυέστου δαῖτα παιδείων κρεῶν| ξυνῆκα καὶ πέφρικα, καὶ φόβος μ'ἔχει| κλύοντ'ἀληθῶς οὐδὲν ἐξηκασμένα.
17 Bouvrie 1988, 61.
18 For a more detailed discussion of the 'history of shudders' in Greek culture, see Douglas Cairns' (2013) stimulating discussion.
19 Haidt (2012) 131.
20 Haidt (2001) 814.
21 Meineck (2012) 7.

War ranks high among the factors that influenced political and social institutions, and left its imprint on art, literature, and culture, thus allowing us to measure the role and importance of feelings, both collective and individual.[22]

The importance of a war-play like the *Seven* lies in the ambiguity of the feelings it reflects: it does reflect feelings of anxiety towards warfare, yet we have Aristophanes' comment in the *Frogs*, which commends the play for arousing in spectators' hearts a warlike spirit, a "desire for destruction".[23] Aristophanes' interpretation, although it attests to the notion that the important question was 'what it felt like' watching the *Seven*, offers only one dimension, focusing solely on the celebration of the warrior ethos.

Indeed, the narrative displays a far more complex web of emotionality. At the other end of the spectrum lies the feeling of fear, embodied in the female chorus, a rather threatening and 'contagious' emotion (237: πολίτας μὴ κακοσπλάγχνους τιθῇς). It has been suggested that, as the most vivid communicator of distress, fear is an essential neurocognitive requirement for generating sympathetic concern.[24] The *Seven* problematizes this mechanism and dramatizes it as an antiheroic emotion, conflicting with and undermining the values of warrior ethos. It is one of the play's most explicit feelings as a self-reported emotional state (203: ἔδεισα, 214: ᾔρθην φόβῳ), and one that is predominantly embodied.[25]

Fear dominates the *Seven* and provides the emotional background, as well as the filter through which subsequent information, including other emotions, is processed.[26] It also takes more than one shape: Eteocles' decision to fight his brother elicits a kind of horror that comes closer to revulsion, a 'moral' emotion (720: πέφρικα 790: τρέω), and the realization that the force behind the events is the family curse represented by the Erinys is equally met with a 'chilling' emotional experience.[27]

Such explicit, often contradictory forms of affectivity, together with all the nonverbal cues in the performance, are essential constituents of theater as a space

---

22 Chaniotis/Ducrey (2013) 9.
23 *Frogs* 1024: ὁ θεασάμενος πᾶς ἄν τις ἀνὴρ ἠράσθη δάιος εἶναι.
24 Marsh (2012) 195.
25 *Seven Against Thebes* 260: ἀψυχίᾳ γὰρ γλῶσσαν ἁρπάζει φόβος; 288–90: φόβῳ δ'οὐχ ὑπνώσσει κέαρ,| γείτονες δὲ καρδίας | μέριμναι ζωπυροῦσι τάρβος.
26 See for example Petrounias' (1976) 33 comment: "the spectator trails the story, participates ever more intensely in the fear felt by the *personae* and deeply experiences the dramatic as such."
27 *Seven Against Thebes* 790–1: νῦν δὲ τρέω μὴ τελέσῃ καμψίπους Ἐρινύς; 832–4: ὦ μέλαινα καὶ τελεία/ γένεος Οἰδίπου ἀρά, /κακόν με καρδίαν τι περιπίτνει κρύος. See also Cairns 2013, 96, who argues that the experience of 'shudders' has often been connected in Greek thought with the divine and the supernatural.

that generates empathetic feelings. Associations of empathy with feelings of fear, pain, and disgust have been very well attested, and to a greater or lesser extent, Greek tragedy deals with representations of all three.[28] I thus want to suggest that all these emotional tensions are present in the language of the *Seven*, in the form of embodied metaphors. The focus of my attention is on Aeschylus' use of such metaphors, particularly gustatory metaphors pertaining to the emotions of anger and disgust, the latter capturing a rather implicit aspect of emotionality.

Both clusters of gustatory metaphors are enmeshed in a wider system of the so-called "agricultural" metaphors, which have been already explored in depth, particularly in relation to the major theme of the earth in the *Seven*.[29] It is not my intention here to review what has been well established; rather, my aim is to discuss these metaphors from a perspective that highlights their role as cognitive and psychological devices, capable of covertly triggering affective intuitions in the listener.[30]

Metaphor was, according to Aristotle, a crucial tool for producing visualization, "bringing before the eyes" (πρὸ ὀμμάτων), particularly "to see things while they are happening rather than what is going to happen".[31] The emphasis lies on internal vision, which, as Munteanu argues, "implies a transfer of emotion";[32] indeed, visualization is an essential aspect of tragedy, considering the fact that spectators had to give a visual content to all the verbal descriptions of the horrific events taking place off-stage.

The audience's emotional attunement, their ability to capture the internal psychological states of the characters on stage, partly hinges on what Vittorio Gallese calls "the synesthesia of embodied metaphor," namely the "imagined bodily experience standing in for affective states and dispositions".[33] By making sense of metaphorical language through imaginative simulation processes, we are in tune with, and gain access to the internal reality shared by the author and

---

28 The study of theater as a sociocultural environment that, among other things, fosters empathetic feelings seems to be all the more relevant nowadays, since empathy has been widely recognized as a mechanism crucial for "regulating social interactions, coordinating behavior, and promoting cooperation among individuals" (Marsh 2012, 192). Generally speaking, empathy and the ability to create representations of others' emotional states, in order to recognize them and respond appropriately, are associated with moral development and prosocial behavior.
29 For example, Cameron (1964) 1–8; Thalmann (1978) 38–49.
30 On metaphor's capacity to shape and act covertly in reasoning, see Thibodeau/Boroditsky (2013).
31 *Rhetoric* 3.1410 b 34–35.
32 Munteanu (2012) 90.
33 Gallese/Wojciehowski (2011) 27.

his audience that would be otherwise unknown. Aeschylus produces such a vivid effect in conspicuously staging Eteocles' internal turmoil, his maddening anger, through both metaphor and spectacle.

> τί μέμονας, τέκνον; μή τί σε θυμοπλη-
>
> θής δορίμαργος ἄτα φερέτω· κακοῦ δ'
>
> ἔκβαλ'ἔρωτος ἀρχάν. (*Seven Against Thebes* 686–8)
>
> "What are you eager for, child? Let not spear-loving lust fill your *thumos* and carry you away. Cast from yourself the beginning of an evil *eros*."

The conceptualization of Eteocles' *menos* is effected through a fairly common ontological metaphor, by which human beings conceptualize emotional experiences as substances that are 'in' them ('container' metaphor).[34] More often than not, these substances are also conceptualized as external, hostile forces that take hold or seize one, which seems to be the case here. The adjective θυμοπληθής, 'filling the *thumos*,' is attested only here and marks Eteocles' anger as a force that enters inside him, overflowing his body, indicating his loss of control. Aeschylus exploits conceptually as well as thematically this type of metaphor, to tie Eteocles' internal state with the driving force of his madness, the δαίμων haunting the family: *νῦν ἔτι ζεῖ* (708); *ἐξέζεσεν* γὰρ Οἰδίπου κατεύγματα (709). We are thus invited to keep visualizing this maddening force as 'seething' within the body of Eteocles, 'boiling up,' to the point where it becomes externalized and overflows, 'boiling out' the curse of Oedipus.

The metaphor is also conceptually consistent with Eteocles' anger as ὀργή (678), a "passionate" concept whose etymology captures what Danielle Allen called the iretic and erotic phenomena, namely "an emotional and cognitive experience associated with fertility, sweetness, and the "melting moods" of sexual desire".[35] Such use of metaphor, unique in its affectivity but also culturally conditioned, namely being neither "superficial" (ἐπιπόλαιον) nor "strange" (ἀλλότρια), meets Aristotle's criteria, as it can both elicit an empathic response (πάσχειν) and induce the listener/spectator to "see in one view" (συνιδεῖν).

When commenting on the play's impact, through the pointed use of ἐράομαι (*Frogs* 1024) Aristophanes captures the language of desire (*eros*) not only as a theme that permeates the narrative of the *Seven*, but also as the feeling state that

---

[34] See Kövecses (2005).
[35] Allen (2008) 59. For the etymology of ὀργή, see Beekes (2010): IE * *uerg̑-* 'swell of juice, strength, anger.'

also 'infects' the audience.[36] Quite frequently, the desiderative aspect of anger is cross-culturally conveyed through a metaphor that has at its basis the physiological force of hunger ('desire-as-hunger'). It is already present in Homeric discourse, often in the form of 'devouring' metaphors, markers of what stands outside culture and threatens to subvert it.[37]

Such emotional metaphors abound in contexts of non-institutionalized violence, an illustration of the conceptual opposites that underlie the Homeric discourse of anger: the raw and the cooked, human and non-human, nature and culture. The same opposites abound in the language of the *Seven*:

ὠμοδακὴς σ'ἄγαν ἵμερος εξοτρύ-

νει πικρόκαρπον ἀνδροκτασίαν τελεῖν

αἵματος οὐ θεμιστοῦ. (692–4)

"Raw-eating desire drives you to manslaughter of bitter fruit, unsanctioned blood-sacrifice."

Gustatory metaphors have as their source domain desire (to taste flesh and blood), which is also a marker of the Argive leaders' monstrosity, instantiated in the warriors' bloodlust. In fact, one of the most dramatic scenes in the myth of the Seven Against Thebes is the duel between Tydeus and Melanippus, which is also beautifully illustrated on the pediment of the Pyrgi Temple in Etruria, depicting the mortally wounded Tydeus eating the brain of his enemy. Aeschylus thus visualizes a familiar myth through the language of desire. The 'animalistic' Tydeus (381; 393–4) is μαργῶν καὶ μάχης λελιμμένος (380), ἐρῶν (392).

In particular, the participle μαργῶν is associated with gluttony, which is also suggested in the adjective δορίμαργος; ὠμός is also characteristic of both Parthenopeus (536) and the Sphinx, who is ὠμόσιτος (540), whereas Eteocles' ὠμοδακής ἵμερος signifies his own mostronsity. These connotations recall the familiar Homeric image of the warrior as raw-meat –eater, which, as Redfield remarked, "catches an aspect of the impurity of war".[38]

Furthermore, weapons in the *Iliad*, as extensions of the Homeric warrior's self, are "material agents ... full of intentions", "desiring to have their fill

---

36 Sexual desire as *Eros* together with *Thanatos*, are, according to Zeitlin (2009) 23, "the two transgressions that engendered the two brothers".
37 Most notable instances are *Iliad* 4. 35–6; 22. 34–5; 24.213.
38 Redfield (1975) 197. Indeed, the emphasis on this 'impurity of war' lies in the repetition of μιαίνω, lines 343–4: μιαινομένοις δ'ἐπιπνεῖ λαοδάμας| μιαίνων εὐσέβειαν Ἄρης.

in human flesh", as Malafouris observes.³⁹ He sees the weapon as a part of the warrior's physical body, arguing that, "[I]f the body shapes the mind then it is inevitable that the material culture that surrounds the body will shape the mind also." Perceiving the weapon as a material instantiation of the warrior's ethos so prevalent and celebrated ever since Homeric poetry, we come to understand that expressions like that of Eteocles: τεθηγμένον τοί μ'οὐκ ἀπαμβλυνεῖς λόγῳ (715) are manifestations of cognitive processes grounded in experiences shaped by war culture. Hutchinson further notes that these two stems "are very often used with regard to passion, even in prose".⁴⁰ Jennifer Lin LeMeSurier posits that "the body is a conduit for remembered knowledge"⁴¹; such extended metaphors are crucial for the production of emotionality, as they revive remembered embodied experience in both the performer's and spectator's consciousness, namely that of war and its resulting violence.

These internal states of maddening, violent turmoil, take on a concrete visual aspect on stage: the qualities of Eteocles' emotional disposition are also those of the iron, *the* symbol of violence in the play (730: ὠμόφρων 944: θηκτός); Schadewaldt suggests that Eteocles puts on his armor during his exchange with the chorus, an act that indicates his "visual and verbal equation with the iron", as William Thalmann observes:

> The audience watches Eteocles become less and less human with every piece of armor he puts on. When he is fully armed and speaks of himself as if he were a weapon, he is no longer a man.⁴²

Such representation is also consistent with the seven leaders' δάιος θυμός at the beginning of the play: **σιδηρόφρων** γὰρ θυμὸς ἀνδρεία φλέγων¦ ἔπνει λεόντων ὣς Ἄρη δεδορκότων (53–4). Moreover, fire as a source domain for both the warriors' θυμός and the female chorus' fear (290: μέριμναι ζωπυροῦσι τάρβος) underscores the violence of these contradictory emotions, which permeates the entire play.⁴³

---

39 Malafouris (2008) 116. Cf. Hector's retort to Ajax, αἴ κε ταλάσσῃς/μεῖναι ἐμὸν δόρυ μακρόν, ὅ τοι χρόα λειριόεντα/δάψει (13.830); ἐγχείη ... ἱεμένη χροὸς ἄμεναι ἀνδρομέοιο (Il.21.70); λιλαιομένη χροὸς ἆσαι (Il.21.168); τὰ δοῦρα ... λιλαιόμενα χροὸς ἆσαι (Il.11.570; 15.317).
40 Hutchinson (1985) *ad loc.* Cf. e.g. *Supp.* 186, X.*Cyr.*2.1.120; *Pr.* 866, Th.2.87.3.
41 LeMesurier (2014) 363.
42 Schadewaldt (1961); Thalmann (1978) 96.
43 It is also worth mentioning that the use of fire as a source domain to convey the violent nature of such psychological states must not be coincidental, considering the subsequent association of fire with the iron, one of the narrative's central symbols of violence: ἐκ πυρὸς συθείς,¦ θηκτὸς σίδαρος (943–4).

Embodiments of this sort, based on practices and habits shaped by a warrior culture, are the outcome of a bodily habits and (martial) training that both spectators and actors have in common. The use of metaphors derived from such embodied states not only evokes them in the audience, but also allows us, as LeMesurier noted, "access to the ideological, political and affective ties formed in the original performance".[44] Importantly, one of the most remarkable features of the *Seven* is that the reactivation of such embodied experience conflicts with, and concurrently works with opposing embodiments, represented by the chorus, in such a way that ultimately creates deeply unsettling moments.[45]

Attached to both movements and language of ritual lament is another set of gustatory metaphors of 'bitterness' that tend to appear in tandem with those conveying anger. These metaphors are principally captured by the recurring use of the adjective πικρός, which can covertly affect perceptions of violence. Aeschylus incorporates this taste word in a highly affective line, which elicits strong empathic responses:

παντοδαπὸς δὲ καρπὸς χαμαδὶς πεσὼν| ἀλγύνει κυρήσας, πικρὸν δ'| ὄμμα
θαλαμηπόλων (357)

"Fruit of every sort, fallen to the ground as it may chance, gives pain, a bitter sight for maid-servants."

Modalities such as sight and touch are confounded in cognitively unforeseen ways: the fruit 'gives pain', the sight of which is 'bitter'.[46] Ἀλγύνω fuses emotional with physical pain, the feeling of intensified grief that is consistent with

---

44 LeMesurier (2014) 365.
45 See Vernant/Vidal-Naquet (1988) 40: "In *Seven*, the chorus of Theban women appeals to a divine presence in an anguished manner, with frantic impulses, tumultuous cries, and a fervor that directs them and keeps them attached to the most ancient idols"; Thalmann (1978) 103: The lyric rhythms in the choral passages "progress from panic through dread and mantic excitement to sorrow"; Seaford (2012) 159: "[T]he chorus of maidens display a combination of supplication, self-lamentation, and hymenaial flight to public space that presents a danger to the local king".
46 See Pecher *et al.* (2003) 119–24. Individuals simulate objects in the relevant modalities when they use them in thought and language. Experiments in support of the hypothesis that perceptual simulation underlies conceptual processing, show that shifting from processing in one modality to the other involves temporal shifting costs, and the same holds for individuals engaging in conceptual tasks (e.g., they are slower to verify that a 'bomb' can be *loud* when they have just verified that a 'lemon' can be *tart*, than when they have just confirmed that 'leaves' can be *rustling*).

the performance of lamentation, and instantiated in the dochmiac metre, which appears at moments of great pain, expressing violent emotion.⁴⁷

From an embodied cognition perspective, there is a causal relationship between embodying emotions, feeling emotional states, and acquiring and using information about emotions. Accordingly, the processing of the emotion concept of grief would involve simulation in the affective response systems, which would also determine the subsequent processing of the adjective πικρός: bitterness ultimately tastes like pain.⁴⁸ Indeed, this implicit sense of a "painful" taste of bitterness recurs in context with the final act of mourning, performed by the two sisters (861–5: πρᾶγος **πικρόν** ... θρῆνον ... **ἄλγος** ἐπάξιον).

Aeschylus' technique underscores the way language subserves performance in capturing the intensity of all the conflicting emotions in the play: the warriors' maddening anger and bloodlust on the one hand, and the chorus' feelings of agony and fear on the other, the latter enabling the elicitation of empathetic responses. This psychological process is further supported by expressions of disgust intertwined with pain. Physical and emotional pain are fused in the performance of grief, the violence of which is finally captured in the metaphorical extension of verbal expressions related to 'striking, cutting through, rending apart':

προπέμπει δαϊκτὴρ

γόος αὐτόστονος αὐτοπήμων,

δαϊόφρων (916–920)

"our heart-rending wail attends them, a product of unforced pain and sorrow, coming from a distressed mind"

Such expressions appear in context with the brothers' mutual slaughter "by strokes of iron" (911: σιδηρόπλακτοι), through "unloving severance" (934: διατομαῖς οὐ φίλοις), recalling once more the qualities of the iron, which are thus tied to the various emotional states that pervade the narrative.

---

47 Hutchinson (1985) 55. For the semantics of *algos*, see Konstan (2006) ch.12 on Grief; as he observes, words based on the root *alg-*, such as *algos* and *algêdôn*, refer principally to physical pain.
48 Emotions may affect language comprehension: the action systems required in emotion simulation, once adapted, affect comprehension of sentences with emotional content congruent with the adapted action system (Glenberg *et al.* (2009) 152–4). Studies have also shown that temporal processing costs occur when switching from the affective system to sensory modalities, and vice-versa (Vermeulen *et al.* (2006) 183–192).

Importantly, when concrete taste words like πικρός, which rely on gustatory representations in the brain, are intended metaphorically, they not only activate gustatory cortices, but also evoke implicit emotional responses; they are thus more emotionally engaging.[49] In the *Seven*, πικρός extends its meaning to eventually define the seed of fratricide and lastly, it is associated with the iron. Accordingly, the taste of kindred blood is of "bitter fruit" (693: πικρόκαρπος), hence unlawful; and as the agent of fratricide, the flesh-tasting iron is bitter (730: πικρός, ὠμόφρων σίδαρος). 'Bitterness' is gradually converted from a concrete, sensory experience, to an aesthetic ("sight"), and then to an affective- emotional one. I thus want to stress its transition from a gustatory quality to a (moral) judgment of taste, and its significance for the emotional meaning the play communicates and co-produces with us, as its audience.[50]

Studies suggest that gustatory embodied experiences may affect moral processing, highlighting the significant role that sensory and perceptual information plays in human conceptual architecture. The metaphorical extension of πικρός conveys a feeling of distaste qua revulsion, a gut reaction that reflects avoidance tendencies in response to contamination.[51] Among the cluster of 'moral' emotions that reflect a concern for the integrity of social order (for instance anger and contempt), disgust is the most visceral, and most suitable as a mechanism of response to a threat. Indeed, disgust evolved from a food-related emotion to a moral one,

---

[49] Citron/Goldberg (2014); during the comprehension of such metaphorical expressions, the amygdala was activated along with other areas (the left hippocampus and parahippocampal gyrus), all of which form part of the limbic system, known to be involved with emotional processing. See also Desai *et al.* (2011) on the involvement of sensory-motor systems in metaphor understanding.

[50] Current research on moral embodied cognition capitalizes upon the insights of David Hume (2004/1772, *An Inquiry Into Human Understanding*. Mineola, NY: p.123), according to whom moral judgments were comparable to judgments of taste.

[51] In his *Expression of the Emotions in Man and Animals*, Darwin claims that "the term 'disgust,' in its simplest sense, means something offensive to the taste" (1972/1965, p. 256). Empirical findings in social psychology suggest that physical and moral disgust are linked through cognitive, behavioral and physiological processes. Chapman *et al.* (2009) performed experiments showing that similar facial motor activity, which has evolutionary origins in taste preference, occurred in response to disgust in gustatory, visual, and moral domains. Their findings suggest that all three states (gustatory distaste, basic disgust, moral disgust) evoked activation of the levator labii muscle region of the face, characteristic of an oral-nasal rejection response. The aim of their study was to test 'the notion that moral cognition calls on a phylogenetically older system originating in the rejection of hazardous food' (1222). Jesse Prinz and his colleagues, adding to the literature demonstrating that moral reasoning can be affected by embodied, sensory information, performed experiments that specifically targeted taste perception, and confirmed that it does affect moral reasoning (Prinz *et al.* (2011)).

that is, "from physical to social rejection," the Aristophanic Βδελυκλέων being a case in point.[52] Accordingly, Jonathan Haidt posits that, "moral intuition appears to be the automatic output of an underlying, largely unconscious set of interlinked moral concepts. These concepts may have some innate basis which is then built up largely by metaphorical extensions from physical experience".[53] As he goes on to suggest, "metaphors have entailments, and much of moral argument and persuasion involves trying to get the other person to use the right metaphor".

Indeed, taste metaphors used for the formulation of assessments and evaluations abound in Greek prose and poetry.[54] A good instance of the latter case is Sophocles' *Philoctetes*, which capitalizes upon such metaphors to reject the Atreidae as πικροί (510), and dramatizes the tension between physical and moral disgust, its social implications (social rejection and exclusion),[55] and the interplay between physical and moral deformation.[56]

If we accept that in its broadest sense, ancient drama is a form of rhetoric too – produced for and conditioned by a particular social and cultural milieu, and reflecting on the very principles and values that confirm the cohesion of the community – I suggest that in the *Seven*, gustatory metaphors *qua* emotional metaphors are strategically placed at pivotal points in the narrative to evoke certain embodied responses. Feelings of aversion and pollution are marked by the proximity of lines 730 (*πικρός, ὠμόφρων σίδαρος*) and 735–8, as the 'bitterness' of the 'savage-minded' iron is attended by a strong sense of stain and contamination resulting from fratricide:

---

[52] Haidt et al. (2008); see also Moll et al. (2005) on human disgust as a mechanism that encompasses "a variety of emotional experiences that are ingrained in frontal, temporal, and limbic networks".

[53] Haidt (2001).

[54] For instance, there is a longstanding tradition in extant Greek literature that associates persuasive speech with honey metaphors, from the Hesiodic Muses and Homeric Nestor, to Apollonius' Jason and his honey-sweet words. Cf. *Il*.1. 248–9; *Theogony* 83–4; *Argonautica* 3. 458. Plato turns the tables on such tradition when, in the *Republic*, he proposes to admit a poet who is ἀηδέστερος (398b). The adjective occurs in the Hippocratic *On Ancient Medicine* (30 part 10), referring to food that elicits disgust (ἀηδέστερος ὁ σῖτος); cf. also *Laws* 2.659e-660a, and the contrast between ἡδέσι and ἀηδέσι σιτίοις.

[55] cf.1018: ἄφιλον ἐρῆμον ἄπολιν ἐν ζῶσιν νεκρόν; 1031–3: πῶς, ὦ θεοῖς ἔχθιστε, νῦν οὐκ εἰμί σοι χωλός, δυσώδης; Πῶς θεοῖς ἔξεστ', ἐμοῦ πλεύσαντος, αἴθειν ἱερά.

[56] This interplay is best captured in the connotations that the root meaning of αἰσχρός-as-ugly/disfigured bears: Neoptolemus' αἰσχρός φανοῦμαι (on αἶσχος and its relatives, see Cairns (1993) 54–60).

ἐπεὶ δ'ἂν αὐτοκτόνωςǀ αὐτοδάικτοι θάνωσι καὶ γαῖα κόνιςǀ πίῃ μελαμπαγὲς αἷμα φοίνιον, τίς ἂν καθαρμοὺς πόροι; τίς ἂν σφε λούσειεν; (734–6)

"But when they will have perished, each slaying the other in mutual death, and the earth's dust has drunk up the dark-clotted blood, who could provide purifying sacrifice? Who could cleanse their stain?"

Moreover, the father's curse against his sons to divide their posessions "with sword in hand" (789: σιδαρονόμῳ χερί), is of "bitter tongue" (788: πικρογλώσσους ἀράς). Once the theme of kinkilling is introduced, these taste metaphors trigger afffectively valenced intuitions in the listener, feelings of distaste that 'infect' the processing of all subsequent information.⁵⁷ The association of 'distaste' with the 'raw-eating' violence of the two brothers eventually comes full circle, when πικρός is used again in its metaphorical extension in the dirge performed by the chorus. First, it appears in context with the iron, at once the means of fratricide and of reconciliation, to define the cause of the strife, the covetous prize of 'bitter' rule (882–4: πικρὰς μοναρχίαςǀ ἰδόντες, ἤδη διήλǀλαχθε σὺν σιδάρῳ); and lastly, it is attached once more to the iron itself:

πικρὸς λυτὴρ νεικέων ὁ πόντιος

ξεῖνος ἐκ πυρὸς συθεὶς,

θηκτὸς σίδαρος, πικρὸς δ'ὁ χρημάτων

κακὸς διαιτητὰς Ἄρης (941–945)

"a bitter resolver of strife, the stranger from beyond the sea, gushed forth from fire, the whetted iron; bitter the evil arbitrator of property, Ares."

Repetition and alliteration (π..κ..ρ..) bring the adjective into the foreground and elicit a deeply visceral response towards fratricide and the murderous violence of warfare, an implicit reminder of the unresolved tension between the 'raw-eating' nature and culture.

It is also worth noting at this point that when this taste word first appears (357), it does not work in isolation, but is preceded by, and thus works in tandem with, a bold multi-sensory image, namely that of newborns feeding on the blood of their mothers' breast: βλαχαὶ δ'αἱματόεσσαιǀ τῶν ἐπιμαστιδίωνǀ ἀρτιτρεφεῖς βρέμονται (348–50), recalling "blood-tasting" Ares (244: τούτῳ γὰρ Ἄρης βόσκεται, φόνῳ βροτῶν). Aeschylus thus incorporates a traditional, well-known

---

[57] See Thibodeau/Boroditsky (2011): "metaphors were most effective when they were presented early in the narrative and were then able to help organize and coerce further incoming information."

conceptualization of "blood-stained" Ares (μιαιφόνος in the *Iliad*) [58] into his own poetic fabric, stirring a profoundly affective response. Once more, the tastes of bitterness, flesh and blood are confounded as they generate a covert feeling of distaste and revulsion.

Feelings of pollution as a response to kin killing and incest resonate throughout the narrative, most prominently through blood imagery;[59] in conjunction with this imagery, gustatory metaphors, as a subset of the wider nexus of agricultural metaphors, trigger similar psychological processes. To be sure, Girard has already drawn attention to the connection between violence and ritual impurity, while Parker notes, "pollution may be a metaphysical expression of the social disruption of relations between family groups".[60] I want to suggest that such considerations were not merely reflected in but felt through language itself, in a deeply visceral sense. Language comprehension involves simulation and recruitment of neural systems used for perception, emotion and action. Such simulation ultimately shapes people's judgments, affecting moral processing.[61]

In this brief analysis, I hope to have shown how metaphor, theme and culture interact in ways that can be culturally and cross-culturally shared, across time and space, based on the common, pre-reflexive and immediate mechanisms that ground our identification with and connectedness to others. I aimed to argue that metaphors should not be discarded as mere ornaments of a highly stylized poetic composition. Instead, any analysis of poetic discourse and the psychological impact of ancient drama should take into consideration the function of embodied metaphor as a cognitive tool, which allows us to gain insight into the emotional complexities interwoven in the narrative fabric, and to better understand the type of emotional communities these tragic plays addressed. As Ana-Maria Rizzuto nicely put it, "To understand internal reality means to understand a human being who not only knows, but also feels that knowledge".[62]

Acknowledgments: I am grateful to William Thalmann for his generous guidance and ongoing support. My work benefited immensely from the incisive comments of Douglas Cairns and William Short. I am also grateful to Jennifer Devereaux for her invaluable feedback and timely suggestions.

---

58 *Iliad* 5.31; 455; 844.
59 See also Seaford's most recent discussion (2012) 174.
60 Girard (1977); Parker (1983) 120–1. As Padel (1995) 164 nicely puts it, in tragedy "madness, passion, pollution and disease are deeply bound to each other."
61 Foroni/Semin (2009).
62 Rizzuto (2001) 552.

Peter Meineck
5 The Affective Ancient Theatre, a Bio-cultural Cognitive Approach

While we possess very little in the way of accounts of how Athenian fifth-century drama was originally received, what we do have is notable in that these responses almost universally deal with the emotionality and affective power of the theatre upon its audience. Here I outline a methodology derived from cognitive theory and affective/cultural neuroscience that focuses on human affective responses and applies it to ancient Greek drama, with a focus on emotionality. As I focus on the affective properties of the fifth-century Athenian theatre I use the example of one cognitive aspect, mask perception, to demonstrate this approach.

Athenian drama was a physically embodied, highly absorbing and profoundly emotional experience for its audience. For example, in book 6 of Herodotus' *Histories*, written around 440, we hear of a performance of a tragedy called *The Sack of Miletus*, by Phrynichus, based on the real destruction of that city, an Athenian ally, by the Persians. Herodotus tells us that "the entire theatre fell into tears" and as a result the playwright was fined 1000 drachmas and the play banned for reminding the Athenians of such a disaster (6.21.10). By the end of the fifth century the theatre had evidently lost none of its emotional force: in Xenophon's *Symposium* (3.11) we read of the basis for the huge popularity of the actor Callippides – he "could fill a theatre because he could move the entire audience to tears."

Audience reactions were both physical and voluble. We hear of audiences hissing, clapping, banging their heels against the back of the seats and even clucking.[1] In Aristophanes' comedies we even hear about official "rod-holders" who were hired to keep the audience members in line.[2] Aristotle and Plutarch both recount a moment of intense theatrical emotionality from a play called *Cresphontes* (now lost). Merope, the Queen of Messenia, is just about to bring an ax down on the person who she thinks killed her son. The audience knows that this is in fact her son. Plutarch tells us that this caused mass panic in the theatre and

---

[1] Demosthenes, *Against Meidias* 22.6 and *On the False Embassy*, 337; Harpocration s.v. *eklozete*; Theophrastus, *Characters* 11.3.
[2] Aristophanes, *Peace* 734–47 with scholion.

Peter Meineck, New York University

that the audience jumped to their feet in terror.[3] Aristotle cites this scene as one of the finest crafted "discoveries" in tragedy.[4]

We feel emotions, they are manifested physically by an affective state and intense embodied emotional experiences *move* us. Plato, Aristotle and Isocrates all wrote that theatre had the power "to move the soul" of its audiences. According to Plato, the living soul is never at rest but is most moved by three divinely inspired states of madness: one is the frenzied ranting of the prophet; another the whirling and dancing of purification rites such as the Corybantic "frenzies"; and third, the extreme emotions generated by the performance of music and song. He reiterates this in *Minos* where theatre is described as "the most popular, enjoyable and soul-moving psychagôgikos branch of poetry" (321a4). Isocrates, for his part, addressed how dramatists took myths and set them to contests (*agones*) and action (*praxis*), not only for our ears, as with Epic or Lyric, but also in front of our eyes, which led to "soul moving experiences" (*Evagoras* 2.49).

One of the most famous of all ancient comments on Greek drama is Aristotle's statement in *Poetics* that drama is primarily an emotional event capable of producing *catharsis* by eliciting empathetic feelings of pity and fear in the audience (1449b25–30). Aristotle describes two essential elements of drama as soul moving – "reversals" (*peripeteiai*), and "discoveries" (*anagnōriseis*) –, which he cites as the most emotionally affecting parts of the story (1450a33). Additionally, he uses the term *psychagôgia* ("soul-moving") to describe visuality (*opsis*). For Aristotle, the soul-moving powers of *opsis* were the preserve of the mask maker (*skeuopoios*), who had a mastery over the creation of the uncanny and the emotional (1450b.16–21).

As Athenian drama spread throughout the Hellenic world it continued to be regarded as an art form that could move its audiences to intense affective states. As late as the second century BCE, Lucian begins his *How to Write History* with a bizarre story of how the population of Abdera went "theatre-mad" after experiencing a performance of Euripides *Andromeda* by a visiting company. They exhibited marked physical symptoms, such as fevers, uncontrolled shaking and nosebleeds. This reminds us of Gorgias' *Helen* where the performance of dramatic speech and song has the power to force its audiences "to shudder with terror, shed tears of pity, and yearn with sad longing."

The ancient sources' account of the emotional power of drama map well into contemporary theories of cognitive embodiment and distributed cognition: the theory that our minds are not confined inside our craniums but embodied,

---

3 Plutarch, *Moralia* 998E; Nauck, *Trag. Graec. Frag.* 456.
4 Aristotle, *Poetics*, 1454a5; *Nicomachean Ethics* 1.17.3.

embedded, extended and enacted beyond our skin and distributed into the environment around us.⁵

Distributed cognition theoretical frameworks share the common view that the mind is not "brainbound" or "computational" and that human thought is not just a function of biological brain architecture, neural responses and chemical reactions. As Prinz has pointed out, the neo-Cartesian principle of the computational brain can be traced to the proliferation of computers since the 1950s. This has greatly influenced the field of cognitive science and has become the major theoretical underpinning that lies behind a good deal of neuroscientific research.⁶

This clinical separation of the human mind from the body and the surrounding environment has been justifiably criticized. For example, Alva Noë who writes, "we think with computers, but computers don't think: they are tools. If computers are information processors, then they are information processors the way watches are [in that a watch doesn't itself know what time it is, though we use it to track time]".⁷ Noë maintains that the disembodied brain is unable to think: "the world shows up for us thanks to our interaction with it. It is not made in the brain, or by the brain. It is there for us and we have access to it." The brain then is not "on its own, a source of experience or cognition ... what gives the living animal's states their significance is the animal's dynamic engagement with the world around it".⁸ The computational brain theory has many brilliant advocates, but there is now a growing number of influential neuroscientists who have married clinical work on brain imaging, neurochemical research and behavioral studies with theories of cognitive embodiment.⁹

Live drama is an embodied experience and theatre exists in the cognitive space between actor and spectator – its effects and affects are felt and thought. These two cognitive processes are not mutually exclusive. The environmental aspects of the ancient theatre need to be considered as an important part of the total experience of ancient drama. This includes the spatial dynamics of the performance space and how it cognitively and chemically affected the audience, and the multisensory information of sight, sound, smell, and touch, both real and "mirrored" by the brain's neural architecture. Greek drama was presented

---

5 See Clark (2008); Clark/Chalmers (1998); Lakoff/Johnson (1999); Varela/Rosch/Thompson (1992); Ward/Stapleton (2012) 89–106.
6 Prinz (2012) 1–14.
7 Noë (2009) 163.
8 Noë (2009) 164–165.
9 For example, LeDoux (1998) 29; Damasio (2008); Damasio/Carvalho (2013) 143–152; Edelman (2006) 26.

within an environment that promoted altered mental states, through movement, rhythm, kinesthetic mirroring, crowd dynamics, emotional contagion, dissociation and empathy. Important past studies consider Greek drama to be a reflection of the political and social concerns of the day, and so it was in part, but for the audience seated on the southeastern slope of the Acropolis in the fifth century, theatre was primarily an embodied, emotional experience.[10]

Bio-Cultural Emotions

In one sense this approach is somewhat Aristotelian in nature, in that like a modern theatrical production process, it dissects drama into its constituent parts to seek understanding of how they all worked together in performance.[11] The sum of theatrical elements was a visual, aural, kinesthetic and somatic *Gesamtkunstwerk* capable of producing the kind of extreme emotional responses we hear of in the ancient sources. But in order to apply contemporary studies from the affective sciences to antiquity it is vital to reevaluate some basic questions about how emotions are perceived and evaluated. What are emotions exactly and are the emotions we know today the same as those experienced by people from another culture in the distant past?

The study of human emotions has a long history stretching back to Plato, Xenophon and Aristotle, who all sought to categorize and explain affective states.[12] In the modern era, Darwin turned his attention to embodied emotions in his seminal study, *The Expression of Emotions in Man and Animals* (1872). This work is still highly influential today in the research of the so-called neo-Darwinists, such as Paul Ekman. Ekman's theory of "basic emotions" posits that there are a finite number of reductive affective states that can be identified across different cultures.[13] This is one of the most debated positions in affective science today and in part a result of the scientific method's obsession with the quantifiable

---

[10] For a good appraisal of recent political and social approaches to Greek drama, see Powers (2014).

[11] Just as the modern Western way of creating theatre consists of different "departments" (costume, wigs, sound, lights, set, actors, dancers, musicians, etc.) unified by stage management under a director who are working with a text provided by a writer.

[12] For example, Plato, *Republic* 4.437d1-442c7; Aristotle, *Rhetoric* 2.1–11; Xenophon, *Memorabilia* 2.6.21.2–23.7.

[13] Ekman/Friesen (2003).

categorization of an affective process that is probably far more mutable and fluid than most studies seem able to allow.

In addition to the categorization of emotions, there has been a great deal of debate on how emotions are caused, processed, expressed and interpreted. Today, most theories of emotions fall somewhere between two distinct theoretical positions: "constructionists" or "cultural relativists" posit that emotional states are learned products of culture, whereas the "universalists" of the psychological or biological school, propose that at least some emotions are universal across humans and a product of the evolutionary process. There is also a schism between those who view emotions as resulting from judgment ("appraisal theory"), and others who surmise that emotions can be far more instantaneous. For example, if one suddenly falls, fear arises before the mind has had any time to form a judgment; this is known as "embodiment theory". Prinz sets out the two positions succinctly in his 2012 book *Beyond Human Nature,* and I think he is correct to conclude that there is no convincing evidence that we need appraisal judgments to distinguish different emotions, and that "the embodiment theory is probably right".[14]

If emotions are affective expressions of embodied experiences, then evidence of emotional responses in ancient Greek culture can help us to understand more about the function and reception of ancient drama. However, traditional forms of understanding the ancient world, primarily via textual analysis, can be problematic when considering ancient emotions. Chaniotis has pointed out that the basic physical elements of emotional experience "do not exist within the study of written sources," especially when we are "dealing with human beings who died twenty centuries ago".[15] David Konstan's seminal study of the emotions of the ancient Greeks delineates "significant differences" between ancient emotions and our own, the recognition of which is essential for understanding Greek literature and culture. He does concede, however, that there may exist at a deeper level basic universal biological "affects".[16]

A solution to this problem of ethnocentric bias has been proposed by the historian Barbara Rosenwein, who suggested that the affective information gleaned from other cultures, in particular those of the past, should be assessed by collating information about the emotional regime of that society, or what she has called "emotional communities".[17] Rosenwein's approach includes gathering the source

---

14 Prinz (2012) 242–247.
15 Chaniotis (2012) 14.
16 Konstan (2006) 260.
17 Rosenwein (2010) 1–32.

material for the group in question, problematizing their emotional terminology, consulting the theorists of that period, weighing emotional attitudes to assess the relative value placed on each emotion, and then going further and looking for emotions in "silences", metaphors and ironies; considering the social role they play; and then tracing changes in attitudes to emotions over time".[18]

At first sight, Rosenwein's methodology in developing a history of emotions seems entirely constructivist, yet she writes "a history of emotions must not deny the biological substratum of emotions, since it is clear that they are embodied in both the body and the brain." For Rosenwein, the differences between constructionist and biological approaches "are not inseparable." She suggests that any history of emotions must address the distinctive characteristics of the society under scrutiny, and she adds, "even bodies (and brains) are shaped by culture."

This is the rationale for taking a bio-cultural approach to ancient drama. This accepts that there are certain physical and chemical biological commonalities that all humans have shared for the last 80,000 years or so.[19] Additionally, that an evolutionary process that developed to respond to environmental stimuli has honed human affective states. But this does not mean that the human mind is fixed and universal across cultures. On the contrary, human biology is highly plastic – for example, the nascent field of epigenetics has shown how DNA can be altered in as little as one generation in response to extreme environmental factors such as stress.[20] Even within one lifetime, brain networks are adaptable, and individuals can reorder existing brain processes while learning a language, playing a musical instrument, mastering a sport, and so on. Yet, our shared human biology does make many elements of our lives universal, whether we like it or not.

Human cultures are the embodied expressions of shared human minds responding to basic biological needs and environmental stimuli in a constant cognitive feedback loop. Survival, food production, shelter, group dynamics, reproduction, and safety are just a few of the basic cultural factors that mitigate cognition and call for a plasticity of brain function. In this respect, differences in culture stem from environmental disparities and differing cognitive solutions to the same basic underlying needs of survival. Human culture is the manifestation of the extended social mind – put simply, minds make culture and culture makes minds. Human biology and human culture are therefore inextricably linked – we

---

18 For these questions applied to classical material, see now Cairns/Fulkerton (2015).
19 On bio-cultural approaches to literature, see Boyd (2005) 1–23 and (2009).
20 See Elbert/Schauer (2014) 215–227; Roth (2014); Whalley (2014).

are all bio-cultural beings and we share a basic biology with the ancient Greeks; it is our cultures that are different.[21]

Classicists, archaeologists and ancient historians have been studying the cultures of the ancient Greeks since the Renaissance, albeit refracted via their own various social milieus. If we accept that human cognition is bio-cultural and that cultures are created by human minds, then it would only be prudent to take the biological side of human cognition into consideration when considering an ancient culture. What then can cognitive studies and neuroscience contribute to our understanding of the ancient world?

One benefit of this interdisciplinary approach is that the clinical aspects of neuroscience allow us to distance ourselves slightly from our own cultural biases when we examine aspects of antiquity. Another is that by thinking with neuroscience we might approach material from a different perspective and form new conclusions. This is certainly a new methodology for classical studies but several scholars have recently applied neuroscience research and cognitive theory to various facets of the theatre arts with a good deal of success. For example, in the field of theatre studies, Bruce McConachie has produced a groundbreaking cognitive study of theatre spectatorship and Evelyn Tribble has explored the mnemonic features of Shakespeare's poetry through the theory of distributed cognition.[22]

A bio-cultural approach to an important aspect of an ancient culture has been recently advanced by Garrett Fagan, who has applied studies in modern crowd psychology to analyze Roman responses to organized spectacles of violence. He terms his approach "psychobiological" and writes that, "an interdependence between contextual stimulus and psychological propensity shapes behavior".[23] Fagan makes the important point that if there were not basic human universal psychological functions across different cultures then "alien societies ought to remain virtually impenetrable to an outsider" and, with this in mind, "it is possible for modern minds to comprehend, analyze and even empathize with the actions of people in other historical eras" (46). This is certainly true of ancient drama. While modern audiences may not grasp the significance of certain ritual actions, religious beliefs or cultural practice, they can still be moved by the incidents that arise from them.[24]

---

21 See Habinek (2011) 64–83.
22 McConachie (2008); Tribble (2011). See also Lutterbie (2011); Blair (2007); Rokotnitz (2011); McConachie/Blair (2013); McConachie/Hart (2006). See also Chaston (2010) who has applied the reproductive processing theories of Kaufmann and Paivio to tragic props.
23 Fagan (2011) 40–41.
24 See also Konstan (2006) 3–40.

An important bio-cultural theory of affective states has also been used by Robert Kaster to examine Roman texts for affective information. Making it clear that no Latin emotional term maps perfectly onto a corresponding English one, Kaster analyzed the affect "from penetration of a phenomenon, through evaluation and response" in order to understand the emotion "through Roman eyes and not through the filter of our own sensibilities".[25] Still, Kaster's approach remains embedded in textual analysis and cannot divorce us from our own cultural predispositions. Chaniotis has suggested that although clearly useful, a lexical approach such as Kaster's alone cannot be the "sole methodology for a detailed investigation of the emotional concepts of another culture".[26] But we do have much more than only texts, including the remains of the material culture and the wealth of cognitive information that can be gleaned from vase paintings, sculpture, architecture, sanctuary layouts, town planning, and environmental relationships. Distributed cognition asserts that such external stimuli that generated the emotions are as much a part of the human mind as the physical brain itself and that by applying research from the neuro- and affective sciences we can significantly add to our arsenal of resources for understanding the ancient world. Luther Martin has called this kind of trans-historical approach "a cognitive historiography", suggesting that it can provide correctives to traditional historiographical tools by identifying and explaining data that have been produced by ordinary processes of human cognition but that have otherwise been neglected in favor of more explicit forms of evidence that historians have, for one reason or another, come to privilege principally texts, which are themselves, of course, constrained products of human minds to be explained rather than unembellished reservoirs of historical facts.[27]

The cultural side of the bio-cultural equation also requires subtle navigation. Here classicists can learn much from the related fields of cognitive archaeology and ethnography, where the practice of comparative social modeling has been used to learn more about ancient artifacts and the cultures that produced them. This is achieved by comparing what we know of a culture that no longer exists with basic empirical similarities found in a similar one that still does.[28] The basic premise of the general comparative approach is that human groups that share certain basic societal characteristics will also share some similar perceptual functions.[29]

---

25 Kaster (2005) 6–7.
26 Chaniotis (2012) 23.
27 Martin (2012) 168.
28 See Malafouris/Renfrew (2010) 1–12.
29 See Abramiuk (2012) 95–124.

From a psychological perspective, a similar approach can be found in the works of the psychiatrist Jonathan Shay and the ancient historian, Lawrence Tritle, both of whom have famously equated the psychological experiences of the modern combat veteran with ancient Greek warriors.[30] Their work on combat trauma provides a brief case study that highlights some of the issues faced when embarking on cross-cultural comparative psychological research. It is also relevant to our focus on the theatre as there are also close connections between the military culture of classical Athens and the organization, recruitment, funding and narratives of ancient drama.[31]

However, while comparing the psychologies of two distinct cultures may be revealing, we need to be aware of the underlying cultural differences and be very cautious not to impose our own social biases. Shay's and Tritle's work has thus been challenged as "universalistic" and even viewed as part of a wider cultural phenomenon of the globalization of American/Western notions of trauma therapy.[32]

We should also be cautious not to adopt the extreme relativist position either. We see the same types of environmental stimuli producing similar biological and psychological responses. What we now call PTSD was called battle fatigue in WWII; shell shock in World War One; debility syndrome in the Boer War; and in the American Civil War, the physical chest pain that may have been caused by extreme anxiety was named "Soldier's Heart". We hear of distinct emotional responses by ancient Greeks to extreme situations throughout Greek literature and we can still empathize with many of them. Surely, one cannot now read the chilling description of the abandonment of the Athenian wounded at Syracuse, as told by Thucydides (7.75), and not see an expert description of what we now call "survivor's guilt".

Masks

Just as the acts recorded by historiography have an emotional causality so ancient performance was created to produce affective responses in its audiences. To demonstrate how this kind of bio-cultural approach can add resources to how we understand antiquity I focus now on one important aspect of ancient audience cognition – the emotional processing of the dramatic mask.

---

[30] Shay (2010) and (2003); Tritle (2002) and (2014) 87–104.
[31] Pritchard (2004) 208–28.
[32] Crowley (2014) 105–130 and (2012).

In today's Western contemporary theatre the theatrical mask is mostly misunderstood. It is regarded as the accoutrement of an earlier age, a forgotten aspect of ancient ritual, or a prop inherited from carnival intended to disfigure and disguise. This attitude has affected the way the Greek dramatic mask has been viewed and led to many misconceptions about its form, function and use. The mask was included in Stanford's study on Greek tragedy and the emotions completed in the 1980's.[33] This book did set out a useful taxonomy of emotional expressions in Greek drama and examined song, noises, cries and silences, music and the spoken word, and certain visual aspects. One major criticism of Stanford is that he reflected the prevailing view that the dramatic mask was a fixed immovable visage that "distanced" the audience in a kind of Brechtian emotional disengagement. Neuroscience studies on facial processing can help us understand that this was not at all the case and that the mask needs to be seriously reappraised as one of the main conveyers of embodiment and emotionality in Greek drama.

Facial emotional recognition, reciprocal eye contact, and mental connectivity to the movements of others are some of the most important ways in which humans communicate emotional states between themselves. What happens then, when the mask denies the viewer the face, the eyes are hidden and movement is choreographed and heightened? I have showed how the fifth-century tragic mask in tandem with bodily movements provoked the face-recognition and emotional processing systems of the ancient theatre spectator enabling them to perceive distinct changes of emotions in the features of the mask as manipulated by the actor.[34] The mask thus fulfills a number of performative functions, yet I here focus on how comparative cognitive approaches can shed more light on ancient affective responses and emotional contagion.[35]

Up until fairly recently almost all face processing studies assumed there was a universality of biological and evolutionary based brain function when it came to how humans processed faces. This stemmed from research carried out in the 1960's by Alfred Yarbus who developed a means of "eye-tracking". This followed exactly where the human eye scanned by recording the saccades (tiny flickers) of the pupil as it scanned faces. These highly influential studies found that participants looked at the eyes and the mouth, forming an "eye-tracking triangle", and only then paid attention to the outline of the face and head. Subsequent, eye-tracking studies on

---

33 Stanford (1983).
34 Meineck (2011).
35 Emotional Contagion has been described as "The tendency to automatically mimic and synchronize facial expressions, vocalizations, postures, and movements with those of another person and, consequently, to converge emotionally". Hatfield/Rapson/Yen-Chi (2011) 19.

scenic vistas found that people focused on human forms, when observing a scene, before observing the background. When humans were not present, they looked first at the places where humans or other animals were most likely to be.[36]

This universal principle has recently been seriously challenged by a series of cross-cultural eye-tracking studies carried out by Takahiko Musada and Richard Nisbett. Starting in 2001, they found that eye-tracking and visual processing actually differs across cultural groups. Masuda and Nisbett found that participants from Japan and China had a marked tendency to view scenes holistically, whereas those from North America and Northern Europe were more specifically analytical.[37] The people he described as "East Asians" attended to a broader perceptual field, focusing on contextual information and causal attributions.[38]

There is now brain imaging research that shows different neural networks operating between East Asian and Western participants undergoing the same cognitive activities.[39] Eye-tracking studies have also shown how people from different cultures look at artworks differently.[40] Studies like this have posited that culture plays an important, if not predominant, part in many aspects of cognition, including how we process faces and read emotions. This is because each distinctive culture has its own scopic regime, or way in which it perceives objects and surroundings. Humans all share the same biological functions for facial processing and it happens in the same area of the brain. The difference is the order in which things are processed, and the cultural importance given to visual elements in the perception of the world around us. Nisbett proposes that the particular nature of Chinese agriculture, involving mass cooperation, led to a culture where the collective was regarded as more important than the individual. According to him, this led to the development of holistic visual processing.[41]

Eye-tracking studies have now found that "East Asian" participants tend to focus on the nose and center of the face. In East Asian cultures, gaze aversion is a cultural norm, as is holistic visual processing. The center of the face at the nose is therefore the strongest single viewpoint to take in overall facial information (see Figure 1 below).[42]

---

36 Yarbus (1967).
37 Masuda/Nisbett (2001) 922.
38 For a critique of Nisbett's oversimplification of his participants' ethnicities, cultures and personal experiences, see the excellent discussion by Geoffrey Lloyd who calls them "global hypostatizations" in Lloyd (2007) 160–70.
39 Han/Ma (2014).
40 Liu *et al.* (2013).
41 Nisbett (2004).
42 Blais *et al.* (2008).

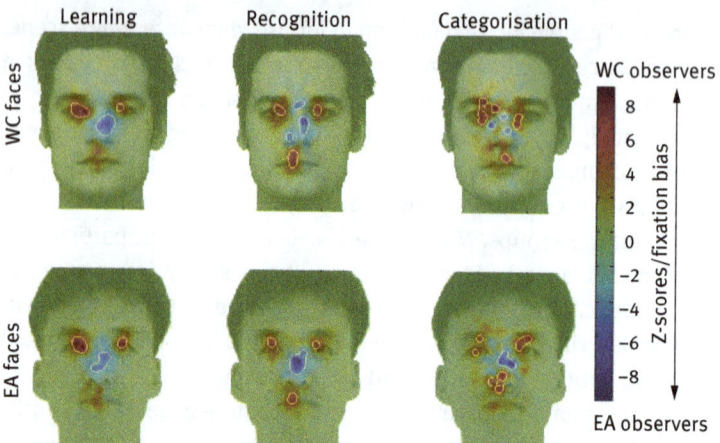

Figure 1: Fixation biases for Western Caucasian (WC – red) and East Asian (EA – blue) observers (Blais, et. al (2008)).

If face processing is culturally predicated, might we be able to apply this to the ancient mask and learn anything of Athenian fifth-century cognition? While we have no surviving Greek dramatic masks to study we do have several research resources available to us. One is what we can generally learn about the scopic regime of the Greeks from their literature in relation to gaze direction. We can also examine the evidence for masks from the iconographic record, and we can use mask research from a culture that uses dramatic masks in a similar way to the Greeks. In this last resource we are fortunate to now have several important studies that have examined the Japanese Noh mask.

Even taking the vagaries of vase painting into consideration, in the fifth-century representations of masks we do see some distinctive commonalities. They all have a relatively small nose, large eyes and a normal-sized open mouth. The facial features are smooth around the eyes and mouth and the bottom lip of the Greek mask tends to be more pronounced. If we compare the Greek masks to Japanese Noh masks dating from the fifteenth to nineteenth centuries we immediately discern some marked differences. The Japanese masks all have very large noses that dominate the mask's face, relatively small eyes and stylized mouths. I suggest that what we are seeing here is not only the aesthetic preferences of the two different cultures but also a physical mimetic representation of their respective cognitive facial processing systems. From the evidence of the Greek mask iconography, it seems, at first sight, that the ancient Athenians processed faces much as Westerners do today, focusing on the eyes and mouth first. Japanese audiences for Noh drama processed faces in much the same way as Nisbett's modern "East Asians", by focusing on the nose in the center of the face, hence the oversize, dominant noses on the masks. It is also notable that the Chinese character that denotes "self" – *ziran*, is made up of the word for "nose" – *zi* and *ran* meaning "correct" or "yes". Furthermore, in Chinese cultural practice, the term *zi* is also used to denote a personal point of view, and many people point to their nose to indicate themselves.[43]

The Role of Literacy

In the facial features of mask representations we may well be able to discern some important cognitive qualities of ancient Greek facial processing, once we establish and identify differing cultural idiosyncrasies. With this in mind one of the most important differences between Western theatre audiences today and fifth-century Athenians was literacy and recent research in this area has indicated that this had a profound effect on how the mask was processed emotionally.

Brain imaging studies have indicated that the processing of faces is performed primarily by what has been named the fusiform face area, part of the brain's fusiform gyrus (ridge) located on the lower part of the temporal lobe between two other long ridges, the occipitotemporal gyrus and the parahippocampal gyrus. This area is associated with high-level image processing and object recognition. This was recently dramatically confirmed by a 2012 Stanford study carried out on a live human subject who had electrodes placed directly on this part of his brain. This was possible because the man in question was undergoing electrocorticography (electrode stimulation of exposed brain tissue) for acute epileptic seizures, and had a section of his skull removed exposing the area where the fusiform gyrus is located. When electrodes where attached to two nerve clusters about half an inch apart (designated pFus and mFus) and stimulated with an electric current, temporarily lobotomizing them, the patient reported that his doctor's facial features "melted away". When the current was stopped, the patient was able to recognize faces instantly.[44]

The fusiform face area shares a good deal of architecture with the fusiform gyrus, in particular what has been called the "visual word form area" (VWFA) and associated with reading. This area is left lateralized in most people and shares networks with the areas of the brain responsible for language processing in the left superior temporal and inferior frontal regions. It has been shown that the

---

[43] Callahan (1989).
[44] Parvizi *et al.* (2012); Rivolta (2014) 19–40.

neurons within this ventral visual pathway tend to respond to basic intersecting forms such as "T", "l" and "X" shapes. Recently, Stanislav Dehaene has proposed that all writing systems make use of variants of these intersecting contoured shapes, to which our primate brain was already "highly attuned". Furthermore, Dehaene posits that the brain is capable of quickly "recycling" the existing neural networks that originally evolved to process similar, but different tasks. In this case, he suggests that when people learn to read, they develop a neuronal "short circuit" between the left ventral visual pathway and the left-hemispheric language areas. In this model, human cultural expression can never be independent of biology and cultural inventions, such as writing can only happen because they utilize preexisting neural architecture. Dehaene calls this "living proof that culture is constrained by brain biology". Antiquity provides an example of the kind of illiterate cognitive processing Dehaene has described. A fragment of the *Theseus* by Euripides includes the character of a herdsman who is reporting (possibly to King Minos) an inscription that reads "Theseus" (ΘHSEUS) and describes the letters he has seen in terms of bisecting lines and curves that resemble naturally occurring objects. Thus the Herdsman's "a circle neatly turned out, as if turned on a lathe with a prominent mark in the middle", *Heta* is described as "two lines first of all and one more in the middle that connects them", and the last letter, *Sigma*, is "a curling lock of hair".[45] Euripides' Herdsman is clearly illiterate and this has an important impact on the way he would have perceived a face. Dehaene has shown that the acquisition of literacy skills involves a reconfiguration of existing brain functionality that creates a lasting difference for facial processing. He concludes:

> The acquisition of reading seemed to induce an important reorganization of the ventral visual pathway, which displaces the cortical responses to the face away from the left hemisphere and more toward the right. This displacement is presumably because the features that are most useful for letter recognition (configurations and intersections of lines) are incompatible with those that are useful for faces, so that one pushes the other away.[46]

In another recent related study, it has been shown that illiterate people process faces far more holistically than literate people, who tend to be much more analytical and adept at recognizing details.[47] The study concluded that brain reorganization induced by literacy reduces the automatic holistic processing of faces.

---

45 Euripides, *Theseus* (*TrGF* 382 = Athenaeus 10.454b-c).
46 Dehaene (2013).
47 Ventura (2013).

To put it simply, both illiterate and literate people react quickly to what they perceive as a face in the visual environment. A literate person, who has reorganized neural networks to be able to read, has an increased ability to call on contextual and analytical cognitive tools. An illiterate person retains a stronger more intensely emotional response to the face for a longer period. Deheane points out that in "recycling" brain function we can perceive the changes in process. For example, he cites the way in which young children learning to read will confuse "b's" and "d's" as they teach their ventral pathways to disable the symmetrical processing systems designed to deal with naturally occurring objects.[48]

With a biological explanation for differences in face processing across literate abilities in place we can now apply the science to what we know about levels of literacy in fifth-century Athens.

Within Greek plays themselves we can detect a distinct cognitive change towards the written word in Athenian culture. Isabelle Torrance has shown how the implements of writing do not appear in any of the extant plays of Aeschylus and Sophocles, and that all references to writing are related to the recording of memory. In this way, writing is perceived as the recording of an important speech act that is enacted again by speaking the written words. This all changes with the plays of Euripides, where letters and inscriptions become agents within the plot structure of the plays, and "for the first time in antiquity writing is internalized and processed as *text*, rather than being read aloud." Torrance concludes "the different ways in which the three great tragedians explore the concept of writing ... suggests a marked development in the perception of writing over the course the fifth century, and suggests that only the elite had the kind of literacy skills capable of reading the text of a play script".[49]

In the fifth century the Athenian elite strove to be literate, composing speeches and controlling the codifications of statutes, laws and trade accounts. The average Athenian citizen probably did not need more than a basic recognition of letters to actively participate in Athenian society, which Thomas suggests might explain the preponderance of lists at this time.[50] The next logical question then, is who was the audience for Athenian drama, the elite, or the same kind of Athenian citizen who attended the assembly and law courts? New archaeological research on the Theatre of Dionysos suggests that the fifth-century *theatron* sat around 5–6,000 people.[51] While not able to accommodate the 30,000 or so

---

[48] Dehaene (2013) 10–12; see also Blackburne *et al.* (2014).
[49] Torrance (2013) 142.
[50] Thomas (1995) 59–74.
[51] Papastamati-von Moock (2014) 20–23; Goette (2007) 116–21.

Athenian voting male population (the *demos*), this was still a larger public space than the Pnyx, the site of the Athenian assembly, which accommodated less than 5000, which by most ancient accounts, included a cross section of the Athenian *demos*. From the wisecracks of the ribald characters of Old Comedy and the political themes lampooned in the plays, we can assume upper, middle and lower class Athenian citizens were all present at the theatre, along with a number of invited ambassadors and dignitaries from allied states. David Roselli has even suggested that non-Athenian citizens such as women, foreigners and slaves could have conceivably also been watching the plays.[52] We can therefore assume that the majority of the spectators were functionally, but not fully, literate.[53]

Even among the Athenian elite there may have been an ambivalent attitude to literacy. Plato, to name but one, was famously suspicious of writing (*Phaedrus* 275a–b). A famous anecdote found in Plutarch (*Nicias* 29.2) may shed some light on this issue as it relates to drama. He writes of a few Athenians who were able to pay their way out of the Sicilian quarries and get home to Athens after being captured in the disastrous Sicilian expedition. This was because they could sing the choruses of Euripides. That Sicilians would pay to hear Athenians come to their homes and sing from the plays suggests that the play script as a transportable text had not yet emerged. When we find depictions of dramatists in comedy they are portrayed composing rather than writing and there is a mention in Plutarch of Euripides teaching his chorus his lyrics by call and response.[54] Thus, even as late as 416 BCE, the spoken and sung word was still the most effective means of communicating drama, and literacy was probably not required to either perform in the plays or watch them.

To sum up, illiterate and semi-literate people process faces more holistically. They rely on more instinctual and emotional processes to parse faces, over analytical or contextual cognitive tools. If we accept that fifth-century audience members were predominantly semi-literate or illiterate, then we can deduce that their perceptual responses to the mask would have been significantly different to most Western theatergoers today: more intensely emotional and far less analytical. Perhaps this is why masks are so very difficult in Western contemporary theatre today: they simply do not provoke the same neural responses they did for the Athenians. Yet masked drama has prevailed in Japan and China in the form

---

52 Roselli (2011).
53 See Pappas (2011) 48.
54 There are references to the act of reading in tragedy but this is not evidence for full literacy. Aesch. fr. 358, is advice to a warrior to fight at close quarters, "like a man reading in old age". See also Sophocles fr. 858.

of Noh, or in the heavy mask-like make up used in Kabuki and Chinese Opera. While it cannot be claimed that Japanese Noh audiences are in any way illiterate, Nisbett's work has shown Japanese people to be more holistic in their visual processing of scenes, objects and faces. Perhaps this is why masked narrative drama remains a thoroughly popular narrative art form in Japan, whereas the mask in the West has become the preserve of the carnival, the mime, the disguised protester, comic superhero, or a child's toy. Though many of the uncanny abilities of the mask are still discernable today, the response of the ancient Athenian was far more emotionally affecting.

Conclusion

The act of creating theatre is an interdisciplinary adventure requiring the considerable skills of writers, directors, actors, dancers, musicians, designers, technicians, producers, marketers, accountants, lawyers, and, of course, the most diverse group of all, the audience. Therefore, we need to arm ourselves with a multiplicity of tools to understand how the theatre of the past might have functioned. In his thought-provoking study of how cognitive theories might be applied to antiquity, G.E.R. Lloyd has written, "There is no single discourse that should have precedence over all others. What we need are different types and levels of analysis allowing indeed that at some points they may be difficult to reconcile as they may relate to different facets of multidimensional phenomena".[55] The theatre is constructed of multidimensional phenomena and while the application of science cannot hope to unravel the simple mystery of the power of actor before an audience, it can help us to begin to understand how Athenian drama came to enthrall its audiences, spread throughout the Greek and Roman world, and become one of the most influential art forms the world has ever known.

---

55 Lloyd (2007) 85.

Gabriel Herman
6 The Sensed Presence as an Analytical Tool in Historical Research

I

Sensed Presence visions (hereafter SP) constitute a special, clearly delineated category of visions that have occurred to people who felt they were on the verge of death. A typical, well-documented case is that of Ron DiFrancisco, who was on the 84th floor of the South Tower of the World Trade Center in New York when it was struck by a Boeing 767 on September 11, 2001. DiFrancisco first considered descending, but the stairwell was suffused with smoke and flames. When he tried to ascend, he encountered even more smoke and flames. He was trapped. At that point he began to panic. Determined that he was "gonna make it out", he turned around, and, unlike the rest, started back down. It was while gasping for air, and realizing that a collapsed wall prevented him from descending further, that the SP vision occurred. This is how he subsequently described it: "Someone told me to get up". The voice, which was male, was insistent. "Get up!" It addressed DiFrancesco by his first name, and gave him encouragement: "It was, 'Hey! You can do this'. But it was more than a voice; there was also a vivid sense of a physical presence".[1] Against all odds, DiFrancesco managed to steer his course through smoke, flames and debris to reach the plaza level. He was one of only four people to escape the building from above the 81st floor.

For a long time SP visions were given short shrift in research. Presumably they were ignored because they usually involved miracles and supernatural beliefs of the sort that stretch the credulity of the rationally oriented researcher. They were also ignored because, mental disease being the central concern of psychologists and psychiatrists, non-pathological mental processes tend to attract less attention. As we shall see, SP events occur to mentally balanced and physically fit people.

The rationale for this neglect has lately been challenged through the publication of a large database of SP events. It would perhaps be no overstatement to say that these works cast the phenomenon into a new perspective.[2] Accounts

---

1 Duffy (2005). For a further interview with DiFrancesco, see Geiger (2009) 10–11.
2 Geiger (2009) and (2013). Geiger notes that ever since the publication of his first book people have approached him with stories of unpublicised events, not all of which qualify as SP. Geiger has collaborated with Peter Suedfeld, an expert in psychological responses to extreme and

Gabriel Herman, The Hebrew University, Jerusalem

https://doi.org/10.1515/9783110482201-007

of miraculous survivals that were hardly believable when related by individuals suddenly acquired credibility when they were repeated, in rough outline, by hundreds. People of diverse vocations and orientations, from all walks of life – mountaineers, sailors, aviators, astronauts, divers, ultra-endurance athletes, soldiers, prisoners of war, shipwreck, air-crash and 9/11 survivors – attested that they had been joined, at a critical moment, by an unexplained supporter who lent them the power to overcome the most dire circumstances and survive. As John Geiger has put it, "All [the narrators] have escaped traumatic events only to tell strikingly similar stories of having experienced the close presence of a companion and helper, and even 'of a sort of mighty person'. This presence offered a sense of protection, relief, guidance, and hope, and left the person convinced he or she was not alone but that there was some other being at his or her side, when by any normal calculation there was none".[3]

II

In an earlier publication on the subject I maintained that we are dealing with a universal mental process that is not affected by differences in time and space.[4] It would seem that throughout history people have experienced similar traumas when confronted with mortal peril. These traumas gave rise to visions which in general outline, if not precise detail, were also similar. It is, therefore, possible to extrapolate from modern cases to historical ones, identifying SP visions in historical documents.

I here reproduce the essence of my argument and also respond to some queries that have arisen since its publication.

Both visions reported in modern times and those recorded in historical documents display unmistakably similar features. These features occur with such striking regularity that they render possible the demarcation of two types of vision, SP and non-SP. The distinction depends on four features which always occur in SP visions but are not all necessarily present in non-SP visions. (The group of non-SP visions is, of course, far larger and less homogeneous than the group of SP visions, and displays a striking variety of sub-divisions).

---

unusual environments. See Suedfeld/Mocellin (1987) and Suedfeld/Geiger (2008). For the identification of SP visions in Messianic Habad (Lubavitch), inspired by Geiger's work, see Bilu (2013).
3 Geiger (2009) 14.
4 Herman (2011).

Feature 1. SP visions usually occur in extreme, life-threatening situations. The visionaries are, as a rule fit, healthy and well-adjusted individuals who are often suffering from stress, fatigue and sleep deprivation and overwhelmed by the feeling that their life is in jeopardy (in other words, we are dealing with visions of non-pathological and non-hallucinogenic aetiology). I shall hereafter refer to this feature as "on the verge of death".

Feature 2. SP visions tend to be superimposed on, and to interfere with those extreme, life-threatening situations while the visionaries are in a conscious or waking state (they are not sleeping or unconscious); the visions are so vivid that they are often mistaken for reality. Non-SP visions usually occur in less dramatic circumstances and do not as a rule interfere with the course of events. I shall hereafter refer to this feature as "superimposed on, and interfering with real-life situations".

Feature 3. SP visions involve either figures, symbolic representations of figures, or vague, indeterminate, 'angelic presences' endowed with supernatural powers derived mostly from the visionary's cultural or religious heritage (i.e. Greek figures or symbolic representations derived from Greek traditions, Christian figures derived from Christian traditions, Jewish figures from Jewish traditions, and so on). I shall hereafter refer to this feature as "symbolic representations" or "angelic presences". This feature may also be present in non-SP visions, but rarely in conjunction with **Feature 4** below.

Feature 4. Stories of SP visions may vary in detail, but they all have an easily recognizable, stereotypic underlying scenario: an angelic presence provides guidance and comfort, urging the visionaries, explicitly or implicitly, to make a final, extraordinary effort. (Most non-SP visions have, at best, a strikingly different scenario). I shall hereafter refer to this feature as "provision of guidance and comfort".

To demonstrate the validity of this claim I present four typical accounts of SP events drawn from diverse time periods and cultures. I assume them to be representative of a much larger group of events sharing the same characteristics.

1. **The battle of Marathon, 490 B.C.:** "... in the battle which was fought at Marathon against the Medes", writes Plutarch (*Theseus* 35), "many soldiers believed they saw an apparition (*phasma*) of Theseus in arms, rushing on at the head of them against the barbarians."
2. **Siege of Antioch by a Christian Army (First Crusade), 1098:** "In addition", writes Peter Tudebode, regarding the Christian army trapped at Antioch "a vast army riding white horses and flying white banners rode from the mountains. Our forces were very bewildered by the sight of this army until they realized that it was Christ's aid .... The leaders of this

heavenly host were Saint George, the Blessed Demetrius and the Blessed Theodor".[5]

3. **Mons, the First World War, in the wake of the battle of Le Cateau (26th August, 1914).** "... by the night of the 27th we were all absolutely worn out with fatigue – both bodily and mental fatigue", commented 'a distinguished lieutenant-colonel', referring to an episode that allegedly occurred during the retreat of British survivors from Le Cateau.[6] "As we rode along I became conscious of the fact that, in the fields on both sides of the road along which we were marching, I could see a very large body of horsemen. These horsemen had the appearance of squadrons of cavalry, and they seemed to be riding across the fields and going in the same direction as we were going ... I did not say a word about it at first, but I watched them for about twenty minutes. The other two officers had stopped talking. At last one of them asked me if I saw anything in the fields. I then told what I had seen. The third officer then confessed that he too had been watching these horsemen for the past twenty minutes. So convinced were we that they were really cavalry that, at the next halt, one of the officers took a party of men out to reconnoitre, and found no one there ... The same phenomenon was seen by many men in our column ... it is an extraordinary thing that the same phenomenon should be witnessed by so many different people".[7] (For further accounts of this vision, see **Section IV**).

4. **Operation "Cast Lead" (January, 2009),** involving house-to-house fighting by Israeli forces in the Gaza strip. Of the versions available of what happened I cite from an interview given to *Channel Seven* by Private Avner Azulay, a (religious) Israeli soldier serving in a supply unit.[8] (For further accounts of this vision, see **Section IV**). "As soon as a group of soldiers attempted to enter a house in the Gaza Strip, we heard a woman's voice saying, 'Don't go into the house, there's death within!' While we were outside the house preparing to enter she repeated this sentence several times. We thought she was

---

5 Tudebodis, Petrus (1866).
6 The 70,000 strong British Expeditionary Force (BEF) landed in France on 14 August 1914. By the end of the year it was almost completely wiped out.
7 *Evening News*, 14th September, 1914.
8 /News/News.aspx/189655, my translation. Channel Seven is an Israeli media network identified with religious Zionism. In Israel's secular media the story of Mother Rachel was generally ignored, in the few cases in which it was referred to it was treated with incredulity and even contempt. No connection has ever been made with the story of the medical officer Avi Ohry, who, after being imprisoned and tortured by the Egyptians in the 1973 war, reported a full-blown SP experience (Ohry (2003)).

possibly a terrorist. This was no ordinary woman, she had no legs or arms, and her face was not visible. This was, in fact, no woman, but an image that emitted white light, ... and she was detached from the ground. Light came out of the image ... She only spoke to me. This was strange. My pals heard her voice but she only wanted to talk to me ... When *they* addressed her she didn't reply. When *I* addressed her she replied. They wanted to shoot her. I told them to wait for a moment while I asked her who she was. She said, in these words, 'I'm Mother Rachel.' As a religious person I know who Rachel was, and that this was no simple matter. I started trembling. It was more than scary."

As indicated in **Table 1** below, the details of all four accounts neatly match the SP paradigm described above.

III

Of course, it can be argued that such accounts are by their very nature extremely unreliable and it is dangerous to base any theories on them. For this reason we will submit each one to more rigorous scrutiny. As I suggested in my article,[9] it is

Table 1: The SP paradigm

Feature	Description of feature	How the feature is manifested in the four cases described above (Marathon, Crusaders, First World War, Operation "Cast Lead")
1	On the verge of death	The soldiers were suffering from sleep deprivation and fatigue. They felt their lives were in great danger.
2	Superimposed on, and interfering with real-life situations	The visions occurred while the soldiers were fighting enemies who apparently were about to prevail; they were not only awake, but highly alert.
3	Symbolic representations or 'angelic presences' drawn from the visionary's cultural heritage	Case 1: Ancient Athenians –> Theseus Case 2: Crusaders –> Christian saints Case 3: British soldiers –> French mediaeval cavalry/angels Case 4: Israeli soldiers –> Rachel the Matriarch
4	Stereotypical scenario: the provision of guidance and comfort	The visionaries in all four cases reported that they had experienced supernatural intervention by virtue of which their lives had been saved.

---

9 Herman (2011).

highly unlikely that the accounts were outright hoaxes, cynically invented with the intention of manipulating public opinion, spreading superstition and fantasies, and capitalizing on the access they afforded to the supernatural. (This does not mean that outright hoaxes do not exist: for example, records of the First World War are replete with 'miracles' showing clear signs of fabrication).[10] The underlying similarity of scenarios, although considerably removed in time and place, argues against such a possibility. Nor it is conceivable that in drafting their stories the visionaries were familiar with the SP paradigm. After all, the SP phenomenon has only recently been identified in scientific literature, and has not filtered down to the general public.[11] Given their unpreparedness for the dire conditions in which they suddenly found themselves, it is also unlikely that the visionaries put together improvised accounts modelled on actual events stored in their minds (that, for example, the Christian besiegers of Antioch drew on the example of Marathon, or that the Israeli soldiers fighting in Gaza were inspired by the Angels of Mons). Unless we believe in miracles, we must conclude that in all four cases the soldiers experienced genuine SP visions, perceiving a virtual reality created by their brain which did not exist in the physical sense. (It is worth drawing attention to a line in the report of the anonymous, 'distinguished lieutenant-colonel': "one of the officers [during the retreat from Mons] took a party of men out to reconnoitre, and found no [French cavalry] there"). To conclude: we are dealing with psychic events triggered by harsh external circumstances; hence the underlying similarities in the accounts.

This inference has been challenged. It has been argued that SP visions are extremely private events. Consequently, if the same vision is reported to have been seen by many, we should suspect a conspiracy and/or fabrication. Put another way, the fact that SP visions are often said to have been shared by many should cast doubt on the veracity of their occurrence.

Indeed, cases abound in which the same vision was supposedly shared by several people. This is what happened in all four cases listed above. The same vision was purportedly shared by entire army units ("many of the soldiers", "our forces", "by many men in our column" and "my pals", in examples 1–4 above),

---

10 See, for instance, Clarke (2004).
11 I have only been able to find the first encyclopaedic reference to SP in Blom (2010) 467. Sacks (2012) makes no mention of the SP. The most authoritative of the earlier books on apparitions (Green/McCreery (1975)) also fails to mention the SP. However, the phenomenon did crop up sporadically in the previous century. For example, see Critchley (1955); Parhon/Stefanescu and Procopiu/Constantinescu (1967); Suedfeld/Mocellin (1987).

and there are many more examples.[12] If reports of SP visions are not the product of colossal conspiracies, then how are we to account for this similarity?

Instead of brushing aside these testimonies, I propose that we accept them as givens. We should use them as the starting point of enquiry. Further research is needed to get to the bottom of the matter, but even at this stage we can suggest that what some, if not all of the participants experienced is a kind of non-verbalized, aniconic trauma, a blinding flash or jolt that passed through their brain, providing encouragement and comfort. Stories and images of what actually happened are only secondary. As soon as the life-threatening situation is past the participants interact, sharing and adjusting their accounts, and convincing themselves through auto-suggestion that they experienced the same vision. A measure of support for this conjecture may be derived from the fact that a) DiFrancesco only heard a voice and vaguely sensed some sort of presence (in other words, he provides us with an early version of his experience, one that was formed before his mind embellished it with imagery and scenario); b) the BEF soldiers reported seeing both mediaeval French cavalry and 'angels', in other words, they agreed that they had experienced something extraordinary but were divided over exactly what they had experienced (see **Section IV**); c) in the Cast Lead example, which is chronologically closest to us and relatively well documented, several versions of the story exist, some diverging considerably from what is assumed to be the 'original', first-hand version (see **Section IV**). In sum, the fact that visions are often reported to have been shared by many should not undermine our belief in the reality of their occurrence.

We are now in a position to trace the causal sequence of occurrences leading up to an SP vision. (a) Harsh, life threatening conditions, combined with fatigue and deprivation reduce the subject to a state of extreme distress; (b) This state stimulates the left temporo-parietal junction of the brain, triggering the image of an indeterminate "shadow person" (remarkably, this shadow person can be clinically reproduced during surgery);[13] (c) The brain processes this vision in ways still unknown to us, adding cultural colouring, adapting to the specific situation, and creating an imaginary episode whose gist is benign intervention on behalf of the subject.

I further argued in my article[14] that, having survived the life-threatening situation, the subject/s (d) describe/s the psychic event as an epiphany or vision, conveying his/her/their conviction that it was "real", and then (e) these reports

---

12 At least five further cases are cited in Herman (2011). To those we could add the case of the Emperor Constantine, described in **section V** below.
13 Herman (2011) 150–51.
14 Herman (2011).

are taken up and amplified by partisan believers, interest groups or (religious) establishments, through skilled manipulation of public opinion. It is these last two points that I now propose to discuss.

IV

The documentation of historical SP events as it has come down to us is rather uneven. (By 'historical' I am referring to cases in which it is no longer possible to obtain information by interviewing living visionaries). We can imagine an entire spectrum of accounts compressed into one and placed, as it were, on the same plane, starting with what might be called 'pure' accounts, those closest to firsthand testimony (as related by the visionary himself/herself right after the event), through mildly embellished ones (as they appear after being told and re-told by those who heard the story from the primary source and are now involved in rumour-mongering), to highly embellished, embroidered and amplified accounts that are taken up and processed by partisan believers, interest groups or, most likely, the religious establishment.

It would be interesting to ascertain how the items of evidence located at different points along that spectrum are interrelated. With that aim in mind I propose to review four cases, three of which we are already familiar with, and one that came to my attention as recently as 2012, during a visit to Portugal.

1. **The apparitions seen during the battle of Marathon (490 B.C.).** In addition to the epiphany described by Plutarch (p. 97), two further epiphanies are reported to have occurred during the battle of Marathon. Herodotus claims to have heard a second, or perhaps even third-hand report of Epizelos' mishap (he lost his sight in the battle) and his vision: "a tall hoplite ... encountered him, whose beard spread all over the shield; this apparition passed Epizelos by, but slew his neighbour in the line" (Hdt. 6.117).[15] The Marathonians, according to Pausanias, "say too that there chanced to be present in the battle a man of rustic appearance and dress. Having slaughtered many of the foreigners with a plough he was seen no more after the engagement. When the Athenians made enquiries at the oracle the god merely ordered them to

---

15 It might be argued that Epizelos' story does not fit into the SP paradigm, which presupposes a benign intervention securing the subject's survival. On closer examination it appears, however, that the story does obey the logic of SP scenarios, integrating as it does the fictitious version of Epizelos' survival with the unfortunate, factual end-result of losing his eyesight.

honour Echetlaios (*He of the Plough-handle*) as a hero" (Paus. 1.32.5).[16] It so happens that the visions of all three heroes (i.e. Theseus, Epizelos and Echetlaios) were depicted in paintings in the *Stoa Poikile* (Aelian *V.H.* 7.38, Paus. 1.15.3 and 1.32.5, respectively), built three to four decades after the battle. These paintings may clearly be regarded as 'processed' versions of visions that the democratic establishment took up and embellished, with a view to spreading and reasserting its growing reputation. As we shall see, SP events provide linkage to the supernatural that few power systems in history can afford to overlook.

If we were to drive home these items of evidence pertaining to the battle of Marathon, the details of the visions would coalesce into two points. First, all the soldiers presumably experienced the same SP event, some interpreting it as the appearance of Epizelos, and others as appearance of Theseus or Echetlos. Second, even if the literary sources had been lost and only the "processed", painted versions of the three incidents had survived (which is not the case: the paintings on the Stoa Poikile have been lost), we would be able to recognise an SP event at the onset of the chain of events leading up to the paintings.

2. **The 'angels' that appeared to British soldiers at Mons (August 1914).** There is another account of the visions allegedly experienced by surviving members of the battles of Mons and Le Cateau between 23rd and 26th August, 1914 (cf. p. 98). This account was published a year after the putative occurrence of the event itself, in August 1915.[17] It was supposedly related by an anonymous 'lance corporal' recuperating in a hospital near Southampton to author Harold Begbie, who was interviewing him for a book. "I could see quite plainly in mid-air a strange light which seemed to be quite distinctly outlined ... I could see quite distinctly three shapes, one in the centre having what looked like outspread wings, the other two were not so large, but were quite plainly distinct from the centre one. They appeared to have a long, loose-hanging garment of a golden tint, and they were above the German line facing us. All the men with me saw them, and other men came up from other groups who also told us that they had seen the same thing ...". When Begbie asked what effect the vision had on the men, the corporal supposedly answered, "... we didn't know what to make of it. And there we all were, looking up at those three figures, saying nothing, just wondering, when one of the chaps called out, 'God's with us!' – and that kind of loosened us.

---

16 *Echetle* in Greek means plough-handle, the verb *echetleuein* signifying "to plough".
17 *Daily Mail*, 18 August, 1915. The story was incorporated in Begbie (1915) 28–30.

Then when we were falling in for the march, the captain said to us, 'Well, men, we can cheer up now; we've got Something with us.' As I tell you, we marched thirty-two miles that night, and the Germans didn't fire either rifle or cannon the whole way".

Despite the crude signs that could indicate fabrication (omitting the names of the sources, belated publication, the (deliberate?) blurring or playing down of the chronological and topological framework), I would classify both accounts (this one and the one on p. 4 above, according to which the soldiers saw a phantom cavalry) as genuine SP events. This is because both accounts display the four features of the SP paradigm outlined earlier. We are seeing versions of genuine SP events[18] that are slightly embellished but not wholly invented or processed to the point where they are unrecognizable, unlike the versions presented by horror-fiction writer Arthur Machen (mixing fiction with reality, Machen wrote that the British troops at Mons were aided by ghostly bowmen from Agincourt),[19] by spiritualist nurse Phyllis Campbell (claiming a superior understanding of the issue by having talked at length with survivors, Campbell published angel stories radically different from the one cited here),[20] or by Reverend Alexander Boddy (who maintained that supernatural angels *really* intervened on behalf of the British forces).[21] In the event that only the 'processed' versions of Campbell and Boddy had survived and the soldiers' accounts had perished, it would have been difficult to identify an SP event at the beginning of the sequence of events leading up to its publication.

3. **The apparition of Rachel the Matriarch according to Israeli soldiers fighting in the Gaza strip.** Here is another account of the vision that Israeli soldiers fighting in the Gaza strip allegedly experienced in January 2009. This version was retold by Rabbi Ovadia Yosef, presumably with a view to bringing it in line with the ideology of the *Shas* party which he headed.[22] I have italicized phrases which are strikingly inconsistent with Azulay's report. "The soldiers arrived

---

[18] The general explanation of the Angel of Mons visions is that they were the product of imagination and hallucination, of popular beliefs intensified by the rumours and fears that pervaded British society during the decade preceding the outbreak of the First World War (Clarke (2002)). Prior to the publication of Geiger (2009), the possibility that they were triggered by SP visions has never been considered.
[19] Machen (1915).
[20] Campbell (1915).
[21] Boddy (1915). The last three examples are cited from Clarke (2004).
[22] http://www.youtube.com/watch?annotation_id=annotation_502569&feature=iv&src_vid=uQ1zHH2cmoO&v=mxDbH-JVwIw. *Shas* is an ultra-Orthodox Israeli political party founded

at a house and wanted to get in. There were *three armed terrorists* waiting for them. And then *a beautiful young woman*[23] appeared and warned: *Don't enter the house, there are terrorists there,*[24] *take care.* – "Who are you?" – "What do you care who I am," said she, and whispered – "Rachel." The rabbi continued to describe how *the soldiers indeed found terrorists inside and killed them. The three were carrying guns, just as the woman said. Mother Rachel was called to the place, 'Go save your sons.'* Ah, praised be His name! God redeems and rescues, and sends angels to save the people of Israel.[25] How we should thank God … Had it not been for that – we would not be alive".

However processed, distorted and embellished this version may be, it nevertheless retains the gist of the original scenario of an SP event. Put another way, for our purposes it is immaterial whether Azulay's or Rabbi Yosef's is the 'correct' version. In both cases we can safely posit an SP event as the basis of the stories. (I have tried to contact Avner Azulay to inquire further about his experience, only to be told that he required rabbinic permission to be interviewed. Rabbinic permission was not available.)

4. **The Nazaré miracle.** In this case we have a straightforward account of an SP event whose memory was preserved, cherished and sanctified by a religious establishment set up specifically for that purpose. The account is presumably the one disseminated by the Catholic Church right after the event itself, apparently in the 12th century. Here it is, quoted verbatim from the Wikipedia article on the legend of Nazaré: "On the early morning of September 14, 1182, Dom Fuas Roupinho of Porto de Mós, was out hunting in his domain, near the coast, when he saw a deer which he immediately began chasing. All of a sudden a heavy fog rose up from the sea. The deer ran towards the top of a cliff and Dom Fuas in the midst of the fog realized he was on the edge of the cliff. He prayed out loud *Our Lady, Help Me*. All of a sudden the lady appeared to him, and the horse stopped miraculously at the end of a rocky

---

by Rabbi Ovadia Yosef in 1984. The primary aim of the party is to represent the interests of Orthodox Sephardic and Mizrahi (Oriental) Jews.

23 According to other versions circulating on the internet the person Azulay encountered was "a good-looking, elderly woman", or, alternatively, "an Arab woman".

24 According to other versions what she said was "get out of that house because it's booby-trapped". The houses, according to those versions, indeed exploded in due course.

25 Another clip, which circulated on the internet for a while in the name of Rabbi Yosef but was subsequently removed, listed the miraculous occurrences which saved the people of Israel since earliest times, starting with the Parting of the Red Sea. The manifestation of Rachel the Matriarch to Azulay figures as yet another item on that list. A rival rabbi has been overheard to reproach Rabbi Ovadia with the words: 'only a sucker would believe that!'.

point thus saving Don Roupinho from certain death. Dom Fuas dismounted and went down to the grotto to pray and give thanks for the miracle. Then he ordered his companions to fetch masons in order to build a small chapel over the grotto so that the miraculous image could be easily venerated by all and as a memorial to the miracle that saved him. Then before walling up the grotto the masons destroyed the existing altar where amongst the stones they found an ivory chest containing some reliques and an old parchment describing the story of the little wooden statue, one palm high, of Our Lady seated breastfeeding baby Jesus seated on her left leg. According to the parchment the statue must have been venerated since the beginning of Christianity in Nazareth, in Palestine ...".[26]

This story, not unlike the one of Rachel the Matriarch, was taken up, monopolized and embellished by a religious establishment (the ivory chest and the old parchment are unmistakably embellishments) without, however, blurring or distorting the four distinguishing features of a classic SP event.

At this point we should note that from the believers' perspective (whether Greek, Christian or Jewish), SP events appear as acts of supernatural intervention, miracles attesting to the propitiousness of the transcendental order. Throughout history power brokers, interest groups and religious establishments have been only too happy to control and cultivate the memory of such events for their enormous propaganda value. SP events, as we have seen, are especially susceptible to interpretation as gateways to the transcendental, to the ultimate sources of human existence.

This feature is especially pronounced in the next example, the story of Constantine's conversion to Christianity.

V

The circumstances of this vision, reported by Eusebius of Caesarea, have been painstakingly scrutinized in two outstanding works by Peter Weiss and Timothy Barnes.[27] I am using Barnes' comments to reconstruct the incident which occurred, supposedly, on the eve of Constantine's battle against Maxentius, on October 28th,

---

[26] https://en.wikipedia.org/wiki/Legend_of_Nazar%C3%A9. I have been unable to find an official website of the shrine.
[27] Weiss (1993) and Barnes (2011). Both authors integrate sources other than Eusebius which need not be cited for the purposes of the present argument.

AD 312, without, however, sharing Barnes' scepticism concerning the mental processes involved in the conversion: "The internal psychological process which led to the 'conversion' of Constantine and his public embrace of the Christian religion", writes Barnes, "is not important to the historian because it is undiscoverable ...".[28]

If we place a passage from Eusebius' *Vita Constantini* within the context of the SP paradigm, we find that Constantine's vision displays all the characteristic features of an SP event (**Table 2**).

> "A most remarkable divine sign was revealed to the emperor (Constantine), which it would perhaps not be easy to accept if anyone else alleged it. However, the victorious emperor himself reported it to the author of this narrative many years later, when we were honoured with knowing him and being in his presence. In the middle of the day, when the daylight was already beginning to fade, he said that he saw in the sky with his own eyes a cross-shaped trophy formed from light above the sun with a picture attached which proclaimed: 'By this conquer' (τούτῳ νίκα). Amazement at the spectacle seized both him and the whole army which was following him on a march somewhere and witnessed the marvellous sight" (Eusebius, *Vita Constantini* I. 28).

On the basis of how Eusebius' story conforms with the SP paradigm, it is thus possible to identify the preliminary incident leading to Constantine's conversion to Christianity as an SP event.[29]

Table 2: The story from Eusebius' *Vita Constantini* from a SP perspective

Feature	Description of feature	How the features manifest themselves in Eusebius' *Vita Constantini*
1	On the verge of death	'*At a critical time*, when he [Constantine] was marching in haste to squash a coup by his father-in-law, *which threatened to end his imperial career and even his life*, ...' (Barnes 2011, p. 80, my italics)
2	Superimposed on, and interfering with real-life situations	*he and his army saw a solar halo* ... (Barnes 2011, p. 80, my italics)
3	Symbolic representations or 'angelic presences' drawn from the visionary's cultural heritage	which they interpreted as a sure sign of victory *under the protection of the sun-god Apollo*' (Barnes 2011, p. 80, my italics).
4	Stereotypical scenario: the provision of guidance and comfort	'he [Constantine] said that he saw in the sky with his own eyes a cross-shaped trophy formed from the light above the sun with a picture attached which proclaimed: "'*By this conquer*"' [Greek: τούτῳ νίκα; Latin: hoc signo victor eris]

---

28 Barnes (2011) 80.
29 It will be noted that his more widely quoted dream only occurred subsequently.

Nor is the underlying mental process indiscernible. Constantine presumably experienced what most people experience when facing death in perilous situations: a blinding flash or jolt that passes through their brain, providing comfort and encouragement and giving them the determination to carry on. As we have seen, people interpret this extraordinary experience as a supernatural intervention, investing it with imagery and a scenario derived from their own cultural or religious heritage. Constantine was no exception. He and his soldiers interpreted the experience as a divine sign, promising victory under the protection of the sun-God Apollo, whom Constantine worshipped. In other words, the vision was not the direct cause of Constantine's conversion to Christianity. It just paved the way.

Nevertheless, there was something remarkable about Constantine's vision. From our perspective it would appear that few SP visions in history have been amplified to such an extent and have generated such a multitude of first, second and third-hand 'processed' versions. Constantine's vision will surely rank as the most influential SP event in history.

VI

We are now in a position to summarise our findings. Generalized from hundreds of individual instances, the SP paradigm offers a convenient analytic tool for identifying SP visions in historical documents. In the first place, it allows us to differentiate SP from non-SP visions. Non-SP visions can hardly be accommodated within the SP paradigm. Take, for instance, the case of Fatima, one of the most influential visions that allegedly occurred in the last century. This is how the vision begins on the shrine's official site: "On the 13th of each month from May to October 1917, the Virgin Mary is said to have appeared to three shepherd children – Lúcia dos Santos (age 10) and her cousins Jacinta (age 7) and Francisco Marto (age 9) – in the fields outside the village of Aljustrel near Fatima. The children later said that her coming had been preceded by an 'angel of peace' who appeared in 1916. Lúcia described her vision of Mary as 'more brilliant than the sun, shedding rays of light clearer and stronger than a crystal glass filled with the most sparkling water and pierced by the burning rays of the sun.' According to Lúcia's account, Mary exhorted the children to do penance to save sinners. They wore tight cords around their waists to cause pain, abstained from drinking water on hot days, and other works of penance. Most important, she asked them to say the Rosary every day. She reiterated many times that devotion to the Rosary was the key to personal and world peace. Many young Portuguese men, including relatives of the visionaries, were then fighting in World War I".[30]

Needless to say, the young shepherds were not under the threat of death when the Virgin Marry appeared to them; nor did the Virgin Mary interfere with what they were doing at the time (herding the sheep); although the vision involved an angelic presence drawn from the young shepherds' Catholic heritage, this angelic presence offered no advice as how to survive, instead exhorting the children to do penance to save the sinners. Clearly, the apparition of the Virgin Mary to the young Portuguese shepherds lacked three out of the four identifying features of SP events.

Furthermore, the SP paradigm enables us to ascertain a category of facts that has by and large been overlooked in discussions of historical method. No agreement exists regarding how to define facts,[31] but there is general agreement on a minimal requirement that should be included in most definitions: for something to be a fact it should impinge on the observer from outside, and be independent of his/her consciousness. In that sense SP visions are no facts at all, since they impinge on the observer from inside and are totally dependent on her/his consciousness. It is mind-boggling that nevertheless, as we have seen, they do interfere with events that impinge on the observer from outside and are independent of his/her consciousness, more or less as if they were 'real'. The SP paradigm allows us to resolve this problem and identify a new category of facts. These facts are *not* virtual realities projected into an imagined space by terror-stricken minds (for instance, neither the phantom cavalry of Mons nor the ghost of Mother Rachel). They are hallucinogenic, chemical and electronic reactions that take place in the brain of the participants in response to harsh external conditions. The SP paradigm helps ascertain the authenticity of such reactions. It can thus be added to the arsenal of tools (such as the evaluation of evidence reliability, cross-examination of witnesses, and detection of biases and falsifications) that historians traditionally employ to ascertain factuality.

---

30 http://www.sacred-destinations.com/portugal/fatima-shrine-of-our-lady-of-fatima.
31 I draw here on Carr (1961) 7–30; Evans (1997) 75–102.

Alex Wardrop, Georgie Huntley and Silvie Kilgallon

7 Transforming Knowledge: Using Arts-based Activity to Explore Classics and Therapeutic Practice

> My purpose is to tell of bodies which have been transformed into shapes of a different kind ...
> – Ovid, Metamorphoses 1.1–2

Introduction

This chapter explores relationships between Classics, arts-based activity, and ideas drawn from art therapy. We take one event – a workshop, *hanging my heart*, held at a museum during an academic conference – to tease out how seemingly different (and potentially oppositional) bodies of knowledge and practice can be transformed by allowing them to touch, even for a moment.[1]

The first part of this chapter provides the background to the workshop, why we chose to concentrate on votive giving, and situates it in a wider community project. It also outlines some of the key themes within art therapy and how such thinking could be utilised by classicists. The second half engages in a discussion of the role that arts-based activity can have in (re)shaping academic methods, practices, and discourse.

For the purpose of inclusivity and interdisciplinarity, we assume no prior knowledge of therapeutic arts-practice, art-based research, or the concept of ancient votive giving, thus in this first section we will also briefly explain these ideas. We then give a short explanation of who MakingLearning (the group who ran the workshop) are, and what the workshop itself entailed, including the practical details of how we prepared for and facilitated it, and, based on our own observations and the feedback we received, the potential benefits for those who participated in it.

---

[1] Thank you beyond words to Dr Sam Thomas without whom this work could never have happened. You are always in our hearts and truly missed. Dr Jen Grove's research and public engagement practice significantly shaped this workshop and chapter, thank you. We would like to thank all of the participants of the workshop and the staff at M Museum, Leuven, in particular Lore, for your support. Last but not least, to Dr Jeroen Lauwers, for taking a risk on us.

Alex Wardrop, Centre for Excellence in Learning, Bournemouth University
Georgie Huntley, University of South Wales
Silvie Kilgallon, University of Bristol

https://doi.org/10.1515/9783110482201-008

After setting the scene, we move to a broader outline of the benefits that arts-based techniques, and a sensibility drawn from the therapeutic arts, can have for academic practice. We argue that the workshop provided a catalyst to transform understandings of ancient votive giving because participants had the opportunity to imbue an object with feeling through the act of making. Engaging in this making process provided some insight into the complex and fleeting emotional and material textures of the ancient practices and artefacts, enhancing understanding in the field. This heightened emotional connection with the material of study (whether texts, ideas, or material culture), we suggest, can transform academic discourse by moving it away from competitive, individualistic and hierarchical models towards a more collaborative, communal sensibility in which cohesion can exist without consensus.

Background

Established in Bristol, UK, during 2013, MakingLearning is a collective of people who have an interest in education, arts-based learning, and community action. Our aim is to explore practice-based ways of learning that make it more inclusive and less intimidating, and provide new insights into how a topic can be taught, understood, and felt. It emerged from a course funded by the UK's Arts and Humanities Research Council which trained Classics and Ancient History doctoral students in public engagement.[2] Since 2013 we have facilitated a number of different activities that include making collaborative patchwork poems, playing around with wool and the words of Nietzsche, reading Aeschylus with dance movement therapy, and making webs for International Women's Day. Each of these sessions paid more attention to learning and art processes than to any outcome. They were not about making beautiful objects but exploring ideas, learning techniques, sharing knowledge and stories, and playing.

The *hanging my heart* workshop fits within this pedagogical sensibility which "brings together academic theory, craft practice, and community engagement to create caring and collaborative learning environments which prioritise creativity and empowerment".[3] We wanted to interrogate how techniques of making could

---

[2] With thanks to Professor Fiona Macintosh and Naomi Setchell at the University of Oxford's Archive of Performances of Greek and Roman Drama for developing this pioneering training programme in the discipline of Classics. See http://www.apgrd.ox.ac.uk/about-us/cagr-phase-2/communicating-ancient-greece-and-rome-cagr

[3] Thomas/Wardrop (2013) "About Us" [blogpost] https://makinglearning.wordpress.com/about-us/

transform understandings of bodies, feelings, pasts, environments, and futures. To do this we re-worked the practice of votive giving in a creative, secular context.

Votive Giving

A votive is a physical object, often left at a specific site or sanctuary, in order to petition a deity for help, health, good fortune, or to give thanks or remembrance. These objects can be made of any material and range from mass-produced pieces to what some might refer to as "found objects" – sticks, stones, bones from cattle, and so forth.[4] Votives, in the present day as much as in antiquity, can also take the form of miniature sculptures of human bodies, or of specific parts of the body relating to the needs and wants of the petitioner.[5] A votive offering, therefore, is an object that represents an act, or attempted act, of communication between a mortal and a divine being. It is the material evidence of an emotive process which draws on the hopes, fears, and feelings of the petitioner.

There have been a number of recent projects that have sought to re-think ancient practices of votive giving, both for academic inquiry and in the public imagination. In 2013 the University of Nottingham and Nottingham Castle Museum ran the *Nemi to Nottingham* project, which saw academics using digital technologies (such as 3D printing) to bring the Sanctuary of Diana at Nemi, and the votive objects discovered there, to a new audience.[6] *The Votives Project* is a blog acting as a network and sharing tool for those interested in votives from any culture or historical period.[7] Such work has aided the progress of traditional academic activity on the topic, and enabled the exploration of votives as a useful tool for artists, educators, and the public.

Part of the work done by *The Votives Project* included the web-based Speculum Dianae resource.[8] Users can build their own virtual temple and send "virtual votives" – images of votives recovered from Nemi – to friends and family by email. Jessica Hughes notes that the act of emailing a photograph of a votive "also potentially restores to the votive some of its empathic, emotional and transactional qualities – qualities that have often been side-lined in academic and antiquar-

---

[4] For an archive of some contemporary votive offerings see the *Archivo de Exvotos* collection, http://archivoexvotos.revista-sanssoleil.com.
[5] For more information about ancient votive practices see Hughes (2008) and Osborne (2004).
[6] See https://nemitonottingham.wordpress.com
[7] See https://thevotivesproject.wordpress.com
[8] See www.speculum-dianae.nottingham.ac.uk

ian discussions".⁹ It also leads to questions around how such technology and techniques could best be utilised for academic purposes. The user of the website enacts votive practice in a quintessentially modern way. It is unique to each site user and different in cultural, theological, and practical ways from ancient practices of votive giving. Nonetheless, it provides the user with an emotional perspective of the process.

The *hanging my heart* workshop is informed by these projects, as we wondered how focusing on part of the process – the actual construction of the votive object – might reveal ways of working with votives that balanced academic understanding and emotional engagement. We were keen to reflect on how the process of making an object enabled a glimpse at the fleeting traces of feeling found in votive hoards excavated in ancient sites and those seen in churches, cemeteries, and roadsides.

Art for Wellbeing

This concern for the emotions led us to think about connections between the workshops we were running and art therapy. It is important to note, however, that the MakingLearning activities cannot be understood as art therapy proper. This is a reserved for a practice with a stringent professional framework and led by a qualified practitioner. However, the workshops we designed are all influenced by the insights and practices drawn from art (psycho)therapy[10] and are rooted in a commitment to the utility of using art-based techniques to explore emotional and personal wellbeing.

When formulating a picture of the history of art therapy Adrian Hill is often cited as an early pioneer.[11] Incarcerated in hospital with tuberculosis, he started to draw and through these drawings he felt a "mental emancipation" from his current illness. Based on his own experience he encouraged other patients to paint and express what they were feeling through their imagery.[12] In 1946, the artist

---

9 Hughes (2013) [blogpost] from https://nemitonottingham.wordpress.com/2013/09/10/dissecting-the-past-writing-the-biography-of-an-anatomical-votive

10 Throughout this chapter we have chosen to use the term 'art therapy' rather than 'psychotherapy', as we felt the former was likely to be more familiar to those outside the field. If there is a difference between the two it is that 'psychotherapy' usually implies a specific type of training on the part of the practitioner.

11 Hill (1945). See also Hogan (2001).

12 See Thompson (1989) for further detail about Hill and his practice.

Edward Adamson opened a studio at Netherne, a long-stay psychiatric hospital. He adopted an approach with his patients that was influenced by humanism and the psychology of Jung and he let them paint, draw, or make what they wanted, rather than teaching them in a traditional style. Adamson thought that artistic process alleviated trauma and stress in his patients. His influence helped initiate the *British Association of Art Therapy* and the formal training process in 1969.[13]

The work of an art therapist is to engage the patient with their own emotional and psychological past.[14] We know from the work of people such as Judith Lewis Herman that sharing traumatic experiences and feelings can help recreate a more meaningful world and provide solace to survivors of trauma.[15] For this to happen, a sense of comfort and safety must be formed in the therapeutic context so that the person undergoing the therapy feels able to disclose anything. Thus, creating a safe space for dialogue – whether verbal or visual – is a key element to art therapy.

Beyond establishing a safe space in which dialogue can occur, art therapy moves the participant into creative making that aims to enable the individual to generate and express thoughts and feelings which may not be immediately present.[16] In her chapter on art and psychoanalysis, Caroline Case further expands this, suggesting that, "Art Psychotherapy is a spontaneous expression which opens up unconscious material to the therapist".[17] In a therapy context, then, art-making can support the uncovering of hidden ideas, thoughts, and memories that are buried under many layers of defences adopted to enable us to survive. In the words of a long-term resident in a psychiatric hospital, "how strange the unconscious flow is. Painting can express it. Painting is there, even if only to tinker away an afternoon in a mental hospital. Painting is real".[18] Working with art materials, skills, and techniques can provide a release for different forms of knowledge, meanings, feelings, and realities.

Art-making in an art therapy context aims to connect participants to their unconscious thought processes and to past events or feelings. One way to make such temporal connections is through play. Playful methods of art-making can arouse kinaesthetic and sensory sensations and through this interaction, connect buried or disjointed concepts and ideas, and generate new feelings and new perspectives on old feelings. Influenced by the pioneering work of psychologist

---

13 For a full history of art therapy, see Hogan (2001). Chapter seven provides a detailed account of the use of art at Netherne and at the Maudsley.
14 Case (1992) 59.
15 Herman (1992) 70.
16 Diggs (2015) 2.
17 Case (1992) 71.
18 Author unknown, "A comment on art therapy by a long-term resident in a psychiatric hospital" from Dalley (ed) (2009) v.

Donald Winnicott, art therapists see play as key to facilitating growth, supporting group cohesion, exploring relationships between one's inner and external realities, and between one's past and present.[19] Play facilitates cohesion and connection in a way that can keep alive different and divergent positions. Art therapy can, therefore, provide techniques and frameworks for making temporal connections that do not elide the difference between past and current experiences, or internal and external realities. That art therapy has the ability to make playful connections, particularly temporal connections between past and present, provides an interesting point of contact with the study of Classics – both disciplines play with relationships between past and present.

Noah Hass-Cohen and Richard Carr make art therapy's ability to create connections clearer by identifying how it "can provide relief by pairing fear-arousing emotions with positive, new sensory experiences".[20] With this in mind, art therapy could be seen as that which transforms the absent (the repressed or hard to voice) into something present (an artwork).

This understanding, combined with Case's explanation of how participants formulate their past *with* their present, allows one to draw further similarities between personal therapeutic inquiry and historical exploration. The historian goes in search of evidence, gaining clues about how the ancients expressed themselves that may in some way shape and influence contemporary modes of being. The close association between archaeological, mythological, and historical forms of knowing and the practice, and therapeutic psychoanalysis are well documented and this volume will add to that fertile relationship.[21] The *hanging my heart* workshop sits within this collaborative dialogue by suggesting other ways for creative, and playful, interaction between therapists and classicists.

Hanging my heart and the Leuven workshop

Having provided some context about art therapy and votive giving, we will outline what the *hanging my heart* workshop is. Simply put, it is a workshop in which we invite participants to use basic but effective art and craft techniques to create objects *as* votive offerings representing their personal feelings, concerns or worries. We did not want to re-create the ancient experience of votive giving.

---

19 Case/Dalley (1992) 87.
20 Hass-Cohen/Carr (2008) 33.
21 See, for example, Zajko/O'Gorman (eds) (2013).

Instead, we wanted to use the ancient votive practice – the making and giving of an object as a spiritual experience – as a model for a care-rooted workshop in which the emotional wellbeing and creativity of participants was a primary concern. The transformation of a mundane object into something sacred through the act of giving it up to the gods is reflected in how we were taking disposable, everyday objects and making them otherwise.

After running this workshop several times, during which we tried various materials for making the votives, we reached the conclusion that foil, such as that from disposable baking trays, was the best medium.[22] It was less mess; required no drying period; could be decorated using easily understood, basic embossing techniques; and it was cheap. Essentially, all that was needed for the workshop was the foil itself and some pens or pencils to serve as embossing tools.

The title of the workshop evokes the idea of hanging up your feelings – your heart – in such a way to recognise that some feelings and experiences hang on tighter than others. In this workshop we wanted to create a space where the knowledge of those feelings could become practiced in different ways and provide different connections with ancient material. At the same time, in basing the workshop on the exploration of ancient practices, a space was created which made the material culture and intellectual legacies of antiquity accessible to a broad public audience, who may have had little or no knowledge of votives or the discipline.

In the context of the academic conference at Leuven we found that the act of making an object in a playful and communal setting opened up understandings of antiquity to more personal and emotional connections. Perhaps more important than this, it served to create cohesion among a diverse group of academics in such a way that honoured in participants' personal and disciplinary knowledges and experiences.

In the space at the museum we laid out the tables so that people could sit together and share friendly dialogue. On the tables were images of ancient votive objects, ancient sacred sites, and quotes relating to the theme of votive giving. These enabled participants to situate their making, their sharing of feelings and personal stories, within a dialogue with the material of antiquity.

In terms of what was made, there was great variety, ranging from constructions drawn from ancient myth to body parts, in particular eyes.

The focus on eyes expressed a tension that came to the surface in the group discussion at the close of the session; an anxiety of being watched by colleagues.

---

[22] We have held the workshop at an arts festival in Oxfordshire, a local arts trail and at separate locations around Bristol. At each event, the objects made focused on site-specific concerns (ranging from lack of affordable housing to ear plugs).

Conferences are places that have a highly structured visual protocol – people must be seen, and they must be seen right. The references to eyes in our votive objects could attest to the prevalence of a performance anxiety within academic conferences. Some of this anxiety was specific to the interdisciplinary nature of the Leuven conference, with classicists being keenly aware that there were psychoanalysts in the room. As facilitators we stressed that the workshop was not an analytic session and that no-one must negatively judge anyone's discussions or creativity.

One particular votive elaborates these anxieties in a personal way. Cut out of the thin metal is a figure with a noose-like scarf. Embossed on its belly are the words, "THE PERFECT CANDIDATE". The piece has the words "Job Anxiety" written on its accompanying label.

In addition to such palpable embodiments of academic anxiety are expressions of everyday hopes, while others conveyed personal stories.

There were also exuberant constructions, elaborating a strong sense of emotional feeling, and those that may be touching upon the collaborative sentiment of the conference.

Reflections from the Workshop

From examining the pieces made and listening to the discussions of the participants, we see the workshop presenting an opportunity for some to talk through the pressures and insecurities felt within the academic environment. By encouraging creativity, play, and the expression of everyday emotions, the workshop had the potential to challenge the conventional status-quo of traditional academia, allowing participants to express themselves differently.

As the workshop was held on the opening night of the conference it was important that the session created a sense of cohesion for the participants, particularly given the whole event was framed as "a dialogue across disciplines". Indeed, one participant said that the workshop "set the tone" of the conference by creating an atmosphere within which people felt comfortable sharing their experiences and their feelings – in a way that was not being judged, or disciplined. The act of making provided the participants with an opportunity to converse about issues sometimes outside the academic domain and this could be seen in some of the pieces made. The idea of sharing stories, playing, and engaging in humour whilst sitting side-by-side contrasts with dominant modes of conference dynamics in which an individual presents on stage whilst others listen and critique through verbal discussion.

After the session we reflected on how the objects made each carried multiple layers of meaning and feeling and were intimately tied to the place, and processes, that made them. Any meaning of the objects was fleeting. This offers an interesting hermeneutic frame for understanding ancient votives. The "self evidence" (to borrow from Jessica Hughes) that votive artefacts provide to the classicist, archaeologist, or historian are layered with traces of personal feeling which was not meant to survive in layers of soil or historical memory.[23] Studying ancient votives involves reading the meaning of those objects made by fleeting, complex, emotional traces which are no longer present. By drawing on insights from art therapy, what workshops like *hanging my heart* can offer is a way of making new emotional connections, however complex and fleeting they may be, and honouring the feelings that are lost.

The fleeting texture of meaning possessed by votive objects, and the objects created during our workshop, is connected to the giving (up) of the object. Something becomes a votive because it is given to, and for, the gods; the giving makes the object a votive. In *hanging my heart*, however, the giving (the hanging of the objects on our makeshift shrine) was a rather marginal aspect. These objects were not being crafted with the intent to give them to loved ones, or to dedicate to gods, or even, necessarily, to keep for one's self (though some did take their pieces away with them). It was the making itself and not the idea of giving to a specific, valued person or entity that invested the objects with emotional potential. However, the knowledge that the object would essentially be lost to the maker once the session was over may have helped influence what people made during the session. The act of giving was not central to the workshop, but the knowledge that the object would be given up still influenced the process of making. The disposable nature of the materials, too, almost demanded the disposability of the objects; they could easily be left behind and forgotten.

The making of the object took such a priority in the workshop that any outcome to *hanging my heart* can be found in the act of collective making rather than in the production of an individual object. The artwork of *hanging my heart* was the process of collective making, not the end result. Each participant was involved in the co-creation of that art/spirit/knowledge work. Acknowledging this shapes pertinent questions about the important role of the collective in votive giving, as well as re-affirming the central importance of a fleeting, emotional, transaction to the meaning of the objects. The pieces made in Leuven were objects of personal feeling in a public context; the workshop created a space for that divide to be explored, to be felt. This collective making that acknowledges deeply personal emotions and hopes or fears is what connects the votives that

---

23 Hughes (2015) [blogpost] http://blog.wellcomecollection.org/2015/06/09/self-evidence/

were made in Leuven to those found in ancient sites and those still bequeathed in places of emotional and spiritual significance.

Working with arts-based techniques and drawing on skills from a therapeutic art context allowed participants to encounter materials and ideas from antiquity in ways that they may not have before. In doing so, insights into how meanings are constructed and re-constructed through fleeting feelings were elucidated. Furthermore, the *hanging my heart* workshop created a sense of cohesion without consensus which gave in the conference an atmosphere of belonging, respectful to participants' personal and disciplinary differences.

The process of collective making created the opportunity to think through a reparative and playful understanding of the relationship to the past that is informed by therapeutic arts practice. In the end, making objects of feeling allowed psychologists and classicists alike to remember that they both work in subjects of feeling.

Arts-based Activity and Academic Practice

We now highlight the benefits that art-based approaches can have for academic practice. We argue that they offer an approach which focuses on processes rather than any singular outcome, and that this creates the opportunity to critically engage with orthodox modes of academic practice and ask pertinent questions about who, or what, is excluded when we, as academics, do our work.

The benefit of arts-based knowledge and techniques have for re-conceiving practice have been recognised by socially engaged, qualitative researchers as a key method of academic inquiry.[24] Researchers like Pranee Liamputtong and Jean Rumbold see artistic expression as a way of "knowing differently" which can elaborate less dominant ways of understanding the world.[25] Using artistic making and expression crumples epistemological textures, transforming the purpose and goal of research, and shifts focus away from conclusions, as such, to the emergence of multiple questions for the researcher/artist and participant/reader.

That art-based activity has the ability to transform academic practice in this way lies in the particularity of making. Susan Finley has noted how making art of, or with, one's research enables a glimpse at the reciprocity at the heart of any

---

[24] See, for example, Denzin/Lincoln (eds) (2000); Knowles/Cole (eds) (2008); Reason/Bradbury (eds) (2006); Richardson (2000).

[25] This phrase is taken from the title of the collection edited by Liamputtong and Rumbold which explores collaborative and artistic research methods (2008).

research question or activity.[26] Indeed, Richard Sennett's exploration of "craftsmanship" elaborates how crafting and thinking operate in tandem precisely because they are concerned with our capacity to change things.[27] Recognising thinking in terms of a certain quality for metamorphosis reorients it as an already participatory and reciprocal process because you are working *with* materials, tools, traces, and techniques beyond your own head, and hands. It reminds us that conclusions can be changed, ideas revised, and that these re-visions happen because of the participation – the collaboration – of others. In the words of Amanda Ravetz, Alice Kettle and Helen Felcey, (re)aligning thinking with crafting is to see it as "societal" because you are working *with* something – whether that is fabric, wood, clay, or disposable baking trays.[28]

Finley and Knowles elaborate the material understanding of research by recognising that the very act of doing it transforms the researcher into an artisan, "building up, layer upon layer, detailed knowledge ... seeking the kind of empirical connection that allows the researcher to interpret meaning in the subtle word, phrase, or gesture of those around her".[29] Situating making at the heart of the research *turns* it into a practice attuned to subtleties, silences, and the silenced.

The capacity that craft and arts working has to ask meaningful questions and convey subtler/silenced meanings is borne out by Helen Ball's work with people living with post-traumatic stress disorder, whereby quilting enabled an "intense knowing" which acknowledged "the depth and intensity/complexity of experience".[30] Further, Elsa Barkley Brown saw the structure of quilting as that which allowed her to build a course on African-American women which did not invalidate their experiences in academic assumptions that are so deeply rooted in the racism that silenced them in the first place.[31] Barkley Brown used quilting as the way for all her students to "learn to center in another experience, validate it, and judge it by its own standards without need of comparison or need to adopt that framework as their own".[32] Structuring a course with the "polyrhythmic, 'nonsymmetrical,' nonlinear structure" of African-American women's strip quilts

---

26 Finley (2003).
27 Sennett (2008) 119ff. For a fuller understanding of the word craft – its constellations and contestations – see Adamson (2007).
28 Ravetz *et al.* (2013) 3.
29 Finley/Knowles (1995) 124.
30 Ball (2002) 18ff. For the use of quilting to espouse different emotional and political epistemologies Lewis and Fraser (1996) elaboration of the NAMES Project AIDS memorial quilt. For another elaboration of a quilting as a metaphor for scientific inquiry, see Flannery (2001).
31 Barkley Brown (1989).
32 Barkley Brown (1989) 922.

created a different pedagogical practice "in which individual and community are not competing entities" that validated the experiences of African-American women, empowered the students and the teacher, and "challenged the most basic notions of the academy".[33] In short, making succeeded where mainstream academic approaches could not.

In self-consciously using the materials, structures, or techniques drawn from arts practice in an academic setting, researchers like Barkley Brown and Ball bring into the academy fields of knowledge that have been relegated beyond the walls of the university. Working with craft thus becomes not just a method of academic inquiry but also a political critique about what, and who, counts as knowledge/knowledgeable within the contemporary university.

One of the ways that working with art and craft materials and techniques serves to trouble the boundaries of disciplinary or institutional knowledge is by its collaborative nature.[34] Arts-based research can be characterised as the practical participatory understanding gained through art and craft making reoriented as, and with, epistemological value. It seeks to use "the actual making of artistic expressions ... as a primary way of understanding and examining the experience by both researchers" and the participants involved.[35] By working with materials that one can transform and opening one's method to/as a messy process-driven approach where outcomes are not so neat, the role of the researcher is called into question. Indeed, using art and craft techniques and materials in an academic context can re-orient subject-forming strategies characteristic of communal craft-production – this can include storytelling, sharing skills, memories, and knowledge, and critiquing dominant systems in a playful, sometimes, ephemeral way.[36] Barkley Brown wrote of her desire to empower her students precisely by *disempowering* her position as teacher.[37] That her pedagogical approach was rooted in a craft-based structure is suggestive of how working with craft can disrupt familiar academic practice and ask what, and who, is excluded from that "familiarity".

Making a learning environment which de-centres the role of the academic as the privileged site of knowledge has pedagogical implications, as recognised

---

[33] Barkley Brown (1989) 926.
[34] For a fuller teasing out of the relationship between craft and collaboration see Ravetz *et al.* (eds) (2008).
[35] McNiff (2008) 11. See also Barone/Eisner (2012); Knowles/Cole (eds) (2008); Liamputtong/Rumbold (eds) (2008); McNiff (1998).
[36] Bratich/Brush (2011) 240 highlight how the "risky" knowledge and subject production of the "knitting circle", for example, gets devalued as "gossip."
[37] Barkley Brown (1989) 926–927.

by Barkley Brown. Including some form of active making into the learning space re-makes it a space of belonging because each learner/maker is actively involved in the process and the outcome.

If, as suggested above, the artwork of *hanging my heart* was the process of collective making, each participant was involved in the co-creation of that art/spirit/knowledge work. Fostering a sense of academic belonging, through techniques such as co-creation, has been shown to support the retention and success of marginalised learners.[38] One of the reasons for this is because participatory activity does not seek to dominate but create a community that listens to and works with the knowledge, experiences, and feelings of all those involved in the learning.

However, framing academic inquiry as/with craft is, appropriately, a work of tension. At the same time as providing the opportunity to expose and subvert dominant and oppressive systems, the very fabric of crafting can perpetuate stereotypes, reiterate status-quos and be exclusive. The time and resources associated with art and craft making means that it is not always as accessible as some may like. But, as Ann Cvetkovich has written, crafting can be read as "form of body politics" rooted in a relationship between the body, work, and an everyday sensibility that, precisely because those things are often not seen as political, occupies an urgent political charge.[39]

Part of that politics includes the space to recognise the uncomfortable, reactionary, and potentially exclusory aspects of art and craft working. For instance, when artists and activists use techniques and materials long defined as "women's work" and confined to the home – quilting, embroidery, knitting – in a public space, the histories and the presents that still see labour and value divided along stark gender, racial, and class lines is potentially *affirmed*.[40]

However, this affirmative approach does not seek to reclaim "the home" as a utopian space outside of the strictures of oppressive capitalism.[41] Rather, "making stuff", and in particular making stuff in such a way which may seem out of place for a specific location, can expose the insidious structures of inequality that we all live with/in. It can, therefore, provide the tools for "re-vision", which Adrienne Rich called "an act of survival." By this she meant that "entering an old text from a new critical direction" can unravel old meanings and weave new

---

[38] See Thomas (2012) for an in depth study of improving retention and success in an English higher education context.
[39] Cvetkovich (2012) 168. For the political charge of craft, see also Corbett/Housely (2011) and Greer (2014).
[40] Bratich/Brush (2011) 238–239.
[41] For an elaboration of this aspect of contemporary crafting see Matchar (2013).

ones.[42] In the field of Classics, for example, we can see this each time new theories emerge to support our looking back at old texts, our revisions. Each of these "acts of survival" faces negative criticism from practices and methods which have already survived the discipline and become familiar.

In her book, *Depression: a public feeling*, Cvetkovich outlines the importance of crafting – of using your body to transform something – as an everyday practice that can connect people, ideas, places, and times.[43] Embracing the heterogeneity of contemporary crafting – including the tensions noted above – Cvetkovich writes of its potential to "[give] rise new forms of collectivity and politics".[44] Drawing on interventions by queer and feminist crafters like Sheila Pepe, Alyson Mitchell and Leslie Hall, Cvetkovich maps how the ordinary, the domestic, and the playful can become sites of personal healing and, in so doing, expose the structures and systems which made you hurt in the first place. What is interesting for this project is how the everyday crafting which Cvetkovich outlines is framed as a spiritual practice.[45] The "repetitive and regular motion of the body" required in knitting and textile working, the time it takes to make something, situates crafting, for Cvetkovich, in the embodied and everyday habits of spiritual practice such as meditation.[46] Crafting, like some elements of spiritual practice, is a transformative process, whether that change is emotional, existential, or material.

Conclusions

Allowing space for the everyday, for the personal, for feelings, within spaces of knowledge (academic conferences and academic books) is disrupting, alienating, troubling. Some of the participants of the session spoke about how uneasy they were about it, how they only planned to stay for a short time, how they didn't really want to be there. Some of this dis-ease was healed by situating the workshop in a broader academic and philosophic context; by putting it in its place. That some of the same people who expressed anxiety about the session at the start, commented at the end how relaxed they felt, is testimony to the transformative charge of using making and play in the way we did. Indeed, the majority of the feedback

---

[42] Rich (1972) 18.
[43] Cvetkovich (2012).
[44] Cvetkovich (2012) 173.
[45] See Cvetkovich (2012) part two, chapter three, "The Utopia of Ordinary Habit."
[46] Cvetkovich (2012) 189.

we received from the session focused on feelings, on the emotional, on things resistant to being put in one place.

The practices we used are not so alien from the academy, in particular, from teaching, research, and practice methods in the social sciences and the therapeutic arts. They are not entirely absent from the discipline of Classics. For example, Judith Hallett and Thomas Van Northwick's ground-breaking collection, *Compromising Traditions: The Personal Voice in Classical Scholarship* is over twenty years old. In the introduction, Hallett situates the collection within a disciplinary shift to paying attention to how the stories (whether they be material stories in the form of votive hoards, spatial stories in the form of archaeological sites, or textual stories from manuscripts) of 'Classics' have been re-written, re-read, and read again.[47]

Further, some of the concerns for the role of the body that emerge when one considers arts-based activity align with recent work on dance, dancing, and theatrical performance in the field.[48] Even more pertinent for this project, we have seen Classicists sharing expertise with therapeutic practitioners to build knowledge and create tools for people to use in their everyday lives. The *Stoicism Today* project run by the University of Exeter, for example, sees students and academics working with professional therapeutic practitioners in the creation of a highly successful programme of work that includes academic publications, public courses, and guided meditation.[49]

Paying attention to the personal, to the mindful, to the embodied, even to the ephemeral within, or across, academic disciplines can become a way to shift scholarship, discover new stories, or tell old stories in different ways. Further, as projects like *Stoicism Today* attest, working with ancient material in different ways, creating a productive dialogue across expertise, and encouraging people to actively participate, has positive repercussions for academic outreach and wider public engagement.

Elliot Eisner, one of the pioneers of arts-based research, wrote of how research that focuses on the processes across which meaning is created must be approached artistically.[50] By calling for an artistic approach to research, Eisner was highlighting the role that complex, messy, emotional, political, physical, and personal charges have for a project. When working with material from antiquity these "complex, messy, emotional, political, physical, and personal charges" are not cleaned up by museum cases, dictionaries, classes, or conferences; they

---

[47] Hallett (1997) 1–2.
[48] See, for example, Mackintosh (ed) (2010).
[49] See http://modernstoicism.com
[50] Eisner (1981).

remain an unacknowledged yet vital part of the project. By acknowledging what can be hard to acknowledge in academia, arts-based working like *hanging my heart*, can bring some of those changes, those complex feelings, back to the meaning of an object, however ancient.

Using arts-based research techniques and creating a learning aesthetic that was resolutely playful allowed participants to explore structures of their own academic working. This is most obvious in the presence of imagery relating to academic life and academic anxieties but is also borne out in the sheer variety of pieces made. Taking the time to play, and play with others, can help (re)create an academic practice that is reflexive and accessible to other people's knowledge and understanding.

Recommendations

We end this paper with some recommendations as to how some of the ideas and practices outlined here could be incorporated into broader academic works, and a list of resources which may be of use to those seeking to explore some of the themes highlighted by this chapter further. Talk to colleagues from different disciplines, share skills, listen to different expertise, including therapeutic practitioners. This could provide new insight into your work, find new audiences for your ideas, and ensure that what you do is caring of others, and yourself. Consider 'disempowering' your position as a researcher/teacher. This could be done by shifting chairs in a classroom into a circle or by including elements of co-creation into a syllabus; it may also include writing collaboratively or in different voices. Using techniques, structures, or materials from arts/craft can create learning spaces that are more accessible than "mainstream" teaching/research practices. Including a creative aspect to an academic conference can "set the tone" and work through some anxieties. Sometimes focusing on the process is more important than the outcome. And remember to play.

Here are some links to some organisations and websites which expand some of the themes discussed in the paper.

> **British Association of Art Therapists:** The professional organisation for Art-Therapists in the UK. BAAT provides training and publishes the peer-reviewed journal, *International Journal of Art Therapy: Inscape*:
> http://www.baat.org/
> **European Consortium for Arts Therapies:** ECArTE is a consortium of European universities. It encourages the development of the Arts Therapies at a European level:
> http://www.ecarte.info/

Higher Education Academy: Under the theme 'Students as partners', the HEA provides guidance and support the development of student partnership. This includes the co-creation of teaching and learning material as well as research (UK-based):
https://www.heacademy.ac.uk/workstreams-research/themes/students-partners
National Alliance for Arts Health and Wellbeing: A resource for arts and health activity, highlighting areas of good practice and guides to help project development (UK-based):
http://www.artshealthandwellbeing.org.uk/
National Alliance for Museums, Health and Wellbeing: A hub for information and expertise sharing specifically focused on the role museums have for health and wellbeing (UK-based):
https://museumsandwellbeingalliance.wordpress.com/
Nemi to Nottingham: Nottingham University's web resource for the project about the Sanctuary of Diana at Nemi and the anatomical votives found there. It includes images, blogposts and details of the 2013 exhibition of the artefacts:
https://nemitonottingham.wordpress.com/
The Welcome Trust's Adamson Collection: It features a selection of assembled by Edward Adamson. The collection of works by patients provides valuable glimpses into the private worlds of patients living with mental illness:
http://wellcomecollection.org/adamson-collection
The Votives Project: It is a project dedicated to the study of votive offerings. Through its network, it facilitates dialogue across different academic disciplines, and between academics and people that practice votive offering. It aims to develop cross-cultural understandings of votive material and their different contexts.
https://thevotivesproject.wordpress.com/

2 The Hermeneutics of Psychology

Joel Christensen
1 Learned Helplessness, the Structure of the *Telemachy* and Odysseus' Return

When Zeus laments near the *Odyssey*'s beginning: "Wretches! Mortals are always blaming the gods. They say that bad things come from us but they have grief beyond their lot thanks to their own recklessness (*atasthalia*)",[1] he echoes the proem's description of Odysseus' suffering to preserve his companions.[2] Repeated invocations of mortal *atasthalia*, moreover, set parallel the fate of the sailors with the suitors at the epic's end.[3] Throughout, the epic shows mortals bearing some blame for their own suffering and invites the audience to evaluate the balance of divine intervention and human action.[4] Just as mortal choices are central to both the *Iliad* and the *Odyssey*, how mortals talk about who is responsible is a subtext of Zeus' assertion. Another way to put this is that our epic is intensely engaged with questions of agency and responsibility and in addressing problematic articulations of causality.

Almost any audience might wonder where in this Odysseus' responsibility fits.[5] Though some authors prefer a Homer who does not criticise Odysseus or

---

[1] *Od*. 1.32–34. Heubeck et al. (1988) 77 argue that the function of this passage is "to start the action".
[2] *Od*. 1.6–9. Pucci (1998) 19–20 notes that the proem anticipates Zeus' comments. On the thematic importance of anticipating the *atasthalia* of the suitors, see Danek (1998) 41–42. Cf. Cook (1995); Steinruck (2008); Bakker (2013) 114–118. For minimisation of the companions' guilt, see Clay (1983) 230; Shay (2002).
[3] See Cook (1995) 34–37 for Zeus' assumption between "between human suffering and crime" (34) and the decision to rescue Odysseus. Cf. Steinrück (2008) 65–67. Peradotto (1990) 60 reads Athena's adduction of Odysseus to the discussion of Aigisthos as an exception to Zeus' theology.
[4] For human responsibility in suffering, see Olson (1995) 214; Lowe (2000) 140; Teffeteller (2003) 19. Cf. Louden (2011) 228. For the critical importance of *atasthalia* as marking a "rational" error for which men are wholly responsible, see Finkelberg (1995). The concern is less about fate vs. free will than the significance of human choice: See Greene (1963) 14; Cf. Miller (2009a) 43.
[5] Rose (2012): it is "popular" to blame Odysseus. Cf. Louden (2011) 228. The narrative may allot some responsibility to Odysseus, but it makes him relatively innocent compared to his companions: Clay (1983) 35–37.

Note: Portions of this paper were improved greatly during presentations at the CAMWS annual meeting in Waco, Texas, at Brandeis University, and at the University of Arizona. In addition, I must thank Erwin Cook, Derek Delisi, Eli Embleton, Alexander Forte, Rosanna Lauriola, David Jacobson and Jonathan Ready for generous responses to earlier drafts.

Joel Christensen, Brandeis University

https://doi.org/10.1515/9783110482201-009

see the Homeric epic as more primitive in its presentation of god and man and justice,[6] many have emphasised the programmatic flavor of Zeus' opening lines,[7] sometimes noting as well their formative content for the epic's players and its audiences.[8]

Scholarship on Homeric psychology has focused on theoretical or philosophical questions, such as whether or not Homeric heroes make real decisions, the implications of the lexical range for Homeric expressions of emotions and thought, and the cultural implications of these questions.[9] More recent scholarship has illuminated cultural and social issues reflected in the poem through the application of cognitive psychology.[10] Throughout these studies there has been a sometimes explicit assumption that there is a correlation between the worldviews expressed in the poem and those of their (putative) audiences.[11] Drawing on the essential intercon-

---

6 For the *Odyssey* as a poem of justice, see Kitto (1966); cf. Dietrich (1965) 326. For the limitations of justice in Homer see Adkins (1960) 61–90. See Katz (1991) *passim* for the ethical outlook of the *Odyssey*. Clay (1983) 235 doubts the clarity of any message about justice. For the political character of the *Odyssey*'s justice, see Rose (2012) 147–151. On the contrasting senses of justice explored through Poseidon and Zeus, see Bakker (2013) 132–134.
7 In favor of the programmatic character, see Adkins (1960) 19–20 for whom this speech is a solution to "the problem of evil"; Dietrich (1965) 216; Griffin (1980); Kullman (1985) 14; Burkert (1997) 262; Mueller (1984) 147; Segal (1994) 195–210; Kearns (2004) 67–69; Allan (2006); and Marks (2008) 22–23. *Contra*: Van der Valk (1949) 243; Maronitis (1973) 95; and Clay (1983). Fenik (1974) 208–300 argues that Zeus' comments in book 1 do not cohere intellectually; they are the sentiments of the poet against the tradition; cf. Schadewaldt (1958) who argues that "poet B" adds Zeus' speech as a moral reading of an older belief system. On Zeus' speech as representing "a later stage of moral thought" to some scholars, see Finkelberg (1995) 17. The *Odyssey* has a more "developed understanding of human autonomy", see Gill (1996) 46 n. 59; cf. Russo (1968) 288–295.
8 For the importance of the warning to Aegisthus as a paradigm for the *Odyssey*'s characters, see Rüter (1969) 64–66; cf. Jaeger (1926). See Cook (1995) 32–33 for the philosophical importance of Zeus' emphasis that Aegisthus was *warned*. For this as in reaction to (and improvement upon) the *Iliad*: Cook (1995) 37. Cf. Lloyd-Jones (1971); Lowe (2000) 140 and Bakker (2013) 115. *Contra*: Allan (2006) 14.
9 For Homeric man's limited conception of self and lack of free will, see Snell (1960); Adkins (1960); *Contra*, Lesky (2004); cf. Russo/Simon (1968); Gaskin (1990); Hammer (2002) 49–79; Russo (2012) for discussions. See also Williams (1993); Gill (1996) 29–92 who argues that Adkins and Snell presuppose Kantian and Cartesian conceptions of self and morality; Gill notes that "those concepts whose absence these scholars note in Homer are precisely those whose validity is questioned by many contemporary theorists" (41). For divisions of thought, emotion and soul in Homer, based on lexical distinctions, see Snell (1960); Sullivan (1988); Zieliński (2002) and Zaborowski's discussion of it (2003). I treat the gods as representative of different perspectives on the relationship between the individual and the rest of the world. For the gods as evidence of internal human psychology, see Dodds (1951) 14; Snell (1960) 18–22; *contra*, Austin (1975) 82–86. Cf. Clay (1983) 136–138.
10 For cognitive approaches, see Minchin (2001).
11 See Russo/Simon (1968); Russo (2012).

nection between narratives and their audiences, I suggest that we understand the epics as displaying and performing what Jerome Bruner has called *folk psychology*.[12] And, in this performance, thanks to the dialogic nature of epic,[13] the poem serves as a vehicle for the audience to explore questions of personal agency.[14]

In this paper, I take up some questions of Homeric psychology from a 'clinical' perspective,[15] exploring how the epic 'diagnoses' by connecting problematic behavior with past experience – and perspectives taken on this experience – then implicitly proposes 'treatment' through its presentation of ameliorative steps performed by its characters. The epic acknowledges that the universe can *seem* completely pre-ordained – thus inducing in humans a state of fatalistic powerlessness – while also proposing 'therapeutic' interventions for such a state. These two processes, moreover, are thematically and structurally critical to the epic's first five books. By drawing on modern psychological theories of Learned Helplessness, I suggest that the epic dramatizes the experience of figures whose repeated failures have made them subservient to (a conception of) fate and unable to act, but who achieve a return to agency – a return to what we might call mental health but which the poem positions as returning to life[16] – through various means which we may recognise as therapeutic. First, I will give an overview of these themes, focusing on the deployment of paradigmatic questions about the relation between divine will and human action in the *Telemachy*. Then I will turn to the structural importance of the same thematic pattern in Odysseus' initial return to

---

[12] Bruner (1986) 49: "... folk theories about the human condition remain embedded in metaphor and in a language that serves the end of narrative. And folk narrative of this kind has as much claim to "reality" as any theory we may construct in psychology by the use of our most astringent scientific methods". Russo/Simon (1968) posit a strong equivalence between the form of Homeric poetry (and performance) and its psychological representations, a homology between epic poetry and the psychology of its characters *and* its audiences. Cf. Russo (2012). On the psychological nature of myth and Homeric poetry, see Segal (1994) 62–64.
[13] On the dialogic nature of epic see Peradotto (1990) 53 n. 13 and 62–63; Heiden (1991) 5; and on dialogism in the *Odyssey* in particular, see Felson/Slatkin (2014) for the term, see Bakhtin (1986) 170 on the dialogue's ability to collapse generational and temporal boundaries. Cf. Scully (1986) 135; Thalmann (1989) 14–21; Bakker (1997) 21–25. For analogical cross-currents in ideology in Homer, see Rose (1997); and Thalmann (1988) 3–5. For the *Odyssey*, see Rose (2012) 142–165; cf. Dougherty (2001); Saïd (2011) 354–372.
[14] See Olson (1995) 205; Miller (2009a) 36–39 argues that epic does not offer a theory of "agency and responsibility" but instead raises the relevant questions. Peradotto (1990) 44–45 distinguishes between motivation and function.
[15] For recent clinical perspectives: Shay (2003); Race (2014).
[16] For *nostos* narratives as a return to life and light, see Frame (1978); see Bonifazi (2009) for *nostos* as "salvation, not death".

life and the therapeutic reclamation of agency in his escape from Ogygia. I will close with brief comments on the therapeutic significance of his stay in Skheria.

The Learned Helplessness Perspective

The *Odyssey* presents Odysseus and Telemachus in their narrative debuts as directionless, or helpless; both are visited by gods to initiate action; and each can be said to undergo transformations of will, to put things broadly. Adducing a framework of Learned Helplessness illustrates that this presentation is not one of an intrinsic human state, but that it results instead from experience. Learned Helplessness (LH) and Learned Helplessness Effects are terms that psychologists have used to characterize a steady decrease in performance when animals or humans are exposed to "uncontrollable outcomes".[17] An early experiment demonstrated that dogs given the possibility to stop exposure to electric shock by pressing a lever, perform more slowly and less effectively over time if the lever randomly or rarely produces that outcome.[18] In a simple example available in a short video, a teacher induces LH by presenting students with sets of possible and impossible anagrams – students presented initially with two impossible tasks show a marked unwillingness or inability to complete the third solvable anagram while students with solvable tasks perform equally well.[19]

Although there is some debate about the extent of its importance, LH has been linked to "depression, anxiety, loneliness, victimization, crowding, unemployment, health problems and even death"[20] More substantially, a state of LH

---

[17] For the first use of the term, see Abraham (1911). Mikulincer (1994) 21: "LH effects results from learning that outcomes are independent of responses." Mikulincer (1994) offers six criteria to recognize deficits caused by LH: (1) LH deficits are present when a person displays problems in functioning and task performance; (2) LH deficits follow exposure to uncontrollable bad events that disrupt the equilibrium between the person and the environment; (3) LH deficits occur mainly when the uncontrollable bad event is appraised to be an imminent threat to one's basic commitments; (4) LH deficits occur mainly when exposure to uncontrollable bad events leads to the heightening of self-focused attention; (5) LH deficits are distally mediated by the acquisition of unfavorable expectancies of control during exposure to uncontrollable bad events and the generalization of these expectancies to new situation; (6) LH deficits are proximally mediated by the adoption of off-task coping.
[18] See Seligman/Maier (1967) and Overmier/Seligman (1967); cf. Mikulincer (1994) 4–5.
[19] Https://www.youtube.com/watch?v=MTqBP-x3yR0.
[20] Bibring (1953) places helplessness at the core of depression; see Peterson/Seligman (1983) for victimization. See Peterson (1986) and Mikulincer (1994) 2–6 for overviews of attributions.

has been shown to impede the learning of new skills and effective execution of old ones.[21] Such an incongruence, derived from repeated and uncontrollable failure—called by psychologists a "person environment mismatch"—can prevent plan-making and disrupt basic self-worth, resulting in an overwhelming view of a dangerous and uncontrollable world.[22] A typical cycle of response is to reorganise or re-analyse events rather than offer new solutions, to ruminate excessively on personal circumstances, and then to engage finally in what is called "avoidance coping", "an escapist attitude and the attempt to cut off the current experience from awareness".[23]

Odysseus, Telemachus and Learned Helplessness

Whether or not LH effects are wholly maladaptive – *not* feeling responsible for a situation can potentially liberate people to engage in new activities without coping with past failure[24] – a state of helplessness can be paralysing and require some intervention. When Odysseus first appears in the *Odyssey*, he has suffered many setbacks at sea from violence and shipwrecks and he sits weeping on the shore by day, sleeping with Calypso every night (5.151–158). For seven years he has been paralysed in a loop of escapist pleasure and sorrow. It is not my claim that Homeric singers and ancient audiences had a term that would translate as our Learned Helplessness or that Odysseus' defeated malaise would necessarily be understood as pathological, but rather that ancient folk psychology implicitly understood and recognised the deleterious effects of repeated defeats from the observation of human behavior. Such a recognition of the paralysing effects of repeated failure is implied before Odysseus' appears and can be shown to be central to the structure of our *Odyssey*.

Prior to *Odyssey* 5, there are moments where Homeric characters reflect upon fate and human action that are not consonant with Zeus' initial comments. In book 1, Telemachus blames Zeus for mankind's suffering (ἀλλά ποθι Ζεὺς αἴτιος, ὅς τε δίδωσιν / ἀνδράσιν ἀλφηστῇσιν ὅπως ἐθέλῃσιν ἑκάστῳ,

---

[21] See Lavelle et al. (1979) for LH effects in education and test-taking; cf. Heckhausen (1977). Human subjects who experience repeated lack of control over outcomes transfer expectations of no control to new tasks, see Mikulincer (1994) 6 and 246.
[22] See Maier/Seligman (1976); Feather (1982); Skinner (1985) for expectancy constructions in LH; cf. Mikulincer (1994) 239.
[23] See Mikulincer (1994) 241 and 257; cf. Lazarus/Folkman (1991).
[24] For LH effects in response to uncontrollable situations: Klinger (1975) and Kuhl (1981).

1.348–149).²⁵ Indeed, the elements of Telemachus' unfolding tale critically anticipate Odysseus' amplified narrative and prepare the audiences for his story.²⁶ In book 1, Telemachus is similar to his father in book 5 – the narrative depicts him in a reverie, looking after his father's return for *him* to disperse the suitors and safeguard their place (ἧστο γὰρ ἐν μνηστῆρσι φίλον τετιημένος ἦτορ / ὀσσόμενος πατέρ' ἐσθλὸν ἐνὶ φρεσίν, εἴ ποθεν ἐλθὼν / μνηστήρων τῶν μὲν σκέδασιν κατὰ δώματα θείη, 1.114–116). His world view is one in which he has no possibility of effecting change and so he engages in "state rumination", a hallmark of LH effects – colloquially, self-pity – and avoidance coping, by going half-heartedly along with the suitors in their feasting and games.²⁷

The audience witnesses what I suggest is a therapeutic intervention from Athena's first appearance.²⁸ When the goddess first addresses Telemachus, she assures him that his father is not dead, while also invoking an important double-causation by claiming that the gods ruined his journey, though savage men hold him (1.195–199) before asserting that Odysseus will "figure out how to come home, since he is *polymêkhanos*" (φράσσεται ὥς κε νέηται, ἐπεὶ πολυμήχανός ἐστιν, 1.205).²⁹ In subsequent conversations, Athena equivocates about Odysseus' fate (1.267–270) but insists that Telemachus must himself consider how to be done with the suitors, how to reclaim agency (1.294–297). Lexical terms interweave these themes: Odysseus will plan to save himself (φράσσεται, 1.205), according to Athena, who orders his son to do the same (φράζεσθαι δὴ ἔπειτα κατὰ φρένα καὶ κατὰ θυμόν / ὅππως κε μνηστῆρας ἐνὶ μεγάροισι τεοῖσι / κτείνῃς ἠὲ δόλῳ ἢ ἀμφαδόν, 1.294–297; cf. 1.264)

---

25 Cf. 1.376–80, when Telemachus prays for retributive deeds from Zeus (αἴ κέ ποθι Ζεὺς δῷσι παλίντιτα ἔργα γενέσθαι).
26 See Page (1955) 169–179 for the unity of the *Telemacheia* (2–4); cf. Katz (1991) 29–33 for earlier opinions on Telemachy. Cf. Murnaghan (1987) 165–166; Cook (2015); Christensen/Barker (2015) for how the Telemachy anticipates the plots of Odysseus' narratives. Saïd (2011) 132 notes that we should "consider the beginning of the *Odyssey* as a sort of indirect portrayal of Odysseus: his absence serves to arouse the listeners' curiosity about the rest of the story".
27 For state rumination, see above, n. 24.
28 For Clarke (1963) 44, Telemachus goes to Nestor and Menelaus as surrogate fathers who introduce him into the heroic world.
29 Clarke (1967) 43: among ancient critics the *Telemacheia* was seen as a form of *paideusis*; cf. Heitman (2005) 58–62 and Austin (1969) for the suggestion that to mature Telemachus needed to learn how to deceive (cf. Austin (1975) 132. Telemachus' journey is a version of an initiation ritual, see Felson-Rubin (1994) 67–91 and Thalmann (1998) 206–215 (for a largely negative view). See Martin (1993) 232–239 for lexical indications of Telemachus' maturation. As Thalmann (1998) 207 notes the process is incomplete – his journey is organised by Athena and his maturation is reversed or stunted by his father's return; cf. Murnaghan (1987) 36–37. For a recent discussion of the *Telemachy* see Petropoulos (2011).

balanced against Telemachus' misreading echo of Zeus when he claims that the gods devise evil for Odysseus (νῦν δ' ἑτέρως ἐβόλοντο θεοὶ κακὰ μητιόωντες / οἳ κεῖνον μὲν ἄϊστον ἐποίησαν περὶ πάντων / ἀνθρώπων, 1.234–236) and likewise established evil pains for him (ἐπεί νύ μοι ἄλλα θεοὶ κακὰ κήδε' ἔτευξαν, 1.244). Throughout the opening movement, the thematic investigation of agency is echoed through a lexical emphasis on human planning and thought. This is by no means incidental in a poem about a hero who is marked by his cleverness. Athena emboldens Telemachus to make a plan, evoking a cooperation in agency between god and man that is a positive inversion of Zeus' complaint well-encapsulated in the subsequent description of Telemachus lying awake at night "making plans in his thoughts about the journey which Athena showed him" (ἔνθ' ὅ γε παννύχιος, κεκαλυμμένος οἰὸς ἀώτῳ / βούλευε φρεσὶν ᾗσιν ὁδόν, τὴν πέφραδ' Ἀθήνη, 1.444–445).

This limited summary of the events of book 1 reveals a thematic pattern which examines agency and intervention to respond both to Zeus' complaint and Telemachus' inaction. Here, (1) a character disavows agency with a resigned "gods are in control" statement;[30] (2) a divine or more experienced figure correctively attributes more to human agency; as (3) both figures negotiate the relationship between controllable and uncontrollable outcomes; then (4) Athena expresses an ideal cooperative aesthetic[31] between man and god that inverts (positively) Zeus' initial complaint[32] and (5) builds upon unclear causal connections in doubly motivated events, culminating in assertions about (6) divine guarantee of justice in the human realm.[33] In short, the interplay between Athena and Telemachus

---

[30] For other fatalistic expressions, see for example *Od.* 2.33–34; 3.83–91 (Telemachus ascribes his father's absence to Zeus); 4.127–134, 181–182, 235–237 and 260–264 (Menelaos and Helen seem especially fatalistic); 4.501–520 (Poseidon ends Ajas' *nostos*); 4.722–28 (Penelope blames Zeus for the loss of Odysseus and Telemachus); 6.187–190; 7.196–203; 8.464–468 and 567–571; 14. 39 (Eumaios); 14.262–265 (Zeus caused the Trojan War).

[31] For the cooperative aesthetic, see 2.115–122 (where the suitors blame their fortune on Athena's intervention and Penelope's intelligence); 4.712–714 (Penelope and Medon are unclear whether Telemachus or a god is the author of his actions); 13.365 (shared agency between Athena and Odysseus); 17.243; 17.601; 19.2; 19.137–139; 21.201.

[32] The action of the poem, in a corollary to Zeus' negative comments is positively depicted as a partnership between man and god, where Athena empowers Odysseus to act for himself, see Kitto (1966) 132–133; cf. Atkins (1960) 13. This cooperative aesthetic refers to some of the events described as "double motivation", see Segal (1994) 217; for a bibliography, see Teffeteller (2003) 15.

[33] For the gods as guarantors of justice, see 2.65–68 and 3.205–209; 14.83–84; 24.186–190; 24.442–449. Throughout, the epic experiments with different types of human causality and agency/instrument of the gods.

presents a sophisticated integration of divine power and human choice, offering instead a cooperative and mutually reinforcing approach to action.[34]

The narrative revisits and revises these themes within the Telemachy.[35] Nestor echoes Zeus when he pairs human decision-making and divine wrath: he says that Zeus decreed a grievous homecoming for the Argives who suffered a terrible fate thanks to the rage of Athena, only after he criticizes them for being neither prudent nor just (3.132–136).[36] Here, then, is a critical expression of the relationship(s) between fate and agency – the gods *have to* make things worse when men do not behave properly. But implicit as well is the promise (7) that prudent and righteous men will be rewarded. Nestor's worldview is an additional corrective: for him, (a) bad things happen to bad people rightly (e.g. Aegisthus, 3.194); when bad things happen (b) there is a human cause; (c) the gods may cause evil or make humans instruments of justice. But there is an open question about the final step: sometimes bad things happen to good men like Odysseus (d).

How precisely does Telemachus progress through these steps toward a different view of agency? It is here where the poem offers an initial 'therapeutic' response to Telemachus' state. When he goes on his journey, Telemachus does not subscribe to Nestor's theodicy because of his life experience: his father never returned, the suitors do what they want, and he seems powerless to change his circumstances.[37] His journey consists of remarkably little action: his 'education' consists of changing contexts, observing the behavior of others, and listening to the stories from the past and contemplating their meanings.[38] Although Telemachus' journey is a critical step in preparing him to act, it is incomplete for two

---

[34] For a bleaker interpretation, see Fenik (1974) 212 and 222 for three relationships: man brings his own doom, gods punish; gods encourage men along criminal paths; gods arbitrarily impose suffering.

[35] For the *Odyssey*'s internal audiences, see Doherty (1995) 17–19 and 73–131; cf. Peradotto (1990) 117–118 who sees invited identification with Telemachus and Martin (1993) for Telemachus reflecting the historical audience. Cf. Murnaghan (2002) 139. Pucci (1987) 201 calls Telemachus an "intoxicated reader".

[36] Note the resonance with mental operations in λυγρὸν ἐνὶ φρεσὶ **μήδετο** νόστον and οὔ τι **νοήμονες**. Athena similarly accuses the suitors (τῶ νῦν μνηστήρων μὲν ἔα βουλήν τε νόον τε / ἀφραδέων, ἐπεὶ οὔ τι νοήμονες οὐδὲ δίκαιοι, 3.281–282) and Odysseus maligns the Phaeacians (ὢ πόποι, οὐκ ἄρα πάντα νοήμονες οὐδὲ δίκαιοι, 13.209).

[37] Telemachus attributes agency to the gods (3.205–209). The incompleteness of his 're-education' is why traveling to Pylos is not enough. Menelaos' Sparta furnishes additional contexts that help to change Telemachus in meaningful ways, see Murnaghan (2002) 144–150.

[38] The tales of Nestor, Helen, and Menelaos allow the *Odyssey* to tell other Trojan War narratives, provide further characterization of Odysseus, and seem to sate Telemachus' hunger for knowledge and prepare him, in some way, to act; see Barker and Christensen (2015).

reasons. First, on a narrative level Telemachus' journey functions to prepare the audience for the appearance of his father – and it is his return to agency that is paramount in this tale. Second, both narratives combine sometimes contradictory views of will and fate and weigh them – just as Telemachus learns more sophisticated ways to weigh the progression of events in the world, so too the audience is invited to learn, consider, and debate. In this way, the Telemachy is therapeutic for the audience as well.

Escape from Ogygia

The pattern I sketched out with Telemachus repeats *mutatis mutandis* through the epic's treatment of Odysseus, but in more subtle ways.[39] The epic presents Odysseus at first in a world that is wholly god-dominated: Zeus predicts the narrative, namely that Odysseus will come to Skheria, be honored, and return wealthier than when he left for Troy (5.33–32). Note, that the means by which he accomplishes this is not divulged. In this way, the cooperative aesthetic discussed above becomes the dominant theme in the book: Odysseus is allowed to go home by the gods, but *he* needs to build his raft on his own, a scene which in part anticipates the rebuilding of the man through the subsequent books (5.160–170 and 228–261). At the beginning of the process, Kalypso plans out the journey for him (καὶ τότ' Ὀδυσσῆϊ μεγαλήτορι μήδετο πομπήν, 5.233); but during the building of his vessel, the narrative emphasizes his knowledge and skilled craft (ξέσσε δ' ἐπισταμένως, 5.245; … εὖ εἰδὼς τεκτοσυνάων, 5.250; … ὁ δ' εὖ τεχνήσατο καὶ τά, 5.259). The episode ends with an elegant expression of cooperation: Calpyso sends a favorable wind (οὖρον δὲ προέηκεν ἀπήμονά τε λιαρόν τε), but Odysseus is the one who *knows how* to handle it expertly (γηθόσυνος δ' οὔρῳ πέτασ' ἱστία δῖος Ὀδυσσεύς / αὐτὰρ ὁ πηδαλίῳ ἰθύνετο τεχνηέντως, 5.268–270).

The subsequent events – where Odysseus' prior sufferings are reimagined through the reappearance of Poseidon whose intervention initiates a range of defeatist and recuperative moments – explore the interplay between suffering and agency. Although divine forces are shown acting against Odysseus, the hero's own willingness to act is instrumental in his survival and success. The process, moreover, resonates with studies in Learned Helplessness (see Table 2.1). As studies in LH effects have shown, both humans and animals can be trained to

---

[39] For how Odysseus' journey in book 5 anticipates the themes and structures of the whole epic, see Marks (2008) 36–61.

Table 2.1: Odysseus' Laments in book 5.1[a]

Passage	Situation	Action Type	Outcome
299–312	Onset of Storm	*State Rumination* (wishes he had died at Troy)	Odysseus blames Zeus Odysseus' own effort and divine help keeps him alive
356–364	Uncertainty concerning Leukothea's help	*Yielding*; Surrender of agency	Poseidon sends a wave; Leukothea preserves him
[394–9]	Simile: Sick Father, healed by gods	Cause and relief attributed to gods	
408–423	Odysseus' own effort and divine help keeps him alive	*Deliberation* [narrative says Athena intervenes]	Swimming
465–473	The land is cold and he is naked	*Deliberation* [narrative says Athena intervenes]	Hibernation in the bush and leaves

[a]For the importance of this sequence as "personified interchange" of an internalised mental process, see Russo/Simon (1968) 488. Cf. Gill (1996) 59 and 86–87.

strive against helplessness by being "exposed to controllable events".[40] And in many cases, the ability to make new causal attributions, to map out a path that leaves room for personal agency, is the first catalyst for what researchers call "expectancy change".[41] Poseidon attacks and Odysseus wishes he had died at Troy (5.299–312) blaming Zeus (Ζεύς, ἐτάραξε δὲ πόντον …, 5.304) and expressing again a fatalistic and foreclosed worldview similar to Telemachus' at the beginning of the epic (νῦν δέ με λευγαλέῳ θανάτῳ εἵμαρτο ἁλῶναι, 5.312).[42] In the language of LH, this is state rumination, a pensive self-pitying condition where no action is thought possible; accordingly, at this first lament, Odysseus takes no action.[43]

In the next step, Leukothea intervenes to save him, but he doubts he can trust the gods – the goddess tells him to abandon his vessel (5.357), he insists he will not obey because the land is so far off (ἀλλὰ μάλ' οὔ πω πείσομ', 5.358),

---

[40] See Mikulincer (1994) 6–7.
[41] See Mikulincer (1994) 112.
[42] For the thematic importance of Poseidon's attacks on Odysseus, see Marks (2008) 44–47. For engagement between the language of Odysseus' suffering and scenes in the *Iliad* (and how this assures both audience and hero that the story will go on), see Pucci (1987) 63–66.
[43] For the extent to which internal state rumination causes paralysis in patients, see White (2007) 106.

and he comes up with his own plan (ἀλλὰ μάλ' ὧδ' ἔρξω, δοκέει δέ μοι εἶναι ἄριστον). After deciding that certain suffering awaits if he clings to the vessel, he takes the risk and swims (5.356–364). Then, as he is being washed ashore he is surprised to see land – and his approach to it is limited by steep cliffs and dangerous terrain. While the narrative claims Athena intervenes, the action shows that Odysseus contemplates the scene, sees the safe passage, and then swims for it (5.408–423). The formulaic language throughout this section binds the series together and emphasizes a subtle but important change. The same speech introductory line prefaces each moment of deliberation (ὀχθήσας δ' ἄρα εἶπε πρὸς ὃν μεγαλήτορα θυμόν, 5.299=355, 408, 464) and each speech starts with a lament:

> "ὤ μοι ἐγὼ δειλός, τί νύ μοι μήκιστα γένηται;, 5.299
>
> "ὤ μοι ἐγώ, μή τίς μοι ὑφαίνησιν δόλον αὖτε, 5.356
>
> "ὤ μοι, ἐπεὶ δὴ γαῖαν ἀελπέα δῶκεν ἰδέσθαι, 5.408
>
> "ὤ μοι ἐγώ, τί πάθω; τί νύ μοι μήκιστα γένηται;, 5.465

After his first lament, he is driven, still speaking, by a wave as the raft explodes (5.313–314). After the last three speeches, however, Odysseus is described as deliberating (εἷος ὁ ταῦθ' ὥρμαινε κατὰ φρένα καὶ κατὰ θυμόν, 5.365, 424) and then finally deciding upon action (ὣς ἄρα οἱ φρονέοντι δοάσσατο κέρδιον εἶναι, 5.474). The language and the action recall Athena's prediction to Telemachus in book 1: φράσσεται ὥς κε νέηται, ἐπεὶ πολυμήχανός ἐστιν, 5.205. And this series of actions repeats when he washes up on land to find himself cold and naked (5.465–473): he laments, but then he makes a decision, takes action, and preserves himself in a pile of leaves.

The events of book 5, often sped over in anticipation of arrival in Skheria, present a structure where Odysseus transforms back into the much tossed-about man described in the proem. A helpful action by the gods is met with a harmful one (and vice versa) – the balance of which leaves Odysseus' initiative as critical in bringing him closer to home: *he* builds the raft, steers his ship, clings to the timber, and swims to safety. Although it is clearly possible to attribute the greater importance to the hand of the gods, the actions given to Odysseus himself are instrumental. They are, furthermore, meaningful psychologically as well: in book 5, we find a defeated Odysseus restrained from action by Kalypso, a plot feature which communicates his total loss of agency. The languor inculcated from multiple defeats is briefly treated by success and desperation. One way to immunize against the effects of LH is to expose people – or animals – to events that are within their control, to facilitate successful execution of decision-making and action.⁴⁴ By this process, the epic dramatizes the rebuilding of Odysseus' abilities to cope with the world as part of his process in returning home. When he covers himself on the shore of Skheria, Odysseus is, as many scholars have suggested, re-entering life as something of a mid-life newborn.⁴⁵ Though this may be pressing the point, researchers have compared the traumatised mind to that of a young child – suffering makes it necessary to re-learn how to relate to the world and how to understand and communicate what has happened.⁴⁶

Conclusion – The Next Therapeutic Step

In this paper I have argued that Zeus' comments at the beginning of the *Odyssey* constitute a programmatic statement addressing one possible strand of thought in the epic's audiences concerning man's helplessness in the face of fate. The depiction of Telemachus in book 1 and through his journey in the Telemachy dramatises various responses to such a debate and models an initial rehabilitative approach. The problem – Telemachus' lack of agency – and the treatment I have suggested resonate strongly with modern studies in Learned Helplessness. Just as the structure of the Telemachy anticipates the structure of Odysseus' return home, as Cook (2014) makes clear, so too the theme of helplessness and the epic's therapeutic response is integrated into Odysseus' escape from his Ogygian paralysis. In both, the epic models a shared responsibility – a cooperative aesthetic – between mortals and gods for human failure and success that provides an alternate worldview to Zeus' first comments.

This paper draws on studies in LH to argue that the epic presents Odysseus as going through a rehabilitation that is as much about his defeatist world view – his psychology – as it is about the needs of the narrative. His rehabilitation – his therapy – is not complete, however. When he comes to land in Skheria, he does not tell his name or reveal is story for three books of the epic. In almost every meaningful way, Odysseus still has not returned to himself. Trauma victims are often paralysed by the memory of their suffering;⁴⁷ the stories they tell about the world and their place in it are, in a sense, pathological within and unto them-

---

44 Mikulincer (1994) 6–7.
45 For Odysseus' rebirth, see Van Nortwick (2009) 21–23; for how the language of book 5 anticipates this, see Pucci (1987) 44–49.
46 See Fernyhough (2012) 201.
47 See Fernyhough (2012) 181–185 for PTSD as a disorder of memory.

selves. Therapeutic interventions for this paralysis emphasise the recuperation of agency through the telling of new stories.[48]

Understanding Odysseus as beset by a similar psychological state enriches our understanding of the necessity of the most famous movement in the epic, the *Apologoi*, his telling of his own tale in books 9–12. Here, the Phaeacians function as Odysseus' confessors and his therapists (as William Race has argued); they are both his audience and collaborators as he retells his tale and isolates his own actions within it.[49] Thus, just as the Telemachy anticipates the events of book 5, so too do both movements prepare us for the contents and therapeutic necessity of the hero telling his own tale. As a result Odysseus' *Apologoi* – in the contemplation of causality in the events after leaving Troy – in part reflect a therapeutic process by which the hero's storytelling negotiates the relationship between divine agency and human responsibility in a way that allows him to reclaim his identity and fully commit to returning home.[50] Through his tale, he explores where and how his own efforts influenced his fate (e.g., by telling the Cyclops his name) and articulates a perspective where he is restored as agent. And his exploration of his own culpability and survival engages the audience in an interpretive dialogue whereby the dramatisation of Odysseus' therapy transforms into a therapeutic dialogue between the poem and their lives.

---

[48] See White (2007) and (2011) for the steps of the post-structuralist therapeutic approach of narrative therapy which trains patients to separate narratives of problems and individual identity and then to 're-author' their narratives to recuperate agency and make new plans for the future.

[49] Race (2013). For Odysseus' act of narration pointing not to the Phaeacians but to the external audience, see Wyatt (1989) 256–257; cf. Pucci (1998) 146–147.

[50] In a recent paper, Burgess (2014) 351 emphasizes that a significant contribution of the epic is "raising the question of its hero's responsibility for his actions".

Lilah Grace Canevaro
2 Anticipating Audiences: Hesiod's *Works and Days* and Cognitive Psychology

Introduction

Ehninger in his article 'On systems of rhetoric' claimed that, "hampered by the primitive psychology and epistemology with which they worked ... the classical writers tended either to scant or to present a patently naive account of the relation between the speech act and the mind of the listener".[1] Nisbet describes how Hesiod is cast by Martin West, the poet's most prominent commentator, as "a 'primitive' poet, carried to and fro by the miscellaneous and contrary urges of the Indo-European story-telling tradition".[2] In this chapter I will analyse Hesiod's *Works and Days* using modern psychological research in order to reveal quite the contrary: that the archaic Greek wisdom tradition presents a high degree of cognitive sophistication, and in particular that the poet demonstrates a great deal of audience awareness. I aim not to impose modern thought anachronistically on an ancient poem, but rather to use the cognitive sciences as a tool to tease out some interesting aspects of Hesiod's didactic project. This is not to say that these aspects have thus far gone unnoticed: many have been discussed through different, more established, scholarly traditions. Yet the value of an analysis grounded in psychology is that it foregrounds ways of thinking: as does Hesiod's *didaxis*. Further, in bringing together archaic wisdom and what is considered to be a modern science we can reflect both on the (often underestimated) complexity of early poetry and on the ancestry of a modern discipline. Such an analysis can make us aware of the transmission of knowledge as a constant in human endeavours: of changing content and mechanisms, but a persistent drive to teach, to learn, and to put one's learning into practice.

Hesiod's *Works and Days* was experienced in antiquity in two ways: as a piece of extended instruction performed in its own right, and as a repository of lines that, when detached from their original context, could be applied to almost any scenario. Through selection, structure and formulation of material, through conscious crafting and consistent moral direction, it is a poem that shapes, up to

---

[1] Ehninger (1968) 134.
[2] Nisbet (2004) 150.

Lilah Grace Canevaro, University of Edinburgh

https://doi.org/10.1515/9783110482201-010

a point, its own reception.³ I will argue that part of this shaping involves anticipating multiple audiences: a complex cognitive task. Kroll notes of audience awareness in antiquity: "while the importance of audience was acknowledged, there is little elaboration of the concept of audience among the major Greek and Roman theorists".⁴ I hope to show that whilst the theory may have been lacking (something which modern psychology more than makes up for), the practice was flourishing.

Chafe defines consciousness as "the locus of remembering, imagining, and feeling".⁵ Classics and cognitive psychology have come together in looking at Greek literature in terms of remembering and feeling.⁶ Work between the fields begins to be done on imagining, for example that of Luigi Battezzato on persuasion and deliberation in Greek tragedy as acts of projection of the self.⁷ I would like to pursue the cognitive experience of imagining, in terms of envisaged modes of reading and reception. I will be using Berkenkotter's article "Understanding a writer's awareness of audience", mapping her categories of audience-related considerations onto Hesiod's *Works and Days*.⁸

Audience-Related Activities: Coding Categories

I. Analyzing/Constructing a Hypothetical Audience
    A. Considering facts about the audience given in the assignment (age, grade level)
    B. Constructing hypothetical audience characteristics (demographic location, ethnic background)

---

3 See Canevaro (2015), and further note 38 below.
4 Kroll (1978) 270.
5 Chafe (1994) 38.
6 On remembering, see e.g. Minchin (2001); Bakker (2005); Clay (2011). See also Rubin (1995) on the cognitive psychology of memory in oral traditions. Though my primary focus in this chapter is on imagining, I will also be concerned with memory, and more specifically the different types of memory triggered by the audience-awareness devices used in the *Works and Days*. On feeling, e.g. Konstan (2006), Cairns (2008).
7 Unpublished paper, delivered at the University of Edinburgh January 2014: "Debates and deliberation in Euripides: the *agōn logōn* in context".
8 The application of criteria is never without problems. We need only think of the endless attempts to categorise didactic poetry, to demarcate a genre that is nebulous at best. And yet, as a heuristic tool it can be useful - and indeed, using criteria that are unrelated to the question 'what is didactic?' can have a particularly strong impact on our understanding of the Works and Days. For another reading of Hesiod's poetry through criteria new and different, see Vergados (forthcoming): a reinterpretation of Hesiod as a historian.

C. Making simple inferences from the description of the audience, which may or may not be accurate
  D. Making complex inferences (more than one) from the description of the audience
  E. Identifying self with audience (role-playing)
  F. Identifying audience with self (projecting)
  G. Creating rhetorical context in oral protocol
  H. Creating rhetorical context in written text
II. Goal Setting and Planning for a Specific Audience
  A. Generating audience-related goals
  B. Naming audience-related plans
  C. Generating sub-goals or refinements of the plan
  D. Consolidating several sub-goals to carry out the plan
  E. 'Satisficing' (temporarily eliminating some sub-goals of the plan to carry out others)
  F. Representing oneself to the audience (*persona*)
III. Evaluating Content and Style with Regard to Anticipated Audience Response
  A. Evaluating audience response to content (may be about text being considered or completed text)
  B. Evaluating audience response to style (*persona*)
  Berkenkotter (1981, 398–399, extract)

The context is rather different: Berkenkotter is analysing a writing assignment, and I am dealing with a poem that originated in an oral tradition. Berkenkotter poses questions directly to authors, whereas with the Hesiodic tradition the issue of authorship is hotly debated. However, the article does have a number of things to recommend it. Firstly, the categories are a useful starting point. It is a typology which has since been much used, I think because it does not impose pedagogical theory and its concomitant constraints on the analysis but draws out a number of key issues which are individually addressed elsewhere in the cognitive sciences. Secondly, the study used 'thinking aloud' protocols in an attempt to track what writers are thinking while they are writing. This goes some way towards bridging the divide between writing and orality, and gives us an important insight into the mechanisms of composition. Thirdly, the contexts do have something in common: teaching. Berkenkotter's assignment is to describe one's career choice to a high-school audience. This is essentially both an autobiographical and a didactic task (involving describing, informing and persuading), and so arguably has more relevance to Hesiod's didactic poem with its immanent, ostensibly autobiographical, narrative persona than would a study concerned with writing fiction. Yet fiction leads me to Berkenkotter's first category.

Analysing/Constructing a Hypothetical Audience

"The writer's audience is always a fiction".[9] This does not hold quite so true in an original performance context of an oral poem, as the audience are physically present and their reaction – not to mention their attention span – are immediately evident. However, it does pertain to future envisaged performances or other avenues of reception. Felix Budelmann has recently argued that the complex temporal markers embedded by Pindar in his epinician odes anticipate not just a one-off performance but also future *reperformances*:[10] and I would argue that Hesiod's *Works and Days* does much the same thing.

Hesiod (by which I mean both a persona and a driving force behind the poem, something I shall come back to) is very clear about his ideal audience:

> οὗτος μὲν πανάριστος, ὃς αὐτὸς πάντα νοήσει,
>
> φρασσάμενος, τά κ' ἔπειτα καὶ ἐς τέλος ᾖσιν ἀμείνω·
>
> ἐσθλὸς δ' αὖ καὶ κεῖνος, ὃς εὖ εἰπόντι πίθηται·
>
> ὃς δέ κε μήτ' αὐτὸς νοέῃ μήτ' ἄλλου ἀκούων
>
> ἐν θυμῷ βάλληται, ὁ δ' αὖτ' ἀχρήιος ἀνήρ.

> That man is altogether the best, he who thinks of everything himself,
>
> considering the things which are then better in the end.
>
> He too is good, who listens to one who speaks well.
>
> But he who does not think for himself nor listening to another
>
> considers in his heart, this man is useless.
>
> *Works and Days* 293–297[11]

The audience must have some kind of drive to learn, repeatedly exhorted as they are to "consider" (φράζεσθαι), to "remember" (μεμνημένος) – to work hard for Hesiod's advice, to store it up and use it at another time. This drive to learn is known in cognitive studies as a 'need for cognition'. There is, of course, a questionnaire to quantify this need: Cacioppo and Petty's *Need for Cognition Scale* (1984). Statements with which to agree or disagree include: "I find satisfaction in deliberating hard and for long hours", and "I prefer my life to be filled with puzzles

---

9 Ong (1975) 9.
10 Budelmann (2017).
11 All *Works and Days* text is taken from West (1978); all translations are my own.

I must solve" – and reverse-scored statements such as "I only think as hard as I have to", and "Thinking is not my idea of fun". The *Works and Days* anticipates an audience that would score highly on such a scale. Higher scores have been linked with better verbal reasoning, higher fluid intelligence and even greater life satisfaction, so the active approach Hesiod encourages is set to be a fulfilling one. As Minchin notes (of Homeric epic, but which can be applied equally to Hesiodic didactic), "a story is deemed by its listeners to be more enjoyable if they have been encouraged to play an active role in the storytelling".[12] Furthermore, as Clements argues, "If listeners were made to search hard for the right answer, then, when they got it, they would remember the point clearly".[13] Hesiod is constructing cognitive patterns for his audience to adopt on a long-term basis.

Under this first category, Berkenkotter includes 'role-playing' (identifying self with audience) and 'projecting' (identifying audience with self). Hesiod negotiates both: the former in his anticipating multiple generalised audiences, and the latter in his personal interjections. In his fable of the hawk and the nightingale (202–212), for example, the inconsistencies in any one specific application of the story point towards multiple identifications, allowing the poet to identify with multiple audiences simultaneously.[14] Moreover, potential identifications do not stop at the level of the poem but can be detached and applied by the audience. Whether you are a hawk or a nightingale, as it were, you must consider the implications of the story for yourself. Through role-playing, through mapping Hesiod's advice onto our own lives, we activate a particular modality of memory: kinetic memory. In this modality – not restricted to movement as we might expect, but to do with experience, emotion and personal motivation[15] – the encoding and retrieval technique focuses on a key word, person or event that is meaningful to the learner. The material becomes anchored in memory because the learner has made an affective investment in it.

In terms of projecting, Hesiod twice treats us to his own opinion. With the first interjection, he situates himself explicitly (and discontentedly) within the Iron Age:

μηκέτ' ἔπειτ' ὤφελλον ἐγὼ πέμπτοισι μετεῖναι

ἀνδράσιν, ἀλλ' ἢ πρόσθε θανεῖν ἢ ἔπειτα γενέσθαι.

νῦν γὰρ δὴ γένος ἐστὶ σιδήρεον·

---

12 Minchin (2001) 215.
13 Clements (2000) 28.
14 On this passage and for a survey of the interpretations, see Canevaro (2015) 54–60.
15 Schwartz/Power (2000) 404.

> Would then that I was no longer among the fifth race of
> men, but either died earlier or was born later.
> For now indeed it is a race of iron.
>
> Works and Days 174–176

Hesiod allies himself with his audience, inspiring confidence. Who better to be emulated by the Iron-Age man than one of us? The interjection is a 'rhetorical sigh';[16] an exclamation of dismay at the current state of things, and trepidation about the dire future Hesiod predicts. However, it is not quite an exclamation of despair, as the fact that Hesiod offers so much advice suggests that he believes in his own didactic authority: follow Hesiod's advice and the future *can* change. In the second instance, Hesiod seems to give his opinion on 'current' justice:

> νῦν δὴ ἐγὼ μήτ' αὐτὸς ἐν ἀνθρώποισι δίκαιος
> εἴην μήτ' ἐμὸς υἱός, ἐπεὶ κακὸν ἄνδρα δίκαιον
> ἔμμεναι, εἰ μείζω γε δίκην ἀδικώτερος ἕξει·
> ἀλλὰ τά γ' οὔ πω ἔολπα τελεῖν Δία μητιόεντα.
>
> Now I myself would not be just among men,
> nor would I wish my son to be, since it is evil for a man to be just
> if the more unjust man will have greater justice.
> But I hope that counsellor Zeus will not yet let these things happen.
>
> Works and Days 270–273

He does not want to be part of a world where injustice is rewarded. However, as with the decline of the Iron Race, the situation has not yet come to this, and Hesiod hopes that Zeus will not let it. Again, he offsets his apocalyptic warning with a dose of optimism – which we can extrapolate as being contingent on our own behaviour.

Goal Setting and Planning for a Specific Audience

As well as anticipating multiple unnamed audiences, the *Works and Days* also has two explicit addressees: Perses (Hesiod's wayward brother), and the

---
16 Verdenius (1985) *ad loc.*

corrupt 'gift-swallowing' kings.[17] Indeed, the fable of the hawk and the nightingale is addressed to the kings (202 νῦν δ' αἶνον βασιλεῦσ' ἐρέω), but its moral is directed to Perses (213 ὦ Πέρση, σὺ δ' ἄκουε Δίκης, μηδ' ὕβριν ὄφελλε): Hesiod switches between these named didactic targets, and implicitly includes his wider audience in the process.[18] At this point I would like to return to the issue of fiction, and its role in anticipating audiences, as the invention of an internal addressee is in essence a work of fiction. Up until the late twentieth century, Hesiodic scholars were preoccupied with whether or not Perses was the real brother of a real Hesiod.[19] In recent decades, however, scholarly engagement with the character has shifted towards seeing him as a literary or didactic tool, regardless of whether or not he existed. This is logical, as the fallacy of biographical reconstruction is that even when poets choose to include autobiographical fact in their work, they do so because it makes poetic sense. Therefore the presumed existence of Perses can never fully explain his inclusion in the *Works and Days*. Whether he existed or not, he is constructed as the perfect didactic addressee, exhibiting all the faults Hesiod wants to highlight and acting as a convenient base for Hesiod's teachings.

A narrative thread which runs throughout the poem and which lends the disparate material a degree of continuity is what Jenny Strauss Clay has called 'the education of Perses'. If followed in a linear fashion, the advice given to Perses seems to indicate that he gradually learns from his brother, and changes his behaviour incrementally, meeting goals along the way. Keith Oatley argues of ancient literature that "The first literary characters have traits, very much like personality traits in psychology or reputations in the minds of others: more-or-less unchanging dispositions".[20] Perses certainly has traits, and more specifically flaws as his main role is to act as the negative exemplar with the bad reputation.[21] However, as Clay has shown, he *can* be taught: perhaps Oatley underestimates these 'first literary characters'. Further, Oatley (drawing on Auerbach's *Mimesis*) identifies Dante as "the first writer to depict character in the modern sense", isolating as an important move in European literature the fact that "He transfers action and truth from heaven ... to here on earth. The idea

---

[17] Cf. Berkenkotter's category V.B 'Directly addressing audience in text'.
[18] This addressing of (at least) two audiences fits another of the 'Miscellaneous Audience-related Activities' under Berkenkotter's section V.
[19] See e.g. Latimer (1930); Forbes (1950); Griffith (1983).
[20] Oatley (2011) 89.
[21] On the development of Perses over the course of the poem, see Canevaro (2015) 26–29; on autobiography Canevaro (2015) 41–43, Canevaro (2017); on the importance of the brother-to-brother didactic model for Hesiod's particular project, Canevaro (2017).

of character is not of people whose traits of personality remain unexplained, or of fate which cannot be apprehended. It's of people appraising events for their emotional implication and, as a result, acting on matters that are important to them here on earth." Laying aside the difficulty of terms such as 'writer' and 'literature', that, I would argue, is exactly what the *Works and Days* is all about. Perses' traits are explained: we are told what he has done wrong, why he has done it and what he needs to change to do better. Iron-Age matters take centre stage, with earth-dwelling mortals left for the most part to their own devices, to make their own fate through justice or injustice. Truth is transferred from heaven to earth in line 10:

Ζεὺς ὑψιβρεμέτης ὃς ὑπέρτατα δώματα ναίει.

κλῦθι ἰδὼν ἀιών τε, δίκῃ δ' ἴθυνε θέμιστας

τύνη· ἐγὼ δέ κε Πέρσῃ ἐτήτυμα μυθησαίμην.

Zeus the high-thunderer who lives in the highest halls.

Listen to me, seeing and hearing, and you: make laws straight with justice.

But I shall tell true things to Perses.

Works and Days 8–10

The juxtaposition "you: I" (τύνη· ἐγώ) contrasts Zeus' job which has been prescribed in the previous line (to straighten out the laws) with Hesiod's own, essentially didactic, task: to tell his brother some home truths. Whether Perses is real or fictional, Hesiod is adamant about the truth of his teachings, and this sets the tone of his didactic authority. Oatley writes: "It takes a certain generosity to engage with a new person. In the same way, it takes a certain generosity to enter into a relationship with a poem ... One needs to trust the author".[22] Already here in the proem of the *Works and Days* Hesiod sets out his goals as teacher, plans for and names a specific audience, and by invoking truth gains the trust of internal and external audience alike. One of Berkenkotter's sub-categories is "Representing oneself to the audience (*persona*)": from this early point in the poem Hesiod establishes an authoritative, independent didactic persona, promising to sing a song tangential to that of the Muses,[23]

---

[22] Oatley (2011) 100–101.
[23] On the Muses' song as tangential to Hesiod's own, see Clay (2003) 72–78; Haubold (2010) 21. On the contrasting Homeric model of poet's and Muses' voices blending, see Graziosi/Haubold (2010) 1–8.

to tackle a task different from that of Zeus, and to set his brother back on the straight and narrow.

Evaluating Content and Style with Regard to Anticipated Audience Response

This category, too, might be approached in terms of truth. Oatley writes: "Modern psychology as science has allied itself with only one kind of truth: truth as empirical correspondence ... If psychology is to be fully psychology, there must be consideration of two other kinds of truth as well: truth as coherence within complex structures and truth as personal relevance. Empirical psychology obeys criteria of the first type of truth. Fiction fails this criterion but can meet the other two. One could say, then, that fiction can be twice as true as fact".[24] This is a provocative statement, to say the least, but what I would take from it is to suggest that the *Works and Days* is psychologically ambitious as it tackles all three kinds of truth, and that it is these truths which create a strong "student-teacher constellation" (to use Katharina Volk's term).

Hesiod teaches us about the world as it is, describing the Iron-Age human condition so that we might face it. His truth must, therefore, have empirical correspondence: that is, it must reflect, more or less accurately, the perceivable state of things. One example of this is Hesiod's Calendar (383–617), and in particular Stephanie Nelson's reading of it.[25] This part of the poem is highly descriptive – so much so that sections of it, such as the passage on winter (493–563), have been considered by many scholars to be inconsistent with an ostensibly practical programme.[26] As Nelson has argued, through this description Hesiod presents us with a vivid picture of the seasonally revolving life on a farm and the importance of hard work at the right time, and on the winter passage she notes that "The length of the section reflects not how long the month of January is, but how long it seems to be. There is no task".[27] Hesiod shapes form to fit content, slowing the narrative pace to depict a season lacking in activity. This is a truth which reflects poetically and aesthetically a real-world empirical situation. Another example is Hesiod's penchant for hyper-precision, most evident in his description of

---

24 Oatley (1999) 102–103.
25 Nelson (1996) and (1998).
26 Most nineteenth century editors rejected the winter passage. See further Canevaro (2015) 73–75.
27 Nelson (1996) 50.

woodcutting (414–447).²⁸ In contrast to the winter passage, the woodcutting scene is full of hands-on advice and minute technical detail.²⁹ Much scholarly attention has been given to assessing whether or not the woodcutting is feasible.³⁰ However, as with the debate over Perses, I would argue that what matters is that through such hyper-precision Hesiod emphatically presents us with a kind of truth: this time not autobiographical, but empirical.

I would like to consider the second type of truth, "coherence within complex structures", in terms of how it is mobilised at a structural level through the arrangement of the *Works and Days*. The poem is made up of a multitude of narrative forms such as myths, fables, proverbs, riddles, precepts and calendars. The complex structure does, however, have an internal coherence, and it is this which an audience must work to uncover. Form maps onto content, as poetic structures teach us about the complexity of human existence. With each narrative form comes a different narrative strategy: some tell stories, some inform, some persuade (or dissuade) – some provide a puzzle. Berkenkotter found that "The writers who verbalized the goal of *persuading* their audience exhibited the greatest frequency and widest distribution of audience-related activities ... In contrast, the writers who decided to *narrate* their personal history showed the lowest frequency and narrowest distribution ... Writers who opted to *inform* fell somewhere in the middle of the spectrum".³¹ The type of narrative strategy adopted affects consideration of one's audience. By combining narrative forms and their associated strategies, Hesiod does not limit himself to a small number of audience-related activities but is more likely to engage with the full range.

Each shift in narrative form comes as a novelty: a new generic challenge to which we have to adjust. Research on story comprehension reveals that cognitive processing load is greatest at the beginning and end of a story episode,³² so when Hesiod introduces a ἕτερόν (…) λόγον at line 106 he is presenting his audience with a heavy cognitive task:

εἰ δ' ἐθέλεις, ἕτερόν τοι ἐγὼ λόγον ἐκκορυφώσω,

εὖ καὶ ἐπισταμένως, σὺ δ' ἐνὶ φρεσὶ βάλλεο σῇσιν,

---

28 On Hesiod's hyper-precision, see Canevaro (2015) 202–208.
29 The woodcutting section has often been criticised for a level of detail that might be considered tedious. However, see Minchin (2001) 79–91 for the cognitive underpinning of lists, and the pleasure an audience might take in such feats of poetic memory.
30 For reconstructions see West (1978) *ad loc.*; Richardson/Piggott (1982); Isager/Skydsgaard (1992) 6–9; Leclerc (1994); Tandy/Neale (1996) 99–103.
31 Berkenkotter (1981) 393.
32 Haberlandt/Berian/Sandson (1980).

> If you wish, I shall summarise another story for you,
>
> well and skillfully, and you take it to heart.
>
> *Works and Days* 106–107

Hesiod himself flags up the value of this shift for the need for cognition, as the line begins εἰ δ' ἐθέλεις, if you wish: he will present his audience with another story, but only if they are up for the challenge. His teachings explicitly require active engagement on the part of the audience. That the correspondences between the ἕτερόν (...) λόγον, that is the Myth of the Races, and the story preceding, the Myth of Prometheus and Pandora, are not immediately evident adds further weight to the process. As our text of the *Works and Days* now stands, this nod to audience participation is crystallised as a rhetorical and didactic device. However, in a context of oral performance we might imagine that such invitations had something genuine in them: perhaps the performer would have taken his cues from the audience and in each instance chosen selectively from a broader repertoire. In particular, we might consider scenes like that of woodcutting in this light: perhaps the performer would have judged the audience's attention span and edited accordingly. This hypothesis conforms with Berkenkotter's fourth category, that of "reviewing, editing, and revising for a specific audience". This is not a category with which we can fully engage in terms of the text as we have it, now a *fait accompli*, but it may apply to an oral poem kept fluid in performance.

The third truth, "personal relevance", takes us to Hesiod himself as immanent narrator. In integrating autobiographical elements – anecdotes from his own life, personal interjections, characters such as his foolish brother Perses and their downtrodden father – Hesiod constructs a personal 'hook' on which we can hang his teachings. The audience will remember and reuse snippets from the *Works and Days* not only because of their mnemonic formulations and wide applicability, but also because of their personality. This taps into another modality of memory: episodic memory which is autobiographical in nature, connected with where we were when we heard something, who told us it, and so on. An immanent narrator is important in giving us that episodic backdrop. Schwartz and Power (2000) argue, further, that the memorisation of maxims more often results in adopting wise behaviour when those maxims are taught within the context of a meaningful relationship with a teacher. Therefore the present persona of Hesiod-as-teacher aids not only rote memorisation, but also enactment.

Furthermore, Hesiod sets us an example of thinking for oneself. He rewrites the genealogy of Eris, Strife, which in the *Theogony* was but one:

οὐκ ἄρα μοῦνον ἔην Ἐρίδων γένος, ἀλλ' ἐπὶ γαῖαν

εἰσὶ δύω· τὴν μέν κεν ἐπαινήσειε νοήσας,

ἡ δ' ἐπιμωμητή· διὰ δ' ἄνδιχα θυμὸν ἔχουσιν.

There was not only one race of Strifes on the earth,

but there are two. One a man would praise having seen her,

the other is blameworthy. They have completely different spirits.

Works and Days 11–13

In this and in many other ways, Hesiod self-consciously breaks away from his own *Theogony*. In the *Works and Days* Hesiod recasts his relationship with the Muses, refines his moral landscape and refocuses his myths in order to mark out the poem as a new, independent didactic project – and himself a new, independent man. This is one way in which Berkenkotter's fourth category "Reviewing, Editing, and Revising for a Specific Audience" might be seen to apply, not to the *Works and Days* in isolation but to the Hesiodic *corpus* more widely.[33] The 'revising' Hesiod does takes place in the space between his poems, as he shifts genre, purpose, and persona.[34] Further, in setting himself up as a model, Hesiod not only epitomises the self-sufficient πανάριστος, but also initiates a self-sufficient mode of learning. He teaches not by prescription but by example – and it is up to the audience to follow that example.[35] Horn and Masunaga (2000) posit that wisdom is not merely an intellectual capacity, but also involves expertise. From this perspective, Hesiod is an ideal teacher as he has practiced what he is preaching.

Brown formulates the issue in another way, suggesting that wisdom is 'more broadly encompassing than expertise. Thus, one might seek the advice of a person one considers wise even within a domain in which this person has no previous direct experience ... The wise person is able to see the essence of the problem and suggest meta-strategies for what one should do.'[36] Hesiod embarks on his teachings on seafaring with a caveat:

δείξω δή τοι μέτρα πολυφλοίσβοιο θαλάσσης,

οὔτε τι ναυτιλίης σεσοφισμένος οὔτε τι νηῶν·

οὐ γάρ πώ ποτε νηί γ' ἐπέπλων εὐρέα πόντον,

---

[33] This corpus-wide approach to Hesiodic poetry is advocated most importantly in Clay (2003).
[34] On genre in the *Works and Days*, see Canevaro (2014).
[35] See further Canevaro (2015) 99–114.
[36] Brown (2000) 194.

> εἰ μὴ ἐς Εὔβοιαν ἐξ Αὐλίδος, ᾗ ποτ' Ἀχαιοί
>
> μείναντες χειμῶνα πολὺν σὺν λαὸν ἄγειραν
>
> Ἑλλάδος ἐξ ἱερῆς Τροίην ἐς καλλιγύναικα.
>
> I shall show you the measure of the resounding sea,
>
> though I am experienced in neither seafaring nor ships.
>
> **For I have never yet crossed the wide sea in a ship,**
>
> **except to Euboea from Aulis, where once the Achaians,**
>
> **waiting out the winter, gathered a great host to sail**
>
> **from holy Greece to Troy of beautiful women.**
>
> *Works and Days* 648–653

He admits that he knows little about seafaring, which creates a paradox of the teacher ignorant of what he is teaching. Hesiod's ability to teach about seafaring, then, comes from two sources: the Muses (upon whom he calls at 658–662), and his didactic prowess in analogous matters (namely agriculture). As Hesiod is not experienced in seafaring, he is not depending on procedural memory here, on a skill that has become unconscious. Rather, he uses declarative memory in a very conscious way, combining episodic elements (his short trip from Aulis to Euboea) with semantic information gleaned from his divine teachers and his own ability to extrapolate from other spheres of activity. This has two effects, one related to the content of his teachings and the other to the way in which he conveys this content. First, the degree of distance between teacher and subject matter marked by this emphasis on declarative rather than procedural memory highlights a particular thread that runs throughout the poem: Hesiod's mistrust of seafaring.[37] It is presented as a necessary evil: a supplement to agriculture but not a satisfactory alternative. Hesiod's and Perses' father, forced to take to the seas, is the example not to follow. Second, by marking this out as conscious rather than unconscious knowledge, Hesiod gives his audience a way into his teachings. He does not present a skill which is habitual to him, the process of skill acquisition taken for granted. Rather, Hesiod's admission of ignorance frames this section as a test case for his didactic method. He will set an example for his audience, overcoming his ignorance by thinking for himself (the πανάριστος, using his knowledge of analogous matters) and by taking advice (the ἐσθλός,

---

[37] For more on Hesiod and seafaring in the *Works and Days*, see Rosen (1990); Canevaro (2015) 127–133.

listening to the Muses). Furthermore, in applying knowledge from one field to another he proves his credentials as 'meta-strategizer'.

Gestalt: the Parts and the Whole

Nagler (1978) argued that Homeric type scenes are "an inherited preverbal Gestalt for the spontaneous generation of a 'family' of meaningful details": in other words that the intrinsic whole is embedded *in nuce* in every extraction. I would like to end this chapter by suggesting that the basic underlying idea of Gestalt psychology, namely that the whole is more than the sum of its parts, is something with which Hesiod's *Works and Days* has an affinity on a structural and conceptual level. This takes us back to the initial dichotomy I made between modes of reading the poem – linear and excerpting. In the former, parts are put together to make one coherent poem. However, models of circumstantial development such as Lamberton's (1988) idea of a "string of beads" which stem directly from tradition underestimate the overarching didactic force of the whole. To a certain extent, the *Works and Days* is the product of a pre-existing tradition, but this does not mean that the elements came together as a natural progression of the tradition. As Lardinois (2005) has persuasively argued, Greek proverbial expressions functioned like a hexameter line in an epic performance: stemming from a thematic core and made up of traditional formulae, they could be simultaneously both traditional and newly created. The arrangement of the *Works and Days* as we now have it seems the work of one person with a strong authorial voice and moral direction – or at least one didactic strategy maintained so as to appear to be the work of one person.[38] Each element, whether traditional or not, is selected with regard to the poem's overarching themes and tethered either by a contextualising line or by reference to a character or *topos* of the *Works and Days*.[39] The consistent moral impetus of the poem and the immanent persona of the narrator combine to tether these traditional building blocks together into something more.

---

[38] I have argued at Canevaro (2015) 34–35 that there is a guiding intentionality behind the *Works and Days* – whether or not that force is singular, and called Hesiod. Questions of composition and reception work in tandem here: whilst I explore instances of the poem's reception in Chapter 1 of Canevaro (2015), in Chapter 2 I argue that the seeds of this reception are to be found in the poem itself. In terms of psychology, the introduction of Gestalt theory into the analysis highlights this interaction as it raises issues both of intentionality (the constructed whole, which is echoed in parts) and reception (tracing back to the intended whole from the part).
[39] For more on tethering in the *Works and Days* see Canevaro (2015) 31–82.

In the excerpting reading, just like type scenes, the audience awareness devices I have discussed in this chapter embed the whole poem, its moral impetus and its didactic authority, into excerpts too. The most notable example of this is what I have called elsewhere the Hesiod stamp, the persona of the narrator, which guides our use and reuse of whatever elements we might detach from the poem.[40] Hesiod's teachings are formulated in an open and applicable way so that they can be reused in various circumstances, but because they were once part of Hesiod's project and retain something of his poetic authority even when detached, they are not open to *all* meanings. Hesiod wants everyone to learn something from his poem, but his message is not morally indeterminate. Components of the *Works and Days* may have begun as traditional precepts, but after circulating as part of the poem they become Hesiodic wisdom and acquire the authority associated with the poet. At work here are two related cognitive strategies. On the one hand, there is the cognitive ideals hypothesis, which argues that detachable didactic elements such as proverbs are designed to evoke universal standards, norms and ideals irrespective of the pragmatic particulars of their use.[41] This explains how these elements can be plucked from the tradition for reuse – and rendered again reusable by Hesiod. Honeck argues that "When all of the examples have faded from memory, the proverb emerges as a kind of ruin that symbolizes their passing".[42] From this perspective, proverbs and maxims find their cognitive value in abstraction, as it is in that way that they get into long-term memory. It is in this way, too, that they operate in later reception, and indeed this begins to explain the relevance we still find in ancient wisdom.[43] On the other hand, by activating episodic memory, the Hesiod stamp holds together, either in one place or in a wider network of receptions, the "miscellaneous and contrary urges" Nisbet writes about.

The founding fathers of Gestalt psychology emphasized the difference between pieces and parts, with Wertheimer (1923) arguing that parts are not primary, not pieces to be combined in and-summations, but parts of wholes. Whereas a piece is any random section and may not have meaning in and of itself, a part is part of a whole and, if the whole is sensible, each part must have a sensible interpretation. Hesiod's *Works and Days*, in its diversity of narrative forms and the individual cognitive challenges they pose, naturally falls into parts – but these parts are coloured by the whole, which in turn is shaped by the poet's persona.

---

40 On the Hesiod stamp see Canevaro 2015 (43–50). On Hesiodic reception e.g. Boys-Stones/Haubold (2010), Koning (2010), Hunter (2014), Van Noorden (2014).
41 Honeck (1997) 27.
42 Honeck (1997) 97–98.
43 See Honeck (1997) 36 on the universalist stance of the cognitive view.

Brown writes: "when adding together various contributions to wisdom, we must keep in mind that as an emergent property wisdom is, by definition, more than the sum of its constituent parts".[44] The interplay between parts and whole which is so central to Gestalt psychology and which Brown shows to be characteristic of 'wisdom' (whatever we take that to mean exactly) is key to the complex structure of Hesiod's *Works and Days*, the explicit and implicit audiences it targets, and the reuses and receptions it generates. Minchin comments on the relevance of Nagler's argument to the cognitive sciences: "Although Nagler declared that his reconstruction of composition was "highly speculative", cognitive research ... offers the necessary theoretical underpinning for his proposals; his pre-verbal Gestalt is no more and no less than the cognitive scientist's script".[45] The teachings Hesiod offers, too, operate as a cognitive script. On one level the *Works and Days* is an 828-line poem, which takes us from the mythical past to the present day, from cosmic considerations to details of bodily functions, through the education of Perses and of ourselves alongside him. On another level, however, the *Works and Days* is made up of parts: parts which can be detached and reapplied. These parts, in retaining something of the whole, provide cognitive schemata, teaching us how to think, how to act, how to learn – in accordance with the wider aims of the poem with which they are associated. However, in making his audience work for their lesson, Hesiod prevents such schemata from becoming habitual or automatic. The cognitive challenges presented by the *Works and Days* engage our executive functions, keeping us on our toes. Hesiod anticipates multiple audiences – and he anticipates that these audiences will find in his poetry something to satisfy their Need for Cognition.

---

44 Brown (2000) 311.
45 Minchin (2001) 40.

Marcia Dobson
3 Why Does Orestes Stay Mad?

Aeschylus' *Oresteia* has been a passion of mine ever since graduate school. I wrote my Ph.D dissertation on Oracular Language in The Delphic Oracles and Aeschylus, believing that the dense metaphorical imagery of the *Agamemnon* was a new phenomenon not previously seen in Greek works, which expressed the emergence of the symbolic in language and hence created the possibility for the internalisation of a coherent self. That is, the language of this play embodies a movement away from external forces of destiny, observed through signs, omens, and oracles, and towards a realisation that the exterior world actually represents an interior psychic space. Aeschylus' *Agamemnon*, then, forms a bridge between what we know as conscious and unconscious perception by creating a vital and accessible preconscious world through complex ambiguities of language that remain fully present and perceptible throughout this first play of his Trilogy.[1]

But I never was able to comprehend the second two plays of the Trilogy as leading to a successful reconciliation of the world of familial and talionic law with the Athenian civic state. In the *Eumenides*, in particular, the highly rhetorical and legalistic forms of discourse seemed incapable of encompassing the depths of the psyche in the same way as did the grand overarching symbols of the *Agamemnon*, and hence could not address the psychic tension underlying Orestes' presumed cure from madness through purification and acquittal. Orestes, in the context of the courtroom, appeared to me a pawn of Apollo's, seen by the Furies as a new-fangled Olympian god ungrounded in natural law,[2] whose raison d'etre is to further the ideology of a new civic paternalism. Orestes acts with ambivalence and compliance rather than with passion and agency in murdering his mother.[3] Indeed, Orestes is so reticent about committing this heinous act that it is his virtually mute companion Pylades, in his only line in the whole tragedy, who has to tell him to remember the threats of Apollo and to carry out his commands.

> Orestes' passive obedience to the will of Apollo strongly contrasts with the murderous passions spurring his parents' crimes. Although, like Agamemnon, Orestes has an impossible

---

[1] See Dobson (1976) and Lebeck (1971).
[2] *Eum.*778–779 and 808–809.
[3] Wilamowitz and Zeitlin confirm the above argument. See however Garvie (1986) xxxi; Lloyd Jones (1970) 32 n. 408 for opposing views.

Marcia Dobson, Colorado College

https://doi.org/10.1515/9783110482201-011

choice to make, for he will suffer in either killing or not killing Clytemnestra, as Agamemnon would have whether or not he had killed Iphigeneia, Agamemnon commits an impious act of violence against his own willingly, to satisfy the blood lust of the Greeks to fight and to be victorious in the Trojan war.[4] Clytemnestra goes even further in considering herself not just a mortal queen, but in taking on the persona of an Erinyes, appearing as an embodiment of fate (Moira) itself. In short, Orestes strikes me as a beleaguered, deeply ambivalent son in a double bind, who obediently trusts the command of a patriarchal god representing a new patriarchal world. Indeed, in the presence of the Furies in the first scene of the Eumenides, Orestes' madness appears a result of being unable to escape. He himself is a hunted animal,[5] and there is no final catharsis, unless one identifies purification by Apollo, and acquittal of murder by the Areopagus as such. But these acts appear to be a rational solution absent of divine or ritual elements. The persuasive and charming language of Athena, the great balancer, through which she convinces the Furies to give up their infernal powers and sends them gloriously underground as "Semnai Theai", may provoke a dramatic sense of ritual release in the Athenian audience, allowing them to experience emotionally and persuasively the transition from an older familial order to a new civic world.[6] But even if this is so, Orestes is still left to wander this world as a madman in the dramas of Sophocles and Euripides, neither of whom pay the least heed to Aeschylus' solution in the Eumenides, a solution that is in large part an attempt to exemplify the glory of Athens and its friendly alliance with Argos by re-instating Orestes as prince of his domain, as well as to instantiate the power of the Court of the Areopagus.[7]

One could perhaps infer that Orestes is himself an adolescent on the verge of manhood, an *ephebe*, as Winkler has argued in relation to Greek tragic choruses, and consider that Orestes' ordeal constituted an initiation into manhood and the state, extricating him from his mother's robes and coils.[8] Harrison, in her explication of traditional rites of tribal initiation in her book *Themis*, might agree.[9] If so, we end up with an Orestes tried, tested and purified by an idealized paternalistic god Apollo, nobly having done the right thing in murdering his mother to exonerate his blood father Agamemnon. That his mother, Clytemnestra, is also his blood relation is the agonised charge of the Furies, but this is swiftly discounted by Apollo's legal claim from apparent precedent that Athena had no mother, and was born solely from her father Zeus. That Zeus swallowed Metis, who was

---

[4] *Ag.* 218–221. For Orestes, see Winnington/Ingram (1983) 82–83, 96–97; Vernant (1990).
[5] Cf. Thomson (1941/1980) 260–265, esp. 263: "Orestes is prostrate with terror and fatigue, like a hare (l. 326) that cowers motionless as the hounds close in for the kill."
[6] Seaford understands the final journey of the "Semnai" as a kind of mystical redemption following earlier patterns of comparison with the Eleusinian mysteries. See Seaford (2012) Ch. 2 and esp. Ch. 15, 273.
[7] See Sommerstein (2010).
[8] Winkler (1992) 20–62.
[9] Harrison (1927/1962) Chs. 1–3.

pregnant with Athena inside of him and gave secondary birth through his head, as the "divinely inspired" Hesiod says in the *Theogony*, is a curious complexity that is suppressed by Aeschylus, and apparently brooks no authority with the Areopagus – best to forget it. Clytemnestra herself is a mere basket and therefore not related to her son by blood. And so Orestes is exonerated and acquitted.

I find this solution to Orestes' crime a cover-up of mythopoeic traditions that cannot possibly have been convincing to the contemporary Athenian audience. Despite the claims made by some scholars that the going medical understanding at the time was that the female contributed no part of herself to her offspring, I do not for a moment think the Athenian audience would have bought into the notion that Clytemnestra was not Orestes' mother, nor would they have been incognisant of the fact the Zeus swallowed Metis to produce Athena.[10] So what was this divergence of Aeschylus from the standard tradition meant to do? Can we assume anything other than that this was his own gloriously ideological hope for the transformation of Athens, or more darkly, a riff on the very possibility of such transformation? Or, somehow, both?[11]

I am equally disturbed by the beginning of the *Eumenides* when I hear that Phoebe gave Phoebus Apollo jurisdiction over the Delphic Oracle as a gift, and the story of his killing of the Python to win it is suppressed entirely.[12]

Surely, an author who can use such profound symbolic language to express the depths of the human psyche as it is revealed in the *Agamemnon* is conscious of this propagandistic revision of the myth, and wants us to be as well? Or does he just want us to situate ourselves in the complexities of the social dilemmas of the time? Looked at from the perspective of symbolic layering, we can in fact apprise that Apollo, in directing his arrows at the Furies in the beginning of the *Eumenides*, is carrying out a variation of the act of killing the Python right in front

---

[10] As for the physiological argument, see Winnington–Ingram (1983) 123: "Such a doctrine ... might be welcomed in a masculine society as a counterpoise to the manifest uncertainty of fatherhood. For, if one thing is sure, it is that the mother carries and bears the child, and the intimacy of this relationship confirmed by instinct and emotion."

[11] Cf. Winnington/Ingram (1983) 126: "(Athena is) a god/goddess to Clytemnestra's man–woman, and her masculinity wins her praise and worship, while that of Clytemnestra leads to disaster for herself and others. There is thus a bitter irony, when the goddess, who in all things commends the male and is free to exercise her preference in action, condemns the woman of manly counsel for seeking the domination which her name demanded."

[12] Cf. Harrison (1927/1962) 385. That Apollo was given possession of Delphi by his sister Phoebe as a birthday present (γενέθλιον δόσιν) is not recorded anywhere else in the literature, to the best of my knowledge, and would hence surprise and confuse the Athenians' understanding of their own myths. See Sommerstein (1989) 80–81.

of us, even as the speech of the Oracle proclaims the opposite story. If that is the case, then we are meant to hold this opposition, as well as to understand that Apollo, although he might seem to represent the new Olympian order, is just as closely bound to the talionic law that the Furies represent. Indeed, his request for Orestes to kill his mother is based on this very law, and the way he argues in the court scene is as black and white as that of the Furies in terms of its criteria for judgement and condemnation.[13]

Ritual Views

As my readings of Greek tragedy deepened through psychoanalytic studies, I became aware that the horrific and highly psychosomatic descriptions of the sicknesses that Apollo says Orestes will suffer, whichever choice he makes, hold further implications that consist in the seeming impotence of a patriarchal and democratically just system to heal blood feud and personal agony. Aeschylus' *Eumenides* leaves Orestes acquitted by the *polis* and reinstated at Argos at the end, but his insanity continues in the dramatic mythical consciousness of the Greeks in the remaining extant plays of Sophocles, Euripides, and is mentioned twice in Aristophanes, as well in many of the lost plays, of which a number apparently were devoted to the Orestes/Electra myth.[14] It is this that drew me to explore Orestes continued madness.[15]

A major issue here concerns the symbolic and ritual atmosphere from which many of our tragic heroes drew suffering and sustenance, and which in turn

---

13 The structure of ambivalence that pervades the *Oresteia* is well demonstrated in Winnington-Ingram's (1983) understanding of Apollo as himself torn between earlier and later forms of law. This ambivalence is clearly visible in this scene where Apollo is stretched between embodying the talionic law and advocating through the Oracle's speech a possible new and forward temporal movement. See Goldhill (1984) 208–209. Seaford (2012) makes the claim that the Apollo of *Choephori* is different from the Apollo of *Eumenides*, where he becomes a genuine figure of the Olympian order. I agree that he may stand out as such a figure in the courtroom drama because he serves as a foil for the Furies. But he nevertheless plays their game, and uses their form of legal argument. If we conceive all major symbolic themes to open up into human action in this Trilogy, then one could imagine Orestes as the mortal (and hence less powerful) Apollo. He receives Apollo's horned bow as a gift, together, perhaps, with his winged, flashing snake-like arrows (*Eum.* 180–181). Orestes and Apollo in their dealings with the infernal powers absorb Erinyes-like features and become themselves avengers.
14 Rein (1954) 4.
15 Note, however, that there are extra-dramatic sources that speak of Orestes as cured from madness. For the Orestes myth through the Greek period, see Sommerstein (2010) 1–6.

brought the audience to experience catharsis, as if caught up in a ritual dance of death and rebirth. Despite the fact that Cornford's ritual theory of Greek tragedy has long since been discredited, there is no doubt that ritual moments in Greek tragedy are profoundly important. Jane Ellen Harrison, in her brilliant book *Themis*, suggests that in ritual cultures what people regard as "sacred," basically that which gives them power to survive in a world of bare subsistence, such as their tools, and those mana-filled animals sacred to the tribe that get eaten, eventually evolve into anthropocentric form as gods with magical tools and animal accoutrements. Despite Harrison's Darwinian overtones, it is reasonable to suppose that we worship what we create in order to sustain ourselves and to give us power, and that our early sense of connection with the earth, in which we experience ourselves as not yet individuated selves removed from nature, creates ruptures, because we must kill what we love and are connected with in order to survive. It is this rupture that causes us to sacrifice and to resurrect that which we have destroyed as sacrament into a new semblance of unity.[16]

This same mentality is evident in the character of Clytemnestra who believes, in her distinctive persona as the Head of the Furies, that she will purify the land of evil if she can sacrifice her "bull" husband (as Cassandra later calls him) to the earth, to bring rebirth to the royal house. In persuading Agamemnon to choose to walk on the royal tapestries, a sacrilegious and hubristic act, and then exclaiming that as she killed him his blood fell on her like the drops of dew that bring up the crops in the springtime,[17] the Athenians likely are reminded of the Bouphonia, in which an ox is lured to the altar by his own choice to sample the barley, purposely put there, and then chosen as the divine object to be slaughtered. The ox is slain because in 'choosing' to commit a ritually imposed sacrilegious act of eating off the altar, he becomes the 'chosen' one, who can then be stuffed and resurrected after a sacred meal so that the year can begin again.[18]

The problem with Clytemnestra is that she represents not only a divine personification of the dreaded and revered Furies, who live in a sacred and timeless space, but is also a legendary human figure with a name and a story. In this guise, she is personally vengeful, and the blood that forms this bloody birthgiving dew is no longer regenerative.[19] Rather, it is a deeply polluting sacrifice that will not

---

16 Simon (1978) 101–102 states that murder in the tragedies is typically framed in the language and imagery of a sacrifice. Every sacrifice is ambivalent, given that the attitude toward the victim is one of both love and aggression.
17 *Ag.* 1389–1393.
18 Harrison (1927[1962]) 142–150.
19 See Zeitlin (1965) 463–508.

end the royal stain of familial devouring and killing that has been inherent in this dynasty from the time of Kronos. In Aeschylus, Clytemnestra has become an individual with her own emotional resonances and moral ambiguities. This mimesis of the ritual, enacted not by a community but a single individual who is historical and legendary in time presents a transition in cultures, a horror show, and a polluted sacrifice that in its miasmic and ambiguous grandeur is reminiscent of earlier ritual. It is precisely because of this that it is dramatically cathartic.

Orestes, as suggested above, works outside of this ritual paradigm and hence seems quite diminished. The obvious presence of the Furies, Athena, and Apollo on a horizontal rather than a vertical plane brings the symbolic ambiguity of the grand metaphors of the *Agamemnon* into a lateral world that admits of no mystery, and certainly no grand ambiguity of language. The larger than life statue-like figures of Apollo and Athena, combined with their languages of legalism and persuasion, attain clarity here in a highly conscious and apparently rational and powerful discourse. What this clarity leads to, however, in the resolution of conflict, is madness, the kind of madness that occurs when a world dependent on ritual and polytheistic gods to order its psyche is relegated to an unconscious world of internalised, still conflicting forces that have no symbolic language to integrate them because they have been repressed by a new civic order, whose intent is to create a unified city-state dependent upon the conscience and responsibility of its male citizens. The workings of this system demand an acknowledged agentic self that feels itself less reliant on or controlled by familial or divine demands.

Oracular Language

One might ask more particularly at this point about the nature of the symbolic language in the *Agamemnon* that is lost in the *Eumenides*, and why it is necessary to maintain it for the sake of the coherence and sanity of Orestes. Much oracular language, that is, the language of the Delphic Oracle, is constructed in oppositional linguistic formulas. [20] This kind of oppositional language is taken up in Aeschylus as expressing grand themes in the *Agamemnon*. Oppositional images, such as dark and light, are bound together in the frameworks of the language itself, and hence seem to bind the characters of the drama to unending oscillations of

---

[20] Oracular language and style have set formulas, which grant assurance of the holding of opposites and triadic forms. This style sets the language in much of the Agamemnon. See Dunbar-Soule (1976) *passim*.

retributive justice with no forward movement, and no transgression of the laws of vengeance and revenge. The blood stays clotted to the ground, and there is neither procession of generations, nor the flexibility of judgement such as comes to the fore in the court trial of the *Eumenides*. Seaford and others understand that if one can get out of this binding of oppositions, one can begin to move forward into a new world.[21] However, if one loses the opposition altogether, resting on one side or the other of an argument (e.g. the freeing of Orestes from matricide because he is not a blood son of his mother, or the movement of the Erinyes from evil and good spirits to only good spirits), the metaphorical language that holds the oppositions itself becomes lost. The result is a collapse of sign and signified, what psychoanalysts call "primary process", not yet fully understood as "secondary process", that is, the process through which one can appreciate and interpret the metaphor inherent in the language of dream, myth, or omen. If one does away with this metaphorical language all together, then there is no possibility for one to move from unconscious to conscious interpretations in a way that can promote meaning, and one remains lost in psychotic fantasy that is impenetrable by rational discourse.

The quality of a metaphorical language that rises above human acts by portraying them in symbol, as omen, holds together ambivalence in that, as Lebeck says, in speaking what is to come through omen, the old men of Argos know and do not know what they are saying at one and the same time, "for the language of prophecy knows no sharp distinction between symbol and thing symbolized, between effect and cause".[22] The universal symbol points to a larger collective realm of repetitive fated acts seen as demanded by gods who always, in ancient Greek tragedy, appear to hold together irreconcilable opposites. Moreover, the old men state that Artemis looks upon the omen of the eagles and the hare and is infuriated with the very symbol that holds the fate of the family, as if the omen itself occurring in the sky is equated with the reality of what it symbolizes. This equation, in which symbol and symbolised become one, is seen and acted upon by a divine figure who herself exists on yet another plane of reality. In this way, the actual world has become the dream, and dream/omen/collective symbol that represents the acts of the family attains the level of reality. One might then say that in the *Oresteia*, "realities" are layered and confused in a predictably psychotic way. Simon affirms this when he says: "if the causes of madness could be

---

[21] Seaford (2012) Ch. 15c. Seaford's conceptualizing of the first two dramas of the Trilogy are based in Heraclitean thought, and the last one in Pythagorean thought bears careful reading and might indeed be a potent response to some of the arguments I present in this paper.
[22] Lebeck (1971) 35.

epitomized in a single sentence, it would be this: Madness comes from conflict." Along with conflict, ambivalence plays an important part. "Intense ambivalence is not necessarily located with the individual, but rather is embedded in the very fabric of the play".[23]

I agree with Seaford when he identifies the "coalescing of opposites" in the *Agamemnon* in its many forms as the problem that needs to open out into differentiation so that forward movement can occur. Indeed, such "psychotic" presentations of imagery in the *Oresteia* might lead us to be thankful for the legal and persuasive language of the *Eumenides*.[24] Nevertheless, Aeschylus' erasure of this kind of symbolic language in this last play of the trilogy disallows the possibility for mediating conflicts between conscious acts of will and unconscious forces. The traumatic forces of destiny and the maternal world expressed in the *Agamemnon* become thereby inaccessible, because they are repressed. Since symbolic process is here giving way to legalisms and 'charming' persuasion, the linguistic world that Aeschylus brings to presence in the *Agamemnon* fades away. This repression of language is part of the underbelly of the new democratic state, and it is what leaves Orestes unable to understand his own terrible ambivalence. Looking at the forms of oracular language extant in the *Oresteia*, one can see that opposition in its coalescent or concrete state makes for nothing but psychosis. But on the other hand, the dropping of oppositions entirely to formulate a new rational schema dispenses with a necessary balance of ambivalence that can hold people together if it is permitted to open into conscious, interpretive flow.[25]

If this is to be all solved by the mystical procession of the Eumenides, or "Semnai" at the end, revealing an ultimate Eleusinian-like redemption, then why is it that other authors do not accept Orestes himself as cured? Perhaps Aeschylus' desire is for a new, more civilized Athenian polis. But sadly, this has little to do with the world of Athens that is to come.

---

23 Simon (1978) 101.
24 Seaford (2012) 266.
25 Unless one continues to situate oneself in the language of paradox and ambiguity, there can be no sensed validity to determined resolutions. In analytic work, it makes no sense to analyse a dream as if it had a single or simple interpretation ungrounded in complex psychic forces, if one wishes for healing. The conflict of opposites must be maintained but in an atmosphere of the recognition and acceptance of both sides if there is to be forward progression. One cannot simply repress one side of discourse as Apollo does when he rejects the mother's part in birth, or Athena, when she, as a kind of empathic listener, coaxes the Furies to maintain only one side of a δίκη, that of blessing, relinquishing their power of cursing. It is this kind of move that produces heaven and hell, saints and sinners, rather than goddesses like Artemis whose function is both to protect and to destroy.

Unable to image the multiplicity of the psyche in the external world, in either the ritual or the metaphorical and symbolic world of Aeschylus' language in the *Agamemnon*, means that there is no more place for ritual catharsis to cleanse a populace, and no more language to hold conflict and ambivalence. This may service the new city state, but it also produces in the personage of Orestes the internal agony of a common, isolated individual trying to live in obedience to a new civic order and cut off at the root. Imagine, says Andre Green, how grand the audience felt looking at Clytemnestra arousing the bloody furies, as opposed to the Euripidean Orestes, lying on a bed (not yet a couch!) and hallucinating.

> I know that Euripides has shown us in Orestes his madness. But he is only showing us a dreamer lying on a bed ... subject to hallucinations which are not presented to us. Can we imagine how the Greek audience might have responded to the apparition of Clytemnestra's bloody ghost harshly awakening the black-garbed, snake-haired, gorgon-faced Furies? That was catharsis. A participation in a collective projective identification which could free the individual from its private monsters by a representation of collective exorcism.[26]

Psychoanalytic and Cultural Perspectives

This Euripidean Orestes arouses our interest and perhaps analytic curiousity, but is not cleansing or cathartic in the old sense. What Green is suggesting above is that by 413 B.C., the democratic project to eliminate the horrors of the world of talionic law by transforming the Furies into "Semnai Theai" and sending them to function as part of the legal apparatus of the Athenian Areopagus did not work. The world of family honor, reverence for the mother and family blood despite all its problems was not thereby erased, but disastrously sent underground. To put it succinctly, modern man was being born.

Given the fact that no time-honored Oracle, but only the all-too-human god Apollo destined Orestes' matricide, one might suspect that the advent of the patriarchy brings all this about in order to sanitize its own right to become a political state with a civic rather than a familial legal system. Given the repression and repudiation of the familial structure without integrating it (i.e. the man is the birthgiver, the woman is the basket, despite the new sanctity of marriage which indicates that is there is no equivalence of the parents even in the marriage vow), the Athenian audience at the beginning of its new progressive culture must have

---

[26] Green (1975) 355–364, at 362.

felt somewhat traumatized.[27] As C. Fred Alford states: "Did Aeschylus intend to leave his audience in doubt and confusion? .... Or did he in the end choose to reinforce the audience's manic defenses against their own doubts?" My own opinion is that there is not much difference between Aeschylus' resolution and the deus-ex-machina favored by Euripides. Both impose an actual resolution so implausible and unsatisfying that, quoting Alford again, "the psychological effect is more unsettling than cathartic".[28]

In Sophocles and Euripides Orestes is indeed a modern man. He is overcome with doubt and confusion, suffers existential dread, and the horror of exile. He is perennially entering the stage from having been exiled, lost or orphaned. He is a wanderer, and when he arrives before us on the dramatic stage, he always seems, rather curiously, to be caught up suddenly in a hopelessly dangerous situation involving a woman. In the *Choephori*, it is first Electra who recognizes him and engages with him to kill Clytemnestra through the invocation of the ghost of Agamemnon, and then Clytemnestra herself. In Sophocles' *Electra*, Electra is demanding that Orestes kill their mother, needing him as a tool to do so. No divine causes are invoked; the only driving force is hatred. In Euripides' *Electra*, it is the same. Orestes is needed by Electra to perform a task about which he is hopelessly ambivalent. In Euripides' *Orestes*, Orestes takes responsibility for the murder and suffers profound guilt for it. It is this taking on of responsibility for his own suffering in his sane moments that is driving him mad. He still blames Apollo, but only when he is delusional.[29] Instead of appearing as an external physical punishment then, as in Aeschylus, Orestes' madness appears as internal and psychopathological. In Euripides' *Iphigeneia in Tauris*, Orestes arrives in Tauris only to find that it is a place where any intruder is doomed to be sacrificed, and learns that the sacrifice will be performed by his own sister, Iphigeneia, a priestess of Artemis. Orestes again becomes delusional, seeing a pursuing Erinys carrying his mother, and goes about madly slaughtering cattle, not unlike Ajax in Sophocles' play of the same name.[30] A deus-ex-machina is required to get him out of his fix.

Orestes' problem is always with women, behind whom lurk an absent and overarching father figure about whom he cannot really be sure. This Orestes is not a hero in the old grand sense, but an unfortunate victim with no giant forces in his world to make his actions either brave or glorious. Indeed, he appears eternally broken, driven and indecisive.

---

27 Wieland (1996) 300–313.
28 Alford (1996) 10.
29 Theodorou (1993) 32–46.
30 *IT*, 281–300.

What does this say about the grand event of the judging of the Areopagus and the creation of new laws, administered by the state, which in their creation of a democracy has presumably given to us a modern and just form of governance? Why does Orestes stay mad?

Melanie Klein's object-relations view on Orestes interprets that Apollo is a manifestation of Orestes' paranoid projections of his own rage against his mother, which he cannot tolerate because of his guilt, represented by the external Furies.[31] Klein also sees Orestes moving into a depressive position through the "good father" Zeus, and the "good mother" Athena, whom she understands as whole objects granting Orestes his own wholeness and integration through acquittal.[32] Klein's twentieth-century view makes sense, however, classicists will disagree with her, understanding that it is at this point in ancient Greek culture that the notion of a self with free will and conscience is just being formed. That is, there is nothing inside Orestes that is unconsciously driving him, as Aeschylus understands it. Rather his madness is expressed by external physical manifestations of the flesh, and appears to be a disease externally caused by the Gods. Further, even though the Furies are seen at times by no one but Orestes, as if they were nothing but hallucinations, they still exist on stage and in the eyes of the Greeks as divine and dreadful goddesses, manifestations of the talionic law.

But even if we can condone Klein's twentieth-century views of projection, projective identifications, and paranoid delusions, her view that Zeus and Athena are the good parents that send Orestes off into a settled, (if depressively ambivalent) restored, healed and socially re-integrated state, is simply mistaken. Orestes' "cure" comes perilously close to looking like "manic denial". It rings false, particularly in light of the fact that the collective mythic consciousness of the tragedians continues to see him and all matricides as having to suffer from insanity.[33]

---

31 In Klein/Segal (1997).

32 Klein identifies a number of developmental "positions" in the growth of the person. In the first, "paranoid/schizoid," the infant splits the parent into good and bad parts to protect itself from both inner and outer aggression. In the "depressive position" the child is able to accept the parent as a "whole object," as well as itself, and must therefore endure the ambivalence that comes with understanding that persons as well as itself contain both good and bad parts. Mourning accompanies this stage, as one "pines" for the all-good parent.

33 Please note that my interpretation of Aeschylus focuses on classicists using primarily classically psychoanalytic and object-relational views. They do not include Lacanian perspectives. However, were we to take such a perspective, we might interpret that the work of the first two plays is really to force Orestes to come to grips with his own (and everyone's) castration, marked by the impossibility of the "imaginary" phallus to yield a longed-for wholeness/completion. The final play pretty obviously offers "the name [*nom*] of the father" (aka "the law [*non*] of the father," the law symbolized as prohibition) as the "solution" to the recognition of castration, but

In Sophocles and Euripides, however, we are at a moment in Greek culture where there is a clear shift from outer to inner, exterior to interior. At first, visions are seen that no one else sees, and they come in the form of madness from the gods. But the gods soon become exterior manifestations of an unconscious that will be seen as an inner menace during the fifth century, and will then have to be extrapolated later through the psychoanalytic view of inner forces that get projected outwards as hallucinations. That is we are now fully anthropocentric, and therefore nothing inner appears as living gods that doom us from without. The gods we see have become hallucinatory projections of our inner states.

Alford raises a question that complicates and deepens this question of sanity in a world transitioning from familial to civic law.[34] He suggests that there is much fragility in an age when the belief in immortal familial gods is overridden by a political demand for belief in the effectiveness of the state and state gods. This transitional stage somehow needs to support the tender coming into consciousness of the individual who is attempting to develop a personal conscience and sense of choice and responsibility. As gods too are then gradually internalised, or even given up because they no longer have personal or familial connection or resonance, but are perhaps imbued primarily with state functions, the grounding of former traditional communities that worships agricultural rituals and feels close to the earth and its family gods can no longer serve as a stabilising force. Alford reminds us that "the family in the late fifth century was in a highly precarious situation, since Solon's reforms, among other things, removed judicial authority from the head of the family, the family had declined at the expense of the state".[35] He quotes Glotz, who says: "At one blow the family system was shattered, undermined at its very foundations. The state was placed in direct contact with individual ... Throughout the whole of the fifth century the last traces of family responsibility were being progressively abolished.[36]

I agree with Alford[37] that the attempt of the polis to take over the justice of the familial law and to create citizens of the state exacerbated the fragile self of the heroes, now having to move into a solely civic dramatic space. The threat of disintegration was great, as it reduced any stability or sense of continuity or

---

of course the "solution" is just as "imaginary" and "silly" as was the idea of wholeness that it attempts to replace. From this Lacanian view, the *Oresteia* is a powerful illustration of the basic tragedy that constitutes the human condition. (cf. Lee (1990) – personal communication)
34 See Alford (1992).
35 Alford (1992), 5.
36 Glotz (1929) 107 and 258; cf. Kovel (1988) 220. Vernant/Vidal-Naquet (1988) 33 note that Greek tragedy is all about heroic standards being subjected to those of the state.
37 See Alford (1996).

immortality they might have garnered through strong family and clan connections founded in the soil of their autochthonous gods and heroes, leaving them existentially destitute, and feeling perhaps like living dead. We must remember that there was no grand transcendence for the Greeks in the Homeric or the early Classical Age, hence perhaps the outcropping of hundreds of mystery cults, which tried to give some comfort against the unendingness of death. Such insecurity can give rise to madness.

In sum, Orestes appears to be an unfortunate victim of an age that was just coming into consciousness, but certainly not at all sure of itself or how to manage its own fragmentation. Where on the one hand the state became unified under its laws and therefore the individual citizen in agreeing with the laws could also feel some integration, the creation of self-consciousness and responsibility for one's own actions itself caused disruption, if not insanity.

In a larger and much more hypothetical world view, this lack of a satisfactory solution to matricide and the repression of familial law suggests that contemporary political societies who base their justification in civic law may indeed be glossing over repressed and unresolved conflicts that can hopefully be mitigated by psychoanalytic discourse. If this is so, then Orestes is symbolic victim left holding the bloody and matricidal murder weapon as a concrete symptom expressing the agony of what is repressed in the modern world. We might then say that the civic state is vulnerable to collapse, because it is constructed on the foundation of the Python, still rotting in the stream without being able to transform into good and fruitful compost, and that Orestes' act has left an emotional wound that renders both state and psyche volatile and prone to fragmentation and instability.

The *Oresteia* then might be thought to conclude with a victory cry or with a procession into an Eleusinian, mystical redemption, based in hope and longing alone, because there cannot but be an unsettling, unconscious sense that the grounds for the victory of the laws of the city state is founded on the loss of a language essential for psychic integration, creating thereby a new dark and disowned human unconscious, and built on the bones of matricide.

Kyle Khellaf
4 The Elegiac Revolution: Deleuze, Desire, and Propertius' *Monobiblos*

> "Indeed, what produces statements in each one of us is not ego as subject, it's something entirely different: multiplicities, masses and mobs, peoples and tribes, collective arrangements; they cross through us, they are within us, and they seem unfamiliar because they are part of our unconscious. The challenge for a real psychoanalysis, an anti-psychoanalytical analysis, is to discover these collective arrangements of expression, these collective networks, these peoples who are in us and who make us speak, and who are the source of our statements."
>
> – Gilles Deleuze, "Five Propositions on Psychoanalysis"[1]

Classical philology has often revealed a desire to retrace the ancient world and make it representationally whole again. While staring down the multi-millennial gap that supposedly separates today's philologists from the texts they study, we often imagine an absence or lack. Therefore, all the more readily do we view the classical canon as some ontologically stable entity, a corpus that is always-already, an ideal other yearning to be understood.

However, rather than accept these perspectives as a given, we can instead view them historically alongside hermeneutic threads that influenced our discipline. We would begin with Cartesian ontology premised upon the thinking subject, noting similarities with Richard Bentley's appeal to innate reason when editing texts.[2] We could also examine Linnaean classification and find it in "Lachmann's" taxonomical approach to stemmatics.[3] We might even see the empiricism of Leopold von Ranke encountering the Romantic idealism of the Hegelian subject striving for a differential unity when Theodor Mommsen attempted through autopsy to collate every known Latin inscription *in situ*.[4]

---

[1] Deleuze (2004) 275–276, hereafter abbreviated *DI*.
[2] His famous adage goes, "In my opinion, *both reason and the textual matter itself* (*nobis et ratio et res ipsa*) have more weight than a hundred manuscripts," in Bentley (1826) 228. Earlier, at p. 5, he warns: "Do not, therefore, do obeisance to the scribes alone, but *have the courage to think for yourself* (*sed per te sapere aude*)."
[3] For a useful overview to this deeply rationalist and scientific endeavor, see Most's introduction to Timpanaro (2005) 1–32.
[4] Mommsen gives an account of his painstaking process in *CIL* vol. 1, i–iv.

Kyle Khellaf, Yale University

https://doi.org/10.1515/9783110482201-012

If at present the field of classical studies seems excited by psychoanalysis, we must ask how this will aid us in unhinging our subject matter from its highly idealized status. We may unwittingly be augmenting our readings with theories that actually favor finitude and subject unity given their propensity to dehistoricize, mythologize, and oversimplify. Such was the assertion of the French philosopher Gilles Deleuze and his close colleague, the psychiatric revolutionary Félix Guattari, in *Anti-Oedipus*, their collaborative critique of psychoanalysis.[5] It rings particularly true for Roman elegy, a genre whose numerous voices strive to liberate their subject networks from narrow constructs of identity and to give open rein to their nomadic desires.

After all, over a century has elapsed since a Propertius going by the name of John Swinnerton Phillimore coined the axiom, *quot editores tot Propertii* – now taken to mean, "There are as many Propertiuses as there are editors of him".[6] James Butrica explains its transformation and afterlife.

> In its original context it described not an existing situation but rather the chaos that Phillimore alleged would result if editors began to adopt significant numbers of transpositions. Such chaos, however, does characterize the current state of Propertian studies; every interpreter seems to create a different Propertius, who in the last twenty-five years has been represented as a feminist, a neurotic traumatized by the siege of Perugia, an anti-Augustan iconoclast, an apostle of love oppressed by a quasi-Stalinist principate, a decadent pre-Raphaelite, and most recently as the 'modernist poet of antiquity'.[7]

Butrica's assessment suggests further inquiry. Must we really restrict Propertius to just one of these lives? If we postulate a schizophrenic Propertius, why not embrace them all? We could follow Deleuze's pivotal move in *Difference and Repetition* – not locating identity prior to external difference, but finding instead an internal, repeated difference presupposed and overshadowed by identity.[8] From there we can prioritize multiplicity over fixed ontology, becoming over being, the collective over the singular. Our guides in this endeavor form a long-awaited triumvirate: Deleuze himself, Guattari, and the poet Propertius in his innumerable iterations from antiquity to the present day.

This last member, unbeknownst to him, has been seeking out the other two for quite some time. As early as 1881, before the first Freudian intervention, John Percival Postgate asked, "These contrasts, these extravagancies, these fluctuations and incoherencies, these half-formed or misshapen thoughts, what do they signify?

---

5 Deleuze/Guattari (1983), hereafter abbreviated *AO*.
6 Phillimore (1901) *praef.* (unnumbered).
7 Butrica (1997) 176.
8 Deleuze (1994), hereafter abbreviated *DR*. For an overview, see the Preface, xix–xxii, and Introduction, 1–27. The importance of this concept for *AO* is explained in Holland (1999) 27.

What is the secret of this chaos?"[9] More recently, Micaela Janan has confirmed such suspicions.

> Out of that gap emerges elegy's schizoid subject, dramatizing fracture and upheaval in the cultural discourses that had previously offered less problematic self-confirmation in a more coherent world.[10]

Joseph Farrell agrees: "Elegy was, in other words, a hybrid genre if ever there was one".[11] While Hans-Peter Stahl observes,

> The idea of defining his own position in a multifarious environment is essential to the young poet, and, without showing ourselves receptive to the manifoldness of subjects actually presented in the *Monobiblos*, we cannot verify his intentions in designing the book.[12]

Cynthia Monobiblos, the title attributed to Propertius' first book of poems (meaning roughly, "Cynthia as single book"), is a deceitful misnomer.[13]

Such disarray need not vex readers always searching for cohesion. Nor should we tame its unbridled multiplicity using Freudian mythology or Lacanian metaphor, which, as Eugene Holland notes, "functions to capture and distort free-form desire in fixed images".[14] If anything, Propertian scholarship demonstrates that free-form desire is the lived reality of this poetic corpus. Every attempt to impose a static representation fails by stripping away countless layers of additional meaning. The history of its textual encounters, with each new readership on the threshold of interpretation, encompasses an ongoing series of Propertian becomings: Propertius-becoming-feminist ... becoming-neurotic ... becoming-iconoclast ... becoming-"the modernist poet of antiquity."

In the hopes of unhinging our classical subjects, this paper will schizoanalyze Propertius' *Monobiblos* and highlight the variations on desire which coexist at numerous levels of this textual corpus, from the poetic narratives themselves to their editorial rewritings. Guattari outlines the process.

> Schizoanalysis, rather than moving in the direction of reductionist modelisations which simplify the complex, will work towards its complexification, its processual enrichment, towards the consistency of its virtual lines of bifurcation and differentiation, in short towards its ontological heterogeneity.[15]

---

9 Postgate (1881) lxxii.
10 Janan (2012) 378.
11 Farrell (2003) 397.
12 Stahl (1985) 124.
13 The essential unity reading is given by King (1975–76).
14 Holland (1999) 98.
15 Guattari (1995) 61.

Just as readers have created a vast network of Propertiuses to match *their* desires, so too do the poems generate multiple voices with which our poet sorts through *his own*. Rather than delineate an ever-shifting organization, I instead highlight Propertius' struggles against such unity, notably the monogyny sought by his mistress Cynthia.

Since Judith Hallett's foundational essay, the elegiac mistress has been viewed as offering an alternative lifestyle to traditional Roman *mores*.[16] However, as Deleuze and Guattari elucidate, countercultural movements frequently become reterritorialized entities in the service of existing structures, especially where the unfixed axioms of capital serve as conduit.[17] This, I suggest, is exactly what Cynthia embodies, activating Propertius' productive desires only to withhold or restrict them, tyrannizing his amatory pursuits as the new Augustan trap. The *Monobiblos*, then, is an illustration of the poet's desiring-production in the face of this Cynthia without Organs (CwO),[18] his attempts to transform these drives from repressed, paranoid neuroses to liberated schizophrenic productions.[19]

Schizophrenic Syntheses: From Propertian Paranoia to De-subjected Desire

At the outset of the *Monobiblos*, the schizo begins to emerge. Cynthia awakens in Propertius an affective set of desires, only to repress them by pushing for primacy therein.

---

[16] Hallett (1973). The Roman mistress has since been reduced to metaphor by Wyke (1987, 1989, etc.), a methodology taken up in Kennedy's (1993) representational analysis.

[17] Deleuze/Guattari (1987): "You make a rupture, draw a line of flight, yet there is still a danger that you will reencounter organizations that restratify everything ... Groups and individuals contain microfascisms just waiting to crystallize," 9–10, hereafter abbreviated *ATP*.

[18] Here I am referring to a key concept in schizoanalysis, the Body without Organs (BwO). Borrowed from Antonin Artaud and first appearing in Deleuze (1990) 86–93 to describe the open-surface body of the schizophrenic, it is developed in *AO* (19) to refer to any void–space on which desires traverse and become subsumed by its anti–production whenever the subject reconstitutes itself. In *ATP* (149–166), the scope of the BwO broadens, incorporating cancerous, stratified, and totalitarian types. For its importance as a corrective to Freud's death drive, see Holland (1999) 26–33.

[19] Holland (1999) x–xii emphasizes this schizoanalytic ideal. It occurs throughout Deleuze and Guattari's writings, in the perpetual revolutions between being and becoming, molar and molecular, etc. Because everyone possesses multiplicative and productive desire, schizophrenic liberation becomes a real possibility.

Cynthia was the first (*prima*) to capture pitiful me with her eyes, I who had previously been touched by no desires (*contactum nullis ante cupidinibus*). It was at that time that Love cast down my gaze, with its constant conceit, and pressed my head beneath his superimposed feet, until the bully taught me to hate chaste girls and to live without forethought (*me docuit castas odisse puellas / improbus, et nullo vivere consilio*).[20]

Cynthia's gaze functions as the "Mirror Stage" of Propertius' elegiac self-actualization.[21] However, *Maman* post Melanie Klein is not present to affirm, "*C'est toi, Properce!*"[22] Standing in her place is *Amor* as abusive uncle (stepbrother? estranged cousin? certainly *no father!*).[23] Such maternal/paternal absence should indicate that Oedipal mythologizing is off the table, and that we are entering the world of *Verwerfung*, the unfettered psychosis of the Real *prior to* repression.[24]

Several additional clues reveal this productive desire lurking behind Cynthia's austerity cuts. First, *Amor* does not restrict Propertius' first syntheses of pluralized desire (*cupidinibus*). Rather, he guides them away from chaste maidens (*castas ... puellas*), for whom another passion is reserved (*odisse*).[25] For "chaste girls" are doubly prohibitive to Deleuzian desire: they belong to the nuclear family under paternal and subsequently matrimonial repression, while also serving as the emperor's preferred floral arrangement.[26] Second, *Amor* additionally (*et*)

---

[20] Prop. 1.1.1–6. All Latin translations are my own unless otherwise noted. I follow the Loeb text of Goold (1990).

[21] Just as the infant subject of Lacan's famous 1949 lecture "imagines" himself as a unified whole ("ideal-I") after interacting with the mirror, so too does Propertius experience a primordial self–realization opposite Cynthia's silent gaze. See Lacan (2006) 75–81.

[22] The reference is to Lacan's 1954 seminar, "The topic of the imaginary," wherein Lacan explains Klein's role in introducing the toddler Dick, trapped in a Real-Imaginary equivalency, into the linguistic realm via Oedipal metaphor as he plays with his toy trains, in Lacan (1991) 80–88.

[23] For the schizo's rejection of the socially constructed, restrictive Oedipal code in favor of limitless becomings on the BwO, see *AO*, 13–16 and 84–106. See esp. p. 97: "There is always an uncle from America; a brother who went bad; an aunt who took off with a military man; a cousin out of work, bankrupt, or a victim of the Crash; an anarchist grandfather; a grandmother in the hospital, crazy or senile."

[24] I have in mind Deleuze and Guattari's notion of the Real as *always accessible* via productive desire; see *AO*, 26–29. Contrast this with the Lacanian notion in Miller (2001) 132 and Miller (2004) of the incongruent Real emerging as *a result of* an irreconcilable conflict between the Symbolic (Rome's change in civic regime) and the Imaginary (the inability to reconcile these changes with the *mos maiorum*).

[25] For hatred accompanying love, see Catull. 85.1: "I hate and I love (*Odi et amo*)." Schizoanalysis would highlight the productive desires in the *id* that circulate and cathect for both of these emotions.

[26] Suet. *Aug.* 71.1: "He clung to his desires (*circa libidines haesit*), even in later years, so they say, being keen on deflowering virgins (*ad uitiandas uirgines promptior*), which were collected for him from all over, even by his own wife."

teaches him how "to live without forethought" (*nullo vivere consilio*) – free from a sovereign ego.

Cynthia will recur throughout the Propertian corpus, even undergoing a juxtaposed death and rebirth in his final book.[27] She here serves as the *Urereignis*, *Cynthia prima*, the factor to be raised to the *n*th power of Deleuzian repetition, the recurring festival of difference.[28] For Cynthia is never compulsive repetition *Beyond the Pleasure Principle*, even if Propertius' neuroses sometimes suggest this.[29] In lieu of a static loop, she manifests as a protean variable.

> Cynthia is ... impossible to define in her own terms because she is ... the point around which the relationships between Propertius and Gallus, Tullus, Ponticus, and Bassus are articulated ... She is the symptom of their discontent, the embodiment of their desires, and the medium of their exchange.[30]

Paul Allen Miller's assessment is astute. Cynthia does form a nexus that links these voices within the *Monobiblos*. Yet she functions not merely as a source of "discontent," but rather as a prism through which emerges the full spectrum of their differential desires. Cynthia is indefinable, but not because she herself is the traded commodity. Rather, she is a BwO void-space for Augustan axioms, the NYSE floor, "permeated by unformed, unstable matters, by flows in all directions, by free intensities or nomadic singularities, by mad or transitory particles,"[31] at times neutralizing them so that new ones can take their place.[32] Indeed, our poet will articulate a diverse series of perspectives for embracing Cynthia – namely, the addressees Bassus, Gallus, Tullus, and Ponticus, who are neither friends nor

---

[27] Poem 4.7, where she confronts Propertius for infidelity from her grave, and poem 4.8, where, alive once more, she crashes his party on the Esquiline.

[28] In *DR*, 1, Deleuze uses the festival to introduce repetition of the non–substitutable as distinct from resemblance based upon similarity: "To repeat is to behave in a certain manner, but in relation to something unique or singular which has no equal or equivalent ... This is the apparent paradox of festivals: they repeat an 'unrepeatable'."

[29] Contrary to the dynamic repetition of *DR*, Freud in 1920 hypothesizes a static repetition compulsion ("repetition, the re-experiencing of something identical, is clearly in itself a source of pleasure"), in Freud (1955) 36–57, at p. 36. For its clearest rebuke, viewing repetition as a Nietzschean affirmation ("I do not repeat because I repress. I repress because I repeat"), see *DR*, xix, 8–10 and 14–19 and Deleuze (1983), 8–10.

[30] Miller (2004) 67.

[31] *ATP*, 40.

[32] Cf. Holland (1999) 28–29.

personae, but rather the schizophrenic becomings which offer Propertius more productive ways of dealing with his Apolline noose.³³

Following Propertius' solo attempts with Cynthia, in poem 1.4 Propertius-becoming-Bassus materializes as an alternative to the poet's insulated obsession. Our poet asks, "Why, Bassus, by praising so many girls to me (*mihi tam multas laudando ... puellas*), do you induce me, having become-another (*mutatum*), to abandon my mistress?" (1.4.1–2). That some external Bassus could actually compel Propertius to leave his beloved simply by praising other women is absurd. Such endeavors usually fail. More likely, the voices of our schizoid Propertius have commenced amatory deliberations, with Bassus-*devenu-L'Anti-Œdipe*. Although stopping short of the schizophrenic *régime*, Alison Sharrock offers a telling analysis.

> In fact, it almost seems that contemplating the beloved is something that is better done together, something that has only limited possibilities for the lover alone ... In both cases, although the poems say "leave us alone in our affair," what they *imply* is something more like "join in".³⁴

Propertius' closing words only add to this idea of multivocality. He orders his alter ego to silence his plural voices (*tu tandem voces compesce molestas*, 1.5.1), so that he can remain in an ontological state of "being" with Cynthia (*quo sumus ... pares*, 1.5.2).³⁵ Furthermore, the declaration that Cynthia will discredit Bassus with all other girls as punishment (1.4.19–22) sounds reminiscent of the scolding Cynthia has just given Propertius in the preceding poem for contesting her monopolistic love (1.3.35–40).

If Cynthia imparts anything, it is that schizophrenia is the better option. Thus emerges the multifaceted junction of Propertius-Gallus, whose name recurs throughout the *Monobiblos*.³⁶ Of Gallus' appearances, poem 1.10 offers us the clearest insights into Propertius' schizoid transformation via perversion.

---

33 The name Cynthia (like Tibullus' Delia) points to Mount Cynthus on the island of Delos, the mythical birthplace and an important sanctuary of Apollo. For Apollo's primacy in the Augustan pantheon, see Feeney (1998) 28–38 and 72–74; Miller (2009b). Cynthia's name, then, becomes an Augustan reterritorialization of the elegiac BwO, although it is never quite so simple: "Thus, when there is no unity in the thing, there is at least unity and identity in the word ... The proper name can be nothing more than an extreme case of the common noun, containing its already domesticated multiplicity within itself and linking it to a being or object posited as unique," *ATP*, 27. Cf. Miller (2011) 337–339.
34 Sharrock (2000) 270.
35 Lines 1.5.1–2 are commonly read as the final lines of poem 1.4, including in Goold's edition.
36 For a discussion, see Janan (2001) 33–36; Miller (2004) 78–85.

> O delightful serenity (*O iucunda quies*), when I was there (*affueram*) for the first time (*primo*) as a witness to love (*testis amori*), an accomplice (*conscius*) to your tears! Oh how delightful a pleasure for me to remember that night (*o noctem meminisse mihi iucunda voluptas*)! Oh how often that night ought to be invoked in my prayers, when we saw you (*vidimus*), Gallus, lingering with your girl having been embraced and drawing out each word in long deferral! Although sleep was pressing my sinking eyelids and the moon was blushing with her horses in the middle of the sky, even so I was unable to depart from your amorous sport: so great was the passion in alternating voices (*non tamen a vestro potui secedere lusu: / tantus in alternis vocibus ardor erat*).[37]

By neurotic standards, poem 1.10 seems perplexing. Why would Propertius find immense *jouissance* in watching the successes of a rival with his own beloved, when he has regularly sought her for his own?[38]

There is a better explanation. For Deleuze and Guattari, perversion lies at the juncture of the third synthesis (where the drives meet the BwO), yet closer to the liberated schizophrenic than the paranoid neurotic, since the forces of production prevail over societal taboos.[39] Instead of the *unproductive* neurosis of a jealous lover, the Gallus-synthesis transforms Propertius into a *productive* pervert. Although his dissociative ego imagines himself spectating from the sidelines, a "witness to love" (*testis amori*), he voices this using the poetic plural (*vidimus*) and claims a strong presence (*affueram*). Moreover, his total awareness and intimate cognizance (*conscius*)[40] implies an active role in the process. The result – a remarkable degree of pleasure (*O iucunda quies ... o noctem meminisse mihi iucunda voluptas*) – utterly enthralled for all his exhaustion: "... even so was I unable to depart from your amorous sport: so great was the passion in alternating voices (*tantus in alternis vocibus ardor erat*)." We ought to ask whose *alternating voices* are constituted here. Those of a separate Gallus and his mistress? Or those of the disjunctive, molar poet and the syntheses of his molecular drives becoming-Gallus, all taking conjunctive pleasure with their lady? For a jealous neurotic could hardly delight in watching an acquaintance with his beloved.[41]

---

[37] Prop. 1.10.1–10. Trans. G.P. Goold (with modifications).
[38] This contradiction has also been noticed by Janan (2001) 35, who likewise reads this 'girl' as Cynthia. See also Oliensis (1997) 160.
[39] Holland (2012) 324–325.
[40] The word *conscius* can mean "privy (as) an accomplice" (*OLD* 2); "inwardly aware (esp. of one's own past actions)" (*OLD* 3), and "prompted by guilt or shame" (*OLD* 4).
[41] Given Freud's exclusionary 1905 statement that "*neuroses are ... the negative of perversions,*" (165), psychoanalysis fails to explain a neurotic Propertius. For here, "this pleasure in looking ... becomes a perversion," since "instead of being *preparatory* to the normal sexual aim, it supplants it," in Freud (1953), 157.

The *Monobiblos* closes with a *sphragis* addressed to Tullus. It is free of amatory topics. Rather, it delves into politics, recalling the fratricidal Perusine War alongside questions of schizoid origin. The poem begins, "Of what sort and whence my genealogy, Tullus, and where my ancestral gods, you ask on behalf of our friendship at any given moment" (*Qualis et unde genus, qui sint mihi, Tulle, Penates, / quaeris pro nostra semper amicitia*, 1.22.1–2). Propertius' ego is remarkably unfixed for a closing *sphragis* poem.[42] The interrogative pronouns *Qualis* and *unde* are juxtaposed with words denoting collective pluralism such as *genus* and *Penates*. We therefore stand on the threshold of a delocalized self about to become someones or somethings. As the poem continues, it takes the reader on a pan-Italic flight. It passes over the graveyards of Perugia (*si Perusina tibi patriae sunt nota sepulcra*, 1.22.3), Italy proper (*Italiae duris funera temporibus*, 1.22.4), Rome (*cum Romana suos egit Discordia cives*, 1.22.5), and Etruria (*sic mihi praecipue, pulvis Etrusca, dolor*, 1.22.6) – en route to Umbria, the poet's "shadowy" *omphalos*.

By saying that a land neighboring Perugia bore him (*proxima suppositos contingens Umbria campos / me genuit terris fertilis uberibus*, 1.22.9–10), the poet situates his emergence alongside these plains of rupture and credits multiple Italic groups for his poetic creation.[43] This too is the third synthesis, the meetings of the productive drives on the usurping BwO, the nomadic self in action.

> The fact has often been overlooked that the schizo indeed participates in history; he hallucinates and raves universal history, and proliferates the races ... We pass from one field to another by crossing thresholds: we never stop migrating, we become other individuals as well as other sexes, and departing becomes as easy as being born or dying. Along the way we struggle against other races, we destroy civilizations, in the manner of the great migrants in whose wake nothing is left standing once they have passed through.[44]

Propertius' departure from the amatory world leads him to explain his reasons for being there in the first place: the fascist violence of Octavian that has since congealed into a softer authoritarianism, the Augustan axioms now inhabiting

---

[42] However, as Peirano (2014) 226 notes, Propertius' *sphragis* functions in a liminal, paratextual manner, achieving "a special kind of closure by replaying the origin not just of Propertius, the writer, but also of the genre," (236). Her observation merits a schizoid expansion – the *sphragis*, as BwO rather than death drive, is not about endings repeating static origins, but about newfound beginnings that continually result from those endings.

[43] For the *sphragis* as an autobiographical space dealing with a text's literary reception, see Peirano (2013) 253–55.

[44] *AO*, 85.

Cynthia. Here, then, where the shattered socius begets schizoid poetics, we are to "seek affinity with our ever-plural Propertius" (*quaeris PRO nostra semPER amiciTIa*, 1.22.2).⁴⁵

Social-production, or When Rome Reterritorializes Elegy

The historical flights of the Tullus poem bring us to a central premise of *Anti-Oedipus*: the unconscious has socioeconomic determinants.⁴⁶ In this respect, Deleuze and Guattari develop arguments by Wilhelm Reich,⁴⁷ while simultaneously reworking Freud and Lacan by way of Nietzsche and Marx.⁴⁸ Their synthesis – the Oedipus complex is not a human universal, but rather the historical byproduct of capitalism separating production from the domestic sphere while simultaneously recreating that soft oppression within it. Just as the boss prevents the worker from enjoying the fruits of his labor, so too does this worker, upon returning home as father, restrict his children's access to mommy.⁴⁹ Thus, repression becomes a socioeconomic consequence of capitalism, instead of a universal component of desire; and desire, now extricated from historical circumstances, can finally be understood as *inherently productive* and "revolutionary in its essence".⁵⁰

---

45 Heyworth (2007) 100–101 notes the hidden signature.
46 Hence the term "desiring-production", which connects the Freudian *Treib* with Marxist labor – both inherently productive concepts repressed only when psychic lack emerges from the false idea of economic scarcity; see *AO*, 26–35.
47 "The strength of Reich consists in having shown how psychic repression depended on social repression … Reich was the first to raise the problem of the relationship between desire and the social field"; see *AO*, 118. See Reich (1946), as well as earlier ideas in Reich (2012) 89–249 and 279–358.
48 Holland (1999) details how *Anti–Oedipus* synthesizes the work of these thinkers, 4–24. Fundamental is the book's third section, which explains social–production as psychic changes effected by societal developments (primitive, despotic, capitalistic); see *AO*, 139–271.
49 See *AO*, 262–271. "The family is indeed the delegated agent of this psychic repression, insofar as it ensures 'a mass psychological reproduction of the economic system of a society'"; see *AO*, 118. It reproduces the desiring–producers (children), yet intervenes with Oedipal restrictions; see *AO*, 120–121.
50 Desire is revolutionary because of this inherent productivity, because it wants what it wants, in the face of what society wishes for it – docile subjects who, as per Reich (1946), unconsciously desire their own exploitation and servitude; see *AO*, 116. Cf. *AO*, 25–30 and *DI*, 232–233.

Consider the mid to late Roman Republic and the emergence of the Augustan principate. Although not a capitalistic society per se, it nevertheless features many of the attributes which Deleuze and Guattari use to define capitalism. Numismatic currency had matured amongst the Hellenistic empires, including the development of Rome's silver denarius. With this came "a significant expansion of monetary liquidity in Italy", the result of an economic sea change following Rome's imperial ambitions and profitable Mediterranean conquests.[51] As Philip Kay has recently argued, and William Harris has confirmed, the impact was remarkable.

> Kay is perfectly right, however, that between the third century BC and the late Republic the Roman economy was radically transformed. It became, according to this view, something rare, perhaps unique (before the seventeenth century), a huge and quite sophisticated system characterized by immense public and private wealth, a complex material culture, ample credit money, prolonged per capita growth on a non-trivial scale, and also, to go with these happy conditions, unprecedented atmospheric pollution.[52]

Consequences included Rome no longer needing to tax her own citizens directly, the growth of public works, a population surge in the capital, and the growth of the *publicani* together with extraordinarily wealthy individuals.[53] These men, seeking to maximize profits, offered large sums to financial intermediaries who pooled and loaned it out, creating a boom in available credit and economic growth.[54] Along with an axiom-inducing surplus, this suggests a shift from an economy of exchange to an economy of debt.[55]

The socioeconomic circumstances of this period offer clear paradigms for psychic schism. In highlighting the interconnectedness of desire and capital, calling it "all desire in flux ... a criss-crossing of desires", Deleuze comments on the axiomatic nature of capitalistic *régimes* – that is, their tendency towards "the dissolution of previous codes and powers" while reinscribing those with

---

[51] Kay (2014) 1–2, 4, 6, 43–58, 87–105. For Holland (1999) 67, the " fundamental capitalist axiom" is liquid currency "no longer embodied in landed property" coupled with "deterritorialized flows of 'free' labor." We should apply this idea to the land-displacements from military resettlements that Rome's social and civil wars proliferated.
[52] Harris (2015) 24.
[53] For a summary, see Kay (2014) 1–2.
[54] Kay (2014) 107–28. That late Republican Rome depended especially on credit is convincingly laid out by Harris (2006).
[55] Paranoia becomes an omnipresent threat amidst the infinite debt owed under capitalism. See Holland (1999) 95–96. For the primacy of debt over exchange in capitalistic societies per *AO*, see 61–64.

additional, unfixed meanings.[56] This carries over into their structures of authority, for which "the gears of power" have already settled "in the fissures of previous regimes".[57] Consider the military victories of leaders such as Pompey and Sulla, whom authors decried for bringing lavish amounts of wealth to Rome.[58] From a Deleuzian perspective, the Augustan principate was merely the end result of a continuum of differential repetition, whose emergent victor allowed capital to sway popular opinion, political alliances, and veteran legions.[59]

The years 18–17 BCE mark an additional watershed for understanding elegy. They saw Augustus institute the *lex Iulia de maritandis ordinibus*, which strongly incentivised marriage and childbearing for Roman nobles, and the *lex Iulia de adulteriis coercendis*, essentially forbidding adultery. Besides the Oedipal fundamentals, we should note several particulars preserved for us by Late Antique jurists in the Justinian *Digest*. First, there was a strong prohibition on using one's marriage as a source of profit; men who deliberately prostituted their wives for financial gain were to be prosecuted as adulterers themselves.[60] Second, adultery was expressly forbidden the wives of soldiers, as were agreements between soldiers and their wives' lovers,[61] suggesting that repression now serves the capital-producing empire. Lastly, the charge of adultery could have severer consequences than that of incest,[62] a striking rebuke of the incest taboo in favor of nuclear repression.

In addition to economic prohibitions, we should also note certain financial incentives promulgated by these laws. Business trips out of one's province were a viable reason for delaying an indictment of adultery against one's wife.[63] As

---

[56] *DI*, 267–68 Looming large in this transformation from fixed meaning to endless recoding of abstract values is the Marxist idea of surplus-value in capitalistic societies – "the continuing production of surplus-value for its own sake," Holland (1999) 68.

[57] *DI*, 268.

[58] The resulting devaluation of the *cursus honorum* became emblematic of the fall of the Roman Republic. Notable criticisms include Sall. *Cat.* 10–13, and Hor. *Carm.* 3.6 and 3.24, who connects them to Roman sexuality. See Syme (1939) 154 and Galinsky (1981) 132. For an overview of the complex changes in the Late Republic, including economic factors that significantly transformed the Roman army and its generals, see Beard/Crawford (1999) esp. 1–11 and 68–77.

[59] Syme (1939) comments on financial matters at length. See esp. 125, 169–170, 180–181, 187–196, 222, 243, 257, 322–325, and 349–368.

[60] *Dig.* 48.5.2 (Ulpian) and 48.5.30 (Ulpian). All references to the *Digest* refer to Mommsen, Krueger, and Watson (1985), and are given in the form *Dig.* citation number (Jurist).

[61] *Dig.* 48.5.12 (Papinian).

[62] *Dig.* 48.5.39 (Papinian).

[63] *Dig.* 48.5.16 (Ulpian). Likewise, office holders could postpone the charges until their terms of office had expired, *Dig.* 48.5.39 (Papinian).

Karl Galinsky explains, the inducements were often political in nature. These included the ability to stand for office as many years before the minimum age as the number of one's children, as well as preferential appointments based on having a large family.⁶⁴ We already noted how financial motives for political office increased tremendously in the later Republic. Now, under the *leges Iuliae*, they were reinforcing political economy *within* the nuclear family. Therefore, these juridical compilations not only highlight the Augustan regime's obsession with eradicating adultery. They also underscore the economic motivations that superimposed themselves on the *paterfamilias*' domestic authority, which was previously codified under Roman law (or at least *imagined* to be codified).⁶⁵ Furthermore, if Galinsky and Sharon James are correct to see Augustus already proposing the Julian Laws in 28–27 BCE (the *lex sublata* mentioned in Propertius 2.7),⁶⁶ then we can read virtually all of the Propertian corpora in this light.

The prominent position of capital alongside sexual repression finds immediate response in Propertius' *Monobiblos*, published early in Augustus' reign.⁶⁷ Already in his second poem he illustrates how Cynthia's financial reterritorialization pushes him towards neurotic mono-desire. Propertius' aversion to Cynthia's ornamentation is couched in terms of opulence. He deplores her ornate hairstyle (*ornato … capillo*, 1.2.1), her Coan silk dress (*Coa veste*, 1.2.2), her Syrian myrrh fragrance (*Orontea … murra*, 1.2.3), and her decision "to destroy the beauty of nature with purchased luxury" (*naturaeque decus mercato perdere cultu*, 1.2.5). Even Propertius' mythical exempla went without jewelry (*nullis … gemmis*, 1.2.21).

Cynthia's use of purchasing power to attract – as evinced in words like *vendere*, *muneribus*, and *mercato* (1.2.4–5) – leads nicely into Deleuze and Guattari's critique of capital's role in Lacanian desire.

> The deliberate creation of lack as a function of market economy is the art of a dominant class. This involves deliberately organizing wants and needs (*manque*) amid an abundance of production; making all of desire teeter and fall victim to the great fear of not having one's needs satisfied.⁶⁸

---

64 Galinsky (1981) 129.
65 Cf. Galinsky (1981) 126.
66 Galinsky (1981) 127–128; James (2003) 229–231. A counter-argument by Badian (1985), who argues that the *lex sublata* was actually a tax measure, speaks volumes about the economic axioms of desire. Cf. Miller (2001) 141–144 for discussion of this ambiguity.
67 We find similar denunciations of capital's role in amatory affairs in Tibullus (1.1.1, 1.1.75–78, 1.4.58–62, 1.5.60, and 1.9.17–20, 1.9.31–34) and Ovid (*Am.* 1.10, 1.14.45–50, and 3.8).
68 *AO*, 28.

Here, the axioms fabricated by Cynthia's ornaments push Propertius towards neurotic projections of faithlessness. Such is the Augustan *modus operandi*: Propertius worries that his exclusive beloved will interest other men. Noting chastity as a sufficient form of beauty (*ampla satis forma pudicitia*, 1.2.24), he declares, "If any girl is pleasing to one man alone, this is ornament enough" (*uni si qua placet, culta puella sat est*, 1.2.26). Such instilling of Oedipal desire through wealth is telling, for it affirms that Cynthia is hardly the amatory alternative to Augustan doctrines. Against her anxiety-inducement, in an era when "all sexuality is a matter of economy,"[69] schizophrenia becomes a veritable Rolling Jubilee for repressed desire.

Properce à La Borde: Editorial Conjunctions and Elegiac Assemblages

In conclusion, let us examine that broader site of elegiac schizophrenia, the Propertian manuscript tradition. Following schizoanalysis, Phillimore's anxieties about the state of Propertian editorship hardly seem like a curse to be faced down in paranoid neurosis. Instead, they welcome editorial activists like Postgate, whom Phillimore deemed "guilty of the same unrestrained desire" (*eiusdem libidinis reum*) as A. E. Housman.[70] This *libido* certainly materialized as interventionism flourished, producing – if not *The Invention of Love* – then, at minimum, the reinvention of elegiac textual desire. For even Housman himself was outdone by Oliffe Legh Richmond's 1928 edition, a desiring-chimera that made drastic modifications to the manuscript texts.[71]

Phillimore's apprehensions merit a closer examination. Butrica and Richard Tarrant rightly indicate that our editor, when pronouncing his famous axiom (*quot editores tot Propertii*), feared excessive emendation and line transposition *in the future*; that the *Urtext* would soon become irrecoverable if the Housmans and the Postgates continued to have their way.[72] Yet nowhere does Phillimore articulate this lucidly. Nor is it his only sentiment. In fact, reading him feels like

---

[69] *AO*, 12.
[70] Phillimore (1901) *praef.* (as with all subsequent citations).
[71] See Richmond (1928) 3–87. Tarrant (2006) 45 offers an excellent summary, calling Richmond's production "the most eccentric edition of Propertius thus far seen."
[72] Butrica (1997) 176; Tarrant (2006) 45.

wading through the same incoherencies as those of our elegiac poet, with deeply psychoanalytic undercurrents.

Phillimore recognized that he faced a corpus whose fragmentation rivals the Hieronymus Bosch-like dream states of the conflicted ego (*ita dilaniatum et κατακεκερματισμένον ut disticha passim inter se locum mutaverint*).[73] He even insinuates that the Propertian archetype is hopelessly lost, anticipating postmodern textual criticism by almost a century. However, he still falls back on the possibility of using one's own rational judgment (*suo cuique arbitrio*) to restore a repressed unity, although he differs from Bentley in urging confidence in the authority of the manuscripts. In this respect, Phillimore seems torn between production and repression, just where schizoanalysis would envisage him. More striking still, Phillimore's psychoanalytic apprehensions often leave their intended subject in shadow (poet? scribe? editor?). Whether he is illustrating the imaginative drives behind each individual's text production (*proprium phantasiae tenorem*), highlighting the primacy of innate mental processes (*in quolibet argumento ... propriam ... inventionem ... Quid enim est aliud ingenium?*), or reassuring himself about scribal wolf-men and their potential animalistic drives (*homines enim. At non beluae*), he might as well be describing *anyone* involved with the Propertian corpus.[74]

How then to approach such a nexus of desire? Describing the Propertian manuscript tradition as though it were hit by an F5 tornado,[75] Butrica suggests we continue emending while ignoring our role in this differential repetitive – we are dealing with "a text that has been distorted from its original state by an exceptionally high degree of corruption and ... more extensive emendation is therefore needed to restore it to that original state".[76] Such is the irony of this interventionist dialectic – desiring-production, hermeneutic repression. An unhindered paleographic delirium is permissible, so long as we analysts sit in the asylum running self-actualizing tests on our Propertian patient, confined by our supposedly rational diagnosis which permits *no second opinion*. Meanwhile, let us ignore how we perpetuate that repressed condition, perpetually on the brink of destabilizing our medicated unity.

---

[73] Cf. Lacan (2006) 78.
[74] Following *ATP*, 26–38, we can view these scribes, like Freud's Wolf Man (and everyone else for that matter), as effecting multifarious desires amidst medieval institutional repression.
[75] Butrica (1997) 196.
[76] Butrica (1997) 178. He later adds, at p. 187: "The text of Propertius is so corrupt that an editor must indeed suspect everything, and must go 'hunting' for corruptions rather than wait for them to present a calling card." Cf. Janan (2001) 11.

Why not instead join the inmates and create an experimental clinic for schizoanalytic paleography much like La Borde, where psychiatric patients and staff interacted as equals?[77] We need not suppress these textual strata as they coalesce. Again, Deleuze and Guattari offer a promising solution.

> A book has neither object nor subject; it is made of variously formed matters, and very different dates and speeds. To attribute the book to a subject is to overlook this working of matters, and the exteriority of their relations ... In a book ... there are lines of articulation or segmentarity, strata and territories; but also lines of flight, movements of deterritorialization and destratification ... All this, lines and measurable speeds, constitutes an *assemblage*. A book is an assemblage of this kind, and as such is unattributable. It is a multiplicity.[78]

Our assemblage would subject the unfettered Propertian corpus to schizoanalysis and "work towards its complexification, its processual enrichment".[79] This means going beyond standard editions, which remain "reductionist modelisations,"[80] and reading *all* manuscript and editorial voices as *productive elements* rather than corruptions to be excised or emended (although emendation constitutes *yet another layer* of productive polyphony).

An excellent location for this paleographic clinic would be in the digital world of hypertext.[81] We can envision an open-source multitext whereupon all readers could make and track changes to the ever-evolving/ever-revolving Propertius, something akin to Jerome McGann's Ivanhoe Game.[82] This online elegy would enable the synchronic reading of multiple variants.[83] One could view the same elegiac couplet in all manifestations by desired layout. Or one might examine the entire poem, selecting a focal text and highlighting known variant readings. In addition, one could map texts according to their geographical histories – a rhizomatic quality of manuscripts usually minimized in standard editions. Deleuze and Guattari welcome such an endeavor.

---

[77] For an account of this extraordinary clinic and its impact on Guattari, see Dosse (2010) 40–75.
[78] *ATP*, 3–4.
[79] Guattari (1995) 61.
[80] Guattari (1995) 61.
[81] McGann (2001) 53–74 presents an excellent overview of hypertext's transformations of textual criticism. Moulthrop (1994) 304–5, also following *ATP*, highlights how hypertext, as a site of "active reception," can erode hierarchies and promote "textual promiscuity."
[82] For a description of the Ivanhoe Game – a carefully documented group act of metatextual rewriting, see McGann (2001) 217–31.
[83] McGann (2001) 56–57.

> The ideal for a book would be to lay everything out on a plane of exteriority of this kind, on a single page, the same sheet: lived events, historical determinations, concepts, individuals, groups, social formations.[84]

Furthermore, if we recall Propertius' *sphragis*, this third member of our triumvirate desires similar unfixed collectivity (1.22.1–2). In fact, we appear to be dealing with a playful schizo who taunts those who analyze him monadically at any given moment.[85] It is as though he has shaped the psychic precondition of his numerous receptions and is now schizoanalyzing his subsequent readers.[86] What happens when we entwine these pleas, encouraging the many historical variants to be born and reborn perpetually on this ferocious, yet fertile plain/plane of immanence (*proxima suppositos contingens Umbria campos / me genuit terris fertilis uberibus*, 1.22.9–10)?

One result would be a break from Lachmannian arborescence – branch-by-branch criticism, with its fixed order of *recensio, comparatio, emendatio*. Instead, it would combine these into a continuous process of permanent revolution,[87] where a desire for *variante petit a* could escape castration by paternal manuscripts.[88] McGann highlights this Propertian *déjà vu inédit*.

> First, the specific material design of a hypertext is theoretically open to alterations of its contents and its organizational elements at all points and at any time. Unlike a traditional book or set of books, the hypertext need never be "complete" … It will evolve and change over time, it will gather new bodies of material, and its organizational substructures will get modified, perhaps quite drastically.[89]

We would likewise reverse Bentley's adage, preferring over a hundred manuscript voices to one editor's rationale.[90] This could markedly transform our discipline, wherein an editorial *oligarchia* adjudicates the classical tradition with axioms such as *lectio difficilior potior*. The conservative critic would doubtless charge us with disemboweling centuries worth of philology and launching its duodenal remnants into a democratic hyperspace. Yet reaching escape velocity remains a

---

84 *ATP*, 9.
85 Cf. *AO*, 14.
86 I owe this incisive idea to my anonymous referee.
87 I have in mind the many meanings of the Latin verb *revolvo*, some repressive, others Deleuzian, as well as the schizoanalytic aim of permanent revolution as "a world created in the process of its tendency, its coming undone, its deterritorialization" (*AO*, 322).
88 Cf. Greetham (2010) 152–80.
89 McGann (2001) 71.
90 Butrica (1984) 351–54 furnishes a list of 146 Propertian manuscripts.

formidable challenge, even for a textual BwO, since recension and reproduction of manuscripts remains carefully controlled by institutions. Moving them to an open-source platform would itself be a radical breakthrough.[91]

Meanwhile, we can embrace the frequency with which classical philology produces the "excessive lover of one's own inclinations" (*nimium amator ingenii sui* – to borrow Quintilian's famous characterization of Ovid),[92] discovering desiring-production in every inquiry. We will therefore heed the call of postmodern textual critics "To study texts and textualities" as the "complex (and open-ended) histories of textual change and variance".[93] Yet, if history is any indication, the molar temptation will remain and we will continue prioritizing one reading over another.[94] By recognizing this potential philological despotism, we acknowledge Miller's assessment that textual criticism is always an interpretive act.[95] Finally, as Propertiuses in our own right, we can accept that these *Elegies*, like so many classical texts, are in no way the work of one author, but rather the collective becoming of many authors, scribes, compilers, interpolators, commentators, editors, and readers – all competing for a primacy of voice on a truly schizoid body of desires.[96]

---

[91] Cf. McGann (2001) 68–69.
[92] Quint. *Inst.* 10.1.88.
[93] McGann (1991) 9.
[94] McGann (2001) 71: "Of course it is true that every *particular* hypertext at any particular point in time will have established preferred sets of arrangements and orderings ... The point is that the hypertext, unlike the book, encourages greater decentralization of design."
[95] Miller (2011) 329. He rightly concludes, at p. 350: "In the end, we are not faced with a choice between a self–transparent, centered, rational intending subject and an arbitrary or unreadable text. This is a false dilemma dictated by an assumed and, I would contend, indefensible humanist ontology."
[96] I wish to thank Eugene Holland, Christina S. Kraus, Jeroen Lauwers, and the anonymous reader for their comments on earlier drafts of this paper, as well as audience members at Yale and KU Leuven for their insightful questions and comments. Any remaining errors are entirely my own. This paper was submitted too early to be able to take into account the detailed new study of Richard Tarrant (*Texts, Editors, and Readers;* Cambridge, 2016) and the recent essay, "Love Elegy and Legal Language in Ovid," by Ioannis Ziogas (in *Wordplay and Powerplay in Latin Literature*, De Gruyter, 2016)."

Katerina Ladianou
5 Staging Female Selves in Sapphic Poetry

Discussing Plato's *Symposium*, David Halperin relies on Foucault's theory of sexuality to argue for a feminine identity that serves as an alternate male identity.[1] In his view, the Platonic Diotima is nothing but a trope, a way to speak about women inside the male discourse. Halperin is discussing a well known theoretical position – basically Lacanian and further explored by Luce Irigaray – using Diotima as an example of a ventriloquised female. This is, of course, neither a paradigm limited to Plato, nor an unfamiliar paradigm in classical scholarship in general, where a central issue has been the question whether female-authored, or female-performed poetry can be characterised as 'feminine' and, if so, in what sense.[2] As far as lyric poetry is concerned, Eva Stehle discusses Alcman's *Partheneion* pointing out how lyric poetry can convey male political ideas using women's voices.[3] In this light, 'feminine' voice is seen as subordinated to the predominant patriarchal ideology, helping to sustain it.[4] Rayor, on the other hand, uses the term "woman-identified" to describe a style of writing that avoids "both imitation and protest" in constructing a dialogue with other women's texts. According to her, this is a discourse that "focuses on women's experience, repossesses tradition, and addresses a female audience".[5] Along similar lines, Jack Winkler uses a positive model to discuss Sapphic poetry as an embodied female experience, exploring the poetic dialogue between Sappho and the androcentric vision and values of Homeric epic. Throughout his essay, Winkler emphasises the idea of Sappho's double consciousness: both of her "private", woman-centered, lyric world and the other "public" male-centered, epic world are parts of a unique poetry that is "both subjectively and objectively woman centered".[6]

---

[1] Halperin/Winkler/Zeitlin (1990) 257–308.
[2] For a good overview see the introduction of Lardinois/McClure (2001).
[3] Stehle (1997), esp. Chapter 2, where she discusses Alcman's fr. 1 and 3.
[4] On a similar view also see Arthur (1983). For the appropriation of the feminine voice by the male see also Bergren (1983) and Arthur (1982).
[5] Rayor (1993) 222 borrowing the term from Diaz–Dioscaretz. Her categories are 1. Feminist; 2. Non-feminist; 3. Women-identified. Referring to discussions on Corinna's poetry, she cites Skinner (1983) as arguing for a non-feminist Corinna who "has fully internalized male values".
[6] Winkler (1996) 108.

Katerina Ladianou, University of Crete

Taking this thought one step further, I am going to argue that the doubleness of consciousness that Winkler is referring to is tied to the construction of feminine voice, self and a more importantly feminine poetics. Following Bahktin's description of the polyphonic self as "a conversation, a struggle of discrepant voices with each other: voices speaking from different positions", this paper will attempt to show that this quality of the polyphonic self is an inherent characteristic of feminine voice.[7] In other words, the Sapphic voice is not one: giving voice to many women, being performed by a chorus, and being heard by a female audience (although not exclusively female, I believe), Sapphic poetry can be perceived as a polyphonic poetry.

At this point, it would be useful to explain my use of the term "female" and differentiate it from "feminine". The distinction followed in this paper begins with the common distinction between sex and gender: while the first is biologically determined the second is socially, culturally and – I may add – literarily, constructed.[8] Female voice is therefore, to this study, a voice uttered by a woman, a biologically female subject, while feminine voice is a voice constructed *as* uttered by a woman. This category, then, covers voices constructed as feminine by both female and male authors. Female voice then, *a qua* sex essentially feminine voice, will not be a part of this study. What I will try to show, on the other hand, is that feminine voice as a construction is more than one: it can be a "feminine" voice as constructed by a prevailing ideology, based on the assumption of dichotomies that need positive and negative poles and assign the negative pole to the "feminine". It is the ideology, deeply embedded in Western civilization, which defines "feminine" as other, irrational, object, as silenced in contrast with the masculine, rational, subject position. It will, however, be the main point of this paper that a different place for feminine voice can be found outside this dichotomy, a place from which feminine voice can be spoken and heard. I will then discuss how "feminine", as the negative pole of the dichotomy, can be different from feminine, the non-hierarchical position that creates the possibility for feminine voice to exist.

Within this context, I will argue that feminist criticism can be employed in order to support the possibility of a polyphonic lyric if read as a supplement of the Bakhtinian theoretical framework. Critics like Irigaray and Cixous insist that woman is excluded from dominant structures of representation. Language for them originates with men and excludes women: all that is left to her is the negative pole and the subordinate object position, a definition only in terms of

---

7 Bakhtin (1984) 217.
8 As de Lauretis (1987) 9 would put it, "the construction of gender is the product and the process of both representation and self–representation." For similar concerns, see also Batstone (2002).

her alterity. Is then the very term "feminine voice" impossible? Almost, for they discuss different paths of possible resistance, a way of "feminine linguistic transgression" described in two different ways: for Cixous an active production of *écriture féminine*, and for Irigaray, feminine discourse, *parler-femme*, a "feminine language" in which feminine subjects can express themselves among each other. Those characteristics of women speaking to each other are, I argue, visible in Sapphic poetry. In a close reading of fragments the characteristics of écriture *feminine*, emphasizing the openness, polyvocalism and lack of a totalitarian form of thought and discourse in feminine texts will become apparent.[9]

I will, then, propose reading Sapphic poetry as an exemplary feminine discourse, since it is the only example of a female poet in archaic Greece with a considerable amount of extant work. Reading Sapphic poetry, then, as feminine discourse produced by women talking to each other will elucidate its characteristic as a "dialogical" text in the Bakhtinian sense. Similarly, I will show that Sapphic poetry promotes multiplicity of voices by denying totalisations, avoids the repression of different voices by undoing the extant hierarchy revealing an elusive self and, at the same time, a voice that precludes "any distinction of identities, any establishment of ownership, thus any form of appropriation".[10] In this sense, Sappho's fragmented, elusive self resembles both her corpus but also her text: a never-ending and a never-to-be-read text, forever lost.[11]

Remembering Female Selves: Time, Space, Memory, and Polyphony in Sappho fr. 94

τεθνάκην δ' ἀδόλως θέλω·

ἄ με ψισδομένα κατελίμπανεν

πόλλα καὶ τόδ' ἔειπέ [μοι·

ὤιμ' ὡς δεῖνα πεπ[όνθ]αμεν,

Ψάπφ', ἦ μάν σ' ἀέκοισ' ἀπυλιμπάνω.

---

9 Contra Skinner (1996) 176–182.
10 Irigaray (1985) 134.
11 Similarly see Williamson (1996) 249: "The would-be critic of Sappho cannot avoid the sense of peering through a series of *fragmented* and distorting prisms at a fragile and *ever-receding* text" (my emphasis).

τὰν δ' ἔγω τάδ' ἀμειβόμαν·

χαίροισ' ἔρχεο κἄμεθεν

μέμναισ', οἶσθα γὰρ ὥς <σ>ε πεδήπομεν·

αἰ δὲ μή, ἀλλά σ' ἔγω θέλω

ὄμναισαι ....

ὀσ[-10-] καὶ κάλ'ἐπάσχομεν·

πό[λλοις γὰρ στεφάν]οις ἴων

καὶ βρ[όδων ...]κίων τε ὔμοι

κα [-7-] πὰρ ἔμοι π<ε> ρεθήκαο

καὶ πόλλαις ὐπαθύμιδας

πλέκταις ἀμφ' ἀπάλαι δέραι

ἀνθέων ἐ [-6] πεποημέναις.

καὶ π.....[ ]. μύρῳ

βρενθείῳ. [ ]ρυ [..]ν

ἐξαλ<ε>ίψαο κα[ὶ βασ]ιληίῳ

καὶ στρώμν[αν ἐ]πὶ μολθάκαν

ἀπάλαν παρ [   ]όνοων

ἐξίης πόθο[ν   ] νίδων

κωὔτε τις [οὔ] τε τι

ἶρον οὐδ' υ[   ]

ἔπλετ' ὄππ[οθεν ἄμ]μες ἀπέσκομεν,

οὐκ ἄλσος[   ]. ρος

.........] ψοφος

          ]... οιδιαι

"Honestly, I wish I were dead." She was leaving me, shedding many tears, and saying this among many things: "Alas, what a dreadful thing happened to us, Sappho, I am leaving you, honestly, without my will". And I replied to her thus: "Go, farewell and remember me, for you know how we cherished you. And, if you don't, I will remind you ... that beautiful things happened to us. Many garlands of violets and roses and saffron you put around you, lying close to me, and round your tender neck you put woven garlands made from flowers, and much perfume …. made from flowers … royal … you anointed, and lying on the soft couch you used to kindle the desire of young women … nor shrine … from which we were absent … nor grove … nor dance … sound … song".[12]

The fragment begins with the utterance of a death wish, followed by a description of a separation scene between two women, one of which is named Sappho. Since the beginning of the poem is missing, there is no clear indication of who the speaker is. Scholarly opinions are therefore divided.[13] According to the first edition of the poem in 1902, it was the girl to whom the first line belongs. Soon enough, though, Schubart, the first editor of the poem, changed his mind, attributing the line to "Sappho".[14] Although Schadewaldt argued that the attribution of the death wish to Sappho should not be doubted any more, nevertheless the matter was not settled with scholars challenging his opinion again in the late '60s.[15] Anne Burnett argued that it is the addressee who utters the wish to die in the opening lines, suggesting that the poem is divided between two points of view: the desperate, disconsolate weeping girl and the courageous Sappho who commands her to go remembering the good times they spent together.[16] Along the same lines, Ellen Greene concludes, "attributing the opening line to the other woman heightens the tension of the poem between the two speakers, whose different approaches toward the separation, reflected in their correspondingly *different modes of discourse*".[17]

Attempting to provide a convincing answer to the issue, this reading will then try to explore the question of the speakers *via* the question of self. Is it one or two different selves described in the poem? Are we dealing with two "points of view" of two different people or is it one splintered self this poem is dealing with? The presentation of the lyric self is the main focus of the poem. The fragment accidentally – albeit quite appropriately – opens with a first person singular. Later, the speaking person is named by her interlocutor in an attempt to point to a specific

---

12 All Sappho fragments follow E. M Voigt's edition. The translations are mine and reflect the discussion at hand.
13 For an overview of the scholarly debate see Burnett (1983) 292–293 and esp. n.38; Robbins (1990); Larson (2010) 179 n. 10.
14 Schubart (1902) 195ff; Schubart (1907) 12.
15 Schadewaldt (1936) 364 and Burnett (1983) 292.
16 Burnett (1979) 23.
17 Greene (1996) 239–240 (my emphasis). Snyder (1997) 56 and 58–59, although she does not align with Burnett in attributing the first line to the second person, strongly emphasizes the *polyvocalism* and *openness* of the fr. 94.

self. Now we know it is *Sappho* speaking, it is her own self being exposed and staged.¹⁸ The poem opens with a wish in present, first person singular (θέλω) and the focus to a self is emphasized by the use of the first person singular, nominative personal pronoun (ἔγω – twice). As the poem moves on time shifts and, at the same time, the self is further exposed. Thus, time works in different levels staging the lyric self. It is then, I suggest, this staging of self though time that is important in fr. 94.

The fragment begins with a present utterance of the lyric self in a moment of self-destruction: I wish I were dead.¹⁹ Then the time shifts to the past moment of separation: she was leaving me, shedding tears. Then a dialogue, as present in the past: she was saying "Sappho I leave you unwillingly, and I said, go, farewell, and remember me. A second person emerges not only as a person in a narrative, but as an interlocutor, who addresses, by name, the lyric I.²⁰ Then another time shift, while memory helps to go again back to the past, even before the separation. It is the time of togetherness: "remember how we lived together, and if you don't, I will remind you." Although it is a narration of past times, the future crops up. The lyric I will go on to describe the previous experience of their common life, trying to preserve, store and secure the memory of the past. The self then is preserved in future perfect, as past and future combine. Memory is both "what we were" and "what we will have been". What the speaker wants is both to create and share the created memory to be preserved in the future.²¹

Hence, the self emerges in three different time levels: now, then, and before. Three different selves, three different feelings: desperation, courage, and bliss. Is it a shattered self, torn in three pieces, a disparate self? In *Problems of Dostoevsky's Poetics*, M. Bakhtin suggests that:

> Language imagines self as a conversation, a struggle of discrepant voices with each other, voices speaking from different positions, and invested with different degrees of authority.²²

---

18 By "*Sappho*", I mean the self the poem stages, not the historical person with whom the present discussion is not concerned.
19 For the death wish and Homeric allusions, see Robbins (1990) 118–119, who sees a parallel with Helen. For Larson (2010) 177 the death wish is modeled after Penelope's similar wish.
20 For the use of *apostrophe* see Greene (1996) 240.
21 Schadewaldt (1950) 113 ff. had already pointed at three time levels of the poem, namely present, past and remote past. I am suggesting a slightly more complex schema of the construction of time as following:
Present→ death wish
Past I→ time of departure → future: I will remind you
Past II→time of togetherness → past future: will have been
22 Morson/Emerson (1990) 217–218.

In this poem, I suggest, three different voices of the *same* self struggle: not only from different spatial positions but from different temporal positions as well. Space and time change, as the voice changes: present time of desperation and death wish, first level of past, place of separation, and a second level of past, a time and place of bliss: a *utopia* of togetherness, smells, beautiful sounds, and love. The self then emerges as polymorphic, even changed: it is not the staging of two different selves, two different persons the poem deals with. It is not one unified, desperate self whose feelings the poem expresses. It is the staging of a changing self, or rather a lament for the lost old self, even a lament for a changed self, or selves. For the courageous lyric I of the past has now become the desperate I of the first line, while, or because, the desperate I of the separation scene has also changed. The poem then focuses, with at least 19 out of the 29 preserved lines, on the memory of the past togetherness, in a last desperate attempt to preserve, by memory, the lost selves.

Furthermore, the poem stages two distinctively feminine spaces: the present scene of separation and the memory of past bliss in the framework of the *hetairia*. Sappho's description marks both spaces as feminine. In the beginning, the dialogue between the friends is marked with grammatically feminine endings. During the departure scene the grammar is heavily gendered with the use of participles and pronouns.[23] When the person addressed as Sappho begins talking, she evokes to memory a past female space of female reciprocity, song, smells and female bodies.[24]

Luce Irigaray describes female space as the space in which women are together in a relationship based on nearness rather than ownership. Ownership and property according to her demarcate the master (male) discourse. For woman is traditionally an exchange object, exchange value between men. On the other hand female discourse is based on a nearness, proximity and reciprocity as opposed to the hierarchy of male discourse.[25]

Often being read as a poem of a friend departed in order to get married, thus to be a part of the male hierarchies, the poem brings forth a different, female world, a world opposed to the prevailing male economy.[26] It is a world in which speaking among – and as – women is possible, a world in which female desire

---

[23] Cf. ll. 2–7. Although feminine forms are common in Sappho, this is actually the only extant fragment with such concentration of feminine forms (6 forms in 6 lines).
[24] Similarly in Greene (1996), *via* Irigaray.
[25] Irigaray (1985) 31.
[26] See Larson (2010) 197–199, who reads Sappho 94 through Penelope. For her, the death wish points directly to the Odyssean heroine and thus invites the reading of the poem within a marriage context.

is spoken.²⁷ Sappho then goes on to explicitly stage such a world: descriptions of female singing, a sound of multiple female voices, smells, and touches.²⁸ All senses come into play evoking desire. Lines 21–23 explicitly describe the intimate space of female desire, which is named in line 23. The lines have provoked many scholarly arguments and a great deal of lyric *amēchania* of scholars who tried to conceal any hint of Sapphic homoeroticism.²⁹ It is nevertheless evident that there is an explicit scene of female homoerotic desire, as a marker, I suggest, of female discourse, or rather female *homilia*.³⁰

In female discourse, Cixous argues, female body must be written. Sappho writes (about) the body, the soft neck on which the garlands are placed, the bodies anointed with perfumes, the bodies reclining on couches, feeling soft to the touch. Women are also talking, or rather singing.³¹ As these voices of the past become voices in the present of performance, another function of feminine writing is accomplished:

> In feminine speech, as in writing, there never stops reverberating something that, having imperceptibly and deeply touched us, still has the power to affect us – song, the first music of the voice of love, which every woman keeps alive ... Within woman the first, nameless love is singing.³²

Participating in the aforementioned scholarly controversy regarding the speaker of the first line, it has been my intention to explore the attribution of the first line to Sappho as it can be read within the framework of the construction of a polyphonic lyric self that this paper tries to explore. Seen as polyphonic, fr. 94 discloses not only the Sapphic voice but also the voice of the departing friend. This sense of dialogism does not mean, I argued, that the first line has to belong to another speaker. The poem stages a dialogue between two women bringing forth two female voices, in a discourse marked as feminine. The poem, then, intentionally marks the discourse as such, revealing the construction of a female self and shedding light on feminine poetics.

In that sense, 94 can be read as a process of constructing a feminine self: a disparate, elusive thus polyphonic self, constructed through memory. Constructing a feminine self through different time levels create a unique dialogue

---

27 Irigaray (1985) 137: "the problem of speaking (as) women is precisely that of finding ... that speech of desire."
28 Irigaray (1985) 209: "In all senses. Why only one song, one speech one text at a time?"
29 Burnett (1979) 25, esp n. 31.
30 See also Larson (2010) 190–191.
31 For singing and dancing, see the last fragmented lines.
32 Cixous (1986) 93.

between time, place and selves. It is time and place that shift together with the interlocutors, creating a palimpsest of lyric dialogism. The self in fr. 94 is twofold: there is the self as shown to the other person of the dialogue, the courageous, hopeful self, and the self as shown to the self in the beginning of the poem, the self wishing for its death. Moreover, in the context of a performance, a third self emerges as the self is again shown to others. This unfinished, open-ended self is expecting the audience might finalise and complete the speaker.

Attributing the first line to "Sappho" rather than the second person of the dialogue emphasises the presentation of a disparate, elusive self which dialogism calls for. Furthermore the "indeterminacy" of the speakers, I suggest, adds to the effect of the disparate selves in a female discourse.[33] It is in the moment of separation that the female discourse exercises its power of bringing the interlocutors closer. In a female space, women speak in "nearness so pronounced that it makes all discrimination of identity impossible".[34]

Polyphony in "Absentia": Fr. 96

] σαρδ. [..]

πόλ]λακι τυίδε [.]ων ἔχοισα

ὠσπ.[...]. ὠομεν· .[. . .

σε †θέᾳ σ' ἰκέλαν, ἀρι-

γνώτα†, σᾷ δὲ μάλιστ' ἔχαιρε μόλπᾳ

νῦν δὲ Λύδαισιν ἐμπρέπεται γυναί-

κεσσιν ὥς ποτ' ἀελίω

δύντος ἀ βροδοδάκτυλος < σελάννα >;

πάντα περ<ρ>έχοισ' ἄστρα φάος δ' ἐπί-

σχει θάλασσαν ἐπ' ἀλμύραν

ἴσως καὶ πολυανθέμοις ἀρούραις·

---

33 I borrow the term from duBois (1995) 138 ff.
34 Irigaray (1985) 31.

ἀ δ' <ἐ>έρσα κάλα κέχυται, τεθά-
λαισι δὲ βρόδα κἄπαλ' ἄν-
θρυσκα καὶ μελίλωτος ἀνθεμώδης.

πόλλα δὲ ζαφοίταισ' ἀγάνας ἐπι-
μνάσθεισ' Ἄτθιδος ἰμέρῳ
λέπταν ποι φρένα κ[.]ρ ... βόρηται

κῆθι δ' ἔλθην ἄμμ[..].. ισα τὸ δ' οὐ
νωντα[..]υστονυμ[. .] πόλυς
γαρύει [. .]αλον π[. . . τὸ μέσσον

"Sardis ... often having her mind here ... how we lived together ... (she honored) you as a being a goddess, Arignota, and she rejoiced most of all in your song. Now she stands out among the Lydian women like the rosy-fingered moon after the sunset, surpassing all the stars. And the light evenly spreads among the salty sea and the flowery fields; the beautiful dew is shed, the roses blossom and the soft chervil and the flowery honey-lotus. But she, roaming about far and wide, remembers gentle Atthis with desire and her tender heart is devoured inside, for your fate. ... come there ... shouts ... sea ... middle ..."

The poem, addressed to a female 'you', is talking about the desire of a second female. It is then a poem about feminine desire: Arignota and Atthis, the woman she desires. Desire is not however spoken in the first or second person. It is spoken by a third, narrated or better *read* as the desire of the other. If it is Sappho who speaks the desire of the women involved in the poem, is it then a female desire? Can the discourse of desire be a female discourse? If desire is written in an always masculine poetic discourse, can it be a female desire, can it be uttered by a female voice?

The poem begins with an enigmatic Sardis standing alone in the first line of the fragment. There is no way to know if this is the beginning of the poem, but at the beginning of the fragment Sardis seems to be the place where the poem is set. The setting however quickly moves from Sardis to "here" with a similar movement from present to the past. Being in Sardis now her mind travels to Lesbos and the memory of past life, how we used to live together is the subject matter of the three following lines.[35] The third person narrator talks about her desire: it is here in Lesbos her mind comes back to all the time, it is you whom she saw as a goddess,

---

35 For memory, see Williamson (1996) 255.

it is your song she liked the best. Atthis is addressed directly in the second person as she becomes the object of Arignota's desire. The speaking subject of Arignota's desire, though, is not she. It is Sappho reading her desire, the desire of an absent girl to the one present.

In another shift of time, the next line comes back to the present but the place changes back to Sardis: she is now in Lydia, preeminent among the Lydian women. As time and place shift, so does desire: it is Arignota now who is the object of desire of the Lydian people, it is Arignota who surpasses in beauty all others, as the moon outshines the rest of the stars. Arignota is desired, not only by the Lydians but perhaps by Atthis as well. In describing Arignota the speaker employs a simile: the picture of the moon surpassing the stars gives way to a description of the moonlight spreading over the sea and flowery, dewy meadows. Following the moonlight, desire crosses the sea from Sardis to Lesbos and vice versa. The boundaries of space are blurred, and so are the boundaries of time: for the image of roses and soft grass bring back the times of togetherness. If Sappho's poetry is nothing but "gardens of nymphs, wedding songs and love affairs"[36], as Demetrius assures us, it is then to those gardens of erotic euphoria that the description points. However, it is not clear if the erotic scenery refers to the past, present or future: is it the gardens they used to be together at a past time that their desire was fulfilled? Are the empty gardens the symbol of a paradise lost, or do they serve as a reminder that they can be 'filled' again?

I will come back to the theme of erotic space, but for the moment let me go to the next shift of time and place. After the description of the idyllic gardens, the time shifts to the present time and space (Lydia). There Arignota roams restlessly, remembering Atthis, her heart devoured by desire. She states her desire to go there, she shouts but her voice gets lost at the uproar of the sea. If this is the end of the poem, the image of Arignota in a desperate attempt to project her voice, to utter her desire, then is it a poem about the impossibility of uttering female desire? The words Arignota *tries to* utter are lost both in the sea staged by the poem and because of the corrupted state of the last lines. Moreover, Atthis' desire is not uttered either. Although we hear *about* her, we never hear her. What we do hear are Sappho's words, reading the desire of both, maybe her own desire as well. But if it is impossible for female desire to be uttered, how is it then possible that she, a woman, can utter her own desire and the desire of others? What is then that make her desire possible to utter?

For Sappho, composing and performing a poem about female desire is at the same time an act of reading and writing: reading the desire of others in order

---

[36] Dem. *On Style*, 132.

to write a poem. But while writing is usually taken to be an act to fix a certain meaning, for Sappho it is not. In Sappho's world, stability of a "text" is undone by performance. For every time the poem is performed, the time and spatial marker of the poem (here–there, now–then) change. If the poem itself enforces time and space shifts, permitting fluidity, a blurring of boundaries, performance goes one step further. Space and time become even more fluid since "here" and "now" change at any given performance and the act of saying the words is not an attempt to fix the moment, but the acceptance of the impossibility of its fixed status. By the same token, an attempt to write desire yields to an attempt of reading desire as an acceptance of its unfixed status. Writing the poem then is an act of "fixating" desire by admitting at the same time the impossibility of such a process of fixation.

The desire that Sappho reads is a feminine desire, but the person who desires and is desired is not easy to read. Although Sappho's reading of desire seems to be conceptualised as an ever receding print, a desire that is read but at the same time cannot be uttered, nevertheless the poem stands as an attempt to utter desire: in order to do so Sappho needs to read feminine desire in the framework of masculine discourse. Why is masculine discourse necessary for female desire to be uttered?

Because, I argue, it is the only the male symbolic that poetic discourse is possible. In this sense, writing a poem is by itself an attempt to write female desire within male discourse? Is this possible? Or is the desire going to be transformed into male desire through male discourse? Sappho's attempt to utter female desire is an attempt to "create" female discourse. By using male discourse Sappho is also trying to supply her own female reading of it, a reading that attempts to shake the illusion of fixation that male discourse professes by upsetting the boundaries of time, space and language. In an act of destabilisation, Sappho uses poetic *topoi* and language that evoke epic with a twist of female reading.

The poem begins with a very "Homeric" metaphor, followed by an equally "Homeric" simile. Both figures of speech evoke epic, masculine discourse. Whether Arignota is a name or an epithet, the description of a girl as godlike is full of Homeric undertones: in *Odyssey* 6.149, Odysseus is uncertain whether Nausicaa is mortal or not and decides to play it safe by asking: "Queen, I come here as a suppliant to you. Are you a goddess or a mortal, I wonder?"[37]

---

[37] My discussion benefits from Winkler's discussion in "Gardens of Nymphs". Winkler reads Sappho 31 as a re-creation of the same scene in the *Odyssey*. My reading re-creates both Winkler's reading on Sappho 31 and Sappho's reading of Homer.

This is, of course, a rhetorical question. Odysseus knows Nausicaa is mortal but the question works as a *captatio benevolentiae*. The fact that a mortal might resemble an immortal works as a compliment. It is also a Homeric way to describe outstanding individuals using epithets that mean "similar to gods". Moreover, and quite interestingly, the epithet ἀρίγνωτος does appear in the same scene, even though it does not characterise Nausicaa in this instance.

In an extended simile, Homer compares Nausicaa and her companions with Artemis and 'her' nymphs. Nausicaa is thus compared to Artemis. Again it is not only the fact that Nausicaa is compared to a goddess that brings this close to Sappho, but also the terms of the comparison between the mortal and they immortal: both Artemis and Nausicaa look preeminent among a team of beautiful maidens. Which, of course, brings us back to Arignota, preeminent among the Lydian women. The word used for the preeminence of Nausicaa among the other girls is μετάπρεπε, a term that strongly evokes the Sapphic ἐμπρέπεται.

Sapphic imagery is closely following the Homeric: a mortal is compared to a goddess as a sign of her preeminence. At this point the presence of Homeric diction is also evident. The epithet attributed to the moon is βροδοδάκτυλος, evoking a very well known formulaic phrase. However, it is noteworthy that the adjective is here used to modify the moon, unlike in Homer, where is always used to modify Eos.[38] As a metaphor, the image of rosy-finger Dawn makes a lot of sense since the sunrays look like fingers and the color of the sky in early morning is reddish as a rose. When the epithet is used for moon, though, it is more puzzling: what does it refer to? Since the metaphor is not anchored in the resemblance of the two objects, the metaphor works at a different level of literary resemblance: the comparison is not between two objects, but between two texts that are in dialogue with one another, as the use of the same adjective points toward the traditional Homeric, male, discourse. At the same time, the use of different noun, moon, does not comply with the audience expectation. The result is a defamiliarisation, which seems to point at once to a different, female poetic discourse.

Thus, my suggestion is that this well-known Homeric epithet is here used in an innovative way, immediately marking a different discourse: unlike the Homeric text, the Sapphic reference to the moon must have evoked an evident association with femininity in the mind of the audience. But the Sapphic imagery goes further: the simile is expanded even more, and displays a certain ambiguity. At first it is Arignota who apparently looks like the moon; further on, however, it

---

38 The adjective used in Homer 27 times *always* describes Eos.

is the image of the actual moon, spreading its light over the sea, over the flowery meadows. The figure of speech, like the figure of Arignota, is fluid, changing. What starts as a simile is now a description.

But a description of what exactly? As space and time are unidentified, the (un)epic light shows Arignota like a goddess, or maybe a goddess like Arignota. The space that is created through the playful inversion of epic, male, Homeric speech, I would suggest, is an unfixed, feminine space, a space for feminine discourse.[39]

Luce Irigaray in *When our Lips Speak Together* emphasises the differences between masculine and feminine discourse, explaining that in masculine discourse the spatiotemporal relationships have a definite end; time and place are limited and vertical. On the other hand, feminine space and time are limitless, endless, fluid and horizontal. In this light, the limitless spatiotemporal relations as produced by the poem again point to its visibly feminine quality. The poem, I argued, presents a feminine limitless space, to be contrasted with the confined masculine space.

In addition, the simile of the moon seems to point toward feminine discourse as well. The image of moon is always close to women. Being grammatically feminine, σελάννα is closely connected with feminine fertility and the feminine body.[40] The period of the moon is closely connected to the female cycle. Σελάννα is of course also a mythological person, a Titan, the goddess of the moon.[41] In mythology, there is also a variety of goddesses associated with the moon, all of whom have connections with women's cults.[42] Plutarch, reflecting common ancient belief, connects Hera with the moon and Zeus with the sun. Therefore, he says, Hera is connected with women expecting a child, which clearly affirms the moon's close association with female fertility.[43]

Similarly, Irigaray argues that a male space is vertical, following the idea of rigid hierarchy, while female spaces are horizontal. Returning to fr. 96, the image of moon usually brings to mind a vertical division (heaven-earth). In the Sapphic poem, though, the image of the moon is horizontal, stretching over the earth,

---

[39] Williamson (1996) 255 uses the term 'elision' to describe the way Sappho represents distances between the speaking positions of the poem figured through space and time.
[40] Stehle in Greene (1996) 148, n. 12.
[41] Sappho seems to have written a poem on the love story of Selene and Endymion, according to the ancient scholiast; see Campbell (1982) fr. 199.
[42] Usually Hera, Hekate, Artemis, Eileithyia just to name the most prominent ones. All have connections with female fertility and childbirth. For Hekate as the goddess of the moon and associations of Artemis with the moon see Johnston (1990) 29–48, esp. 31 n. 8.
[43] Plut. *Aetia*, 282c4 ff.

creating a limitless space without fixed boundaries, merging Lesbos and Sardis. The moonlight is spread over the sea; the moon is no longer up in the sky but at sea. The movement of the female voice as a result is not upward:

> Stretching upward, reaching higher, you pull yourself away from the limitless realm of your body. Don't make yourself erect, you'll leave us. The sky isn't up there: it's between us.[44]

The sky in the Sapphic poem is between the protagonists, spread horizontally as, according to Irigaray, it should in all feminine discourse. In addition, is it possible that Sappho's voice is heard in the space 'in-between' that may be alluded to in the last (?) fragmentary line?

Fr 96 can be read, then, as a poem writing feminine space and time, writing feminine desire and a plurality of feminine voices. Sappho stages Fr. 96 not as monologically as it might seem at first sight. The narrator enables and generates a dialogue, creating a discourse blurring time and space, writing desire, writing of a body without fixed boundaries, in an incessant mobility and restlessness. It is a dialogic representation in which one persona enables the presentation of the other; a dialogic discourse that the choral performance will automatically turn into polyphony. Moreover, its discourse is feminine. Unfinalized and open, without boundaries, even literally: another fragment without beginning and end, voicing the fluidity of feminine discourse. A fragment ending in the middle with its last word being μέσσον, not separating but mediating between past and present, enabling a dialogue regardless of space and time, not only between Arignota and Atthis but also between Sappho and Irigaray.

Taking up the discussion of a feminine voice then, I hope to have shown that the voice of Sappho can be considered as a paradigmatic embodiment of feminine discourse: a fragmented, elusive self, a never-ending and a never-to-be-read text, forever lost and impossible to pin down. Sapphic poetry defies closure because it is a feminine text, as Cixous would put it. At the same time, its fragmented quality is not seen as problematic but as expressive. It is not a lack of meaning we are dealing with. On the contrary, the fragmentation of the Sapphic text seems almost organic. Defying closure and singular meaning, it is an open text ready to be re-opened and re-read.

With a close reading of Sappho's texts, this paper attempted to map the feminine poetics of Sappho and to provide answers to matters of lyric construction of selfhood, by emphasising the continuous construction of the feminine self. Writing a feminine self is considered as staging a fragmented, elusive self, a self under construction. Such an understanding of Sapphic poetics points to a very

---

44 Irigaray (1985) 213.

old yet very fresh possibility of a polyphonic lyric, by decoding the inherent and persistent polyphony of feminine poetics and its delicately rebellious relationship with masculine poetics, both in archaic poetry and for a twenty-first-century readership.[45]

---

[45] I would like to wholeheartedly thank Jeroen Lauwers for organising a stimulating and thought provoking conference. I would also like to thank the reader, Anneleen Masschelein, for her feedback and helpful comments. Last but not least, I am grateful to the audience of the conference, especially Glenn W. Most and Vered Lev Kenaan, for comments and fruitful discussion.

3 Reviving Classical Ideas through the Centuries

Luca Grillo
1 Irony in Cicero's *post reditum* Speeches

Early in August 57, Cicero returned to Rome from exile, something from which, as Nisbet points out, "he never recovered, politically or psychologically".[1] Indeed, the illusion that he had regained his old splendour and prestige soon clashed against the realization that his attempts to recover had failed. The orations he composed between August 57 and April 52, broadly known as *post reditum* speeches, duly document such attempts, illusions and failures.[2] Around April 56 Cicero resigned himself to occupying a place in the orbit of Caesar, Pompey and Crassus, who had just re-formed their alliance, the so-called 'first triumvirate'; this milieu limited his freedom (cf. *QFr.* 2.7), and he was forced to take up their cause. With a speech *On the Consular Provinces* in 56 he gave a shocking defence of Caesar's reappointment in Gaul;[3] in 54, pleasing Caesar once more, he unwillingly defended a personal enemy, Vatinius, whom he had publicly and passionately accused before;[4] then pleasing Pompey, he defended Scaurus,[5] and even that same Gabinius he had accused so fiercely in *De Provinciis Consularibus* (9–16); and lastly, pleasing Crassus, he defended Plancius.[6] Moreover, these compromises were perceived as a betrayal of his more conservative ideals,[7] and Cicero himself was dissatisfied with them: in 54, commenting on his recent cases,

---

[1] Nisbet (1961) xvi.
[2] See e.g. the optimistic tone of *Att.* 4.1 (esp. 4.1.3), written in September 57, and the gloomy realization of *QFr.* 3.5 (esp. 3.5.4), written in November 54.
[3] On the historical context of this speech, see Nicholson (1992) 19–29; Grillo (2015) 9–16.
[4] Cicero attacked Vatinius in February/March 56, but defended him in August 54; cf. Alexander (1990) 133–134 and 141–142.
[5] Scaurus, a stepson of the dictator Sulla, was related by marriage to Pompey; cf. Gruen (1974) 148–149. The trial was held in summer 54, cf. Marinone (2004) 132.
[6] Cf. Cassius Dio 39.32.2–3; Taylor (1964) 22; for the date see Alexander (1990) 132; Marinone (2004) 132.
[7] In a letter to Atticus, written in summer 56 (*Att.* 4.5.1), Cicero famously refers to his changed policies as a *palinōdia*, "recantation"; cf. Grillo (2015) 14–16.

Note: I thank the organizers of "Psychology and the Classics," for a very pleasant and productive conference and the participants for helpful feedback. I also wish to thank the Center for Global Initiatives at the University of North Carolina at Chapel Hill, the Dean and the Department of Classics for their support, which helped me to attend the conference. Throughout this paper translations are mine, unless otherwise indicated, and all dates are BC.

Luca Grillo, North Carolina Chapell Hill

he ironically wrote to Atticus that *parantur orationibus indices gloriosi*, "glorious titles for my orations are in store" (*Att.* 4.15.9, July 54). Embittered, he withdrew from the courts to work on his *De Oratore* for a while (55–54).

His bitterness and frustration found expression in the rich irony of the *post reditum* speeches. Some cases fit the definitions by ancient manuals of rhetoric, but some others do not. With this contribution I wish to use both ancient and modern theories to offer a holistic explanation of how Cicero's irony functions. In the first part I analyze some instances in light of ancient theories and in light of Grice's pragmatics. In the second and third parts, I borrow two models which subsequently sprang from Grice's pragmatics, and which help to explain other instances of irony in Cicero. I will argue that each of these models provides helpful hermeneutic tools to appreciate the complexities of the *post reditum* speeches. Seminal contributions by Nünlist and Lloyd on the *Iliad*, by Goldstein on Herodotus' *Histories*, and by Opsomer on the *corpus Plutarcheum* have demonstrated the applicability of these modern theories to Greek texts,[8] but, to my knowledge, less has been done with pragmatics and irony in Latin literature.[9] I also hope to show that although these models lie somewhat beyond ancient definitions of irony, in fact classical texts anticipated some of their discoveries.

Cicero's "Traditional Irony" and Gricean Pragmatics

We can take as a starting point Cicero's revelation to his friend Atticus, quoted above, that "glorious titles for my orations are in store" (*parantur orationibus indices gloriosi*). The context (cf. *Att.* 4.15.7) and other letters (e. g. *Att.* 4.16.6 and 4.17.4) leave no doubt that Cicero was obviously dissatisfied with the inglorious compromises which speeches like *Pro Scauro* document. Clearly he meant the opposite of what he said, and this is precisely the way various ancient manuals of rhetoric define irony, saying one thing and meaning its opposite. For instance, the *Rhetorica ad Herennium* considers irony as a form of 'allegory' (*permutatio*):

> Permutatio est oratio aliud verbis aliud sententia demonstrans ... [permutatio] ex contrario ducitur sic, ut si quis hominem prodigum et luxuriosum inludens parcum et diligentem appellet. (*Rhet. Her.* 4.46).

---

8 Nünlist (2000); Lloyd (2004); Goldstein (2013); Opsomer (1998) and (2000).
9 The one instance I know of is Zoccola (2007), who applies some models from pragmatics to Terence's use of irony in *Hecyra*. I plan further to discuss and use models from pragmatics and cognitive sciences in a monograph I am writing on irony in Latin literature.

"Allegory is a type of speech indicating one thing by the letter and one other by the meaning ... allegory is drawn from contrast when one mockingly calls a spendthrift and voluptuary cheap and restrained." (Trans. adapted from Caplan, Loeb 1968).

This understanding of irony as "a type of speech meaning one thing by the letter and one other by the meaning", finds illustrious forerunners in the Greek tradition and will be very influential.[10] Similarly, for Quintilian irony is found "in that type of allegory by which words and meaning are opposite" (*in eo vero genere [allegoriae], quo contraria ostenduntur, ironia est*, 8.6.54).

Before looking at other examples, it is worth noting that the *Rhetorica ad Herennium* talks about a difference between what is stated and what is meant *aliud verbis aliud sententia*, while Quintilian talks about opposites, *contraria*; these two definitions have shaped our understanding of irony for centuries. For example, the Webster English dictionary diplomatically defines irony as "the use of words to express something other than especially the opposite of the literal meaning". Equally noteworthy is the fact that Latin has no single word for irony: the *Rhetorica ad Herennium* uses *permutatio* while Quintilian, clearly describing the same phenomenon, here opts for *ironia*; but this discrepancy is just the beginning. Cicero and Quintilian use also *illusio*, *fictio*, *simulatio* and *dissimulatio*,[11] and even when they trouble to explain how these terms differ from each other they do not always stick to their own categorizations.[12] One differentiation, however, deserves mentioning: Quintilian specifies that irony can be restricted to a single word or expression, in which case he calls it a trope, or to a whole section or attitude, in which case he calls it a figure.[13] The trope is shorter or easier to understand, and especially it functions differently from the figure: the trope does not *pretend* something different, *non aliud tamen simulat*, while the figure does, *in figura totius voluntatis fictio est* (9.2.45–46).[14]

---

10 Cf. e.g. Anaximenes (*Rhet. Alex.* 1434b, 21) and Tryphon (*On Tropes*, Spengel 3.205.1 and West (1965) 243 = Spengel 3.222).
11 E.g. *illusio*, Quint. 8.6.54; *fictio*, Quint. 6.3.90; *simulatio*, Quint. 6.3.85; *dissimulatio*, Cic. *De or.* 2.269.
12 For instance, Quintilian, dismayed at the confusing proliferation of vocabulary, suggests dismissing Latin translations altogether and just using εἰρωνεία (9.2.44); but in fact he uses *ironia* more often than εἰρωνεία; also his definition of *dissimulatio* (9.2.9 and 9.2.95) as 'faking misunderstanding' is inconsistent with his use at 9.1.29 as synonym for εἰρωνεία.
13 On Cicero's use of irony as a trope and as a figure, cf. Canter (1936), who focuses on the latter, and Haury (1955) 23–25.
14 *Igitur* εἰρωνεία *quae est schema ab illa quae est tropos genere ipso nihil admodum distat (in utroque enim contrarium ei quod dicitur intellegendum est), species uero prudentius intuenti diuersas esse facile est deprendere: primum quod tropos apertior est et, quamquam aliud dicit ac sentit,*

The following passages represent instances of irony as a trope, also known as verbal or rhetorical irony. *Pro Caelio* displays many examples of this type, which constitutes another 'instrument of persuasion'.[15] For instance, Cicero over and over again calls Clodia a whore without saying it:

> nihil iam in istam mulierem dico; sed si esset aliqua dissimilis istius ... (*Cael.* 38).
>
> "here, I say nothing against this woman; but if there were one, different from this one ..."

Clearly, *dissimilis istius* means the opposite, and the audience appreciates the irony easily concluding that this 'different' *mulier* is precisely Clodia. And similarly Cicero later promises not to name any specific woman (*mulierem nullam nominabo* ... 48; cf. 50), but it is not hard to guess which *mulier* he is talking about. This use of *ironia ex contrario* fits the definitions by the *Rhetorica ad Herennium* and by Quintilian; but ancient manuals provide further guidance to explain it. For instance, the *Rhetorica ad Alexandrum* attributed to Anaximenes uses εἰρωνεία of two different phenomena: "εἰρωνεία means saying something pretending not to say it" (εἰρωνεία δέ ἐστι λέγειν τι μὴ λέγειν προσποιούμενον, 1434a, 21), a form of *praeteritio*, as when we say "not to mention that ...;" but it also means "calling things by their opposites" (τοῖς ἐναντίοις ὀνόμασι τὰ πράγματα προσαγορεύειν, 1434a = 21). Cicero's irony in this passage reconciles the two definitions by Anaximenes. Moreover, writing after Cicero, Quintilian specifies that irony, among other things, allows one elegantly to pass over something unpleasant (8.6.55–56), as Cicero pretends to do here.

These precepts from ancient manuals of rhetoric can productively be put in conversation with some modern theories. As a point of departure into the proliferating bibliography on irony by psychologists and cognitive scientists, we can take Paul Grice's pragmatics of conversation and in particular his theory of the Cooperative Principle. Seeking a rational foundation for the general conditions of communication, Grice identified four maxims which speakers are expected to observe in order to communicate successfully: 1. Quantity: "make your contribution as informative as is required (for the current purposes of the exchange)." 2. Quality: "Try to make your contribution one that is true ... Do not say what you believe to be false ... Do not say that for which you lack adequate evidence." 3. Relation: "Be relevant."

---

non aliud tamen simulat ... Ergo etiam breuior est tropos. At in figura totius uoluntatis fictio est, apparens magis quam confessa, ut illic uerba sint uerbis diuersa, hic sensus sermonis ... Quint. 9.2.44–46.

15 On Cicero's understanding of irony see Haury (1955) 7–25; see Albrecht (2003) 65 on his use for persuasion.

4. Perspicuity: avoid obscurity of expression and ambiguity; be brief and orderly".[16] For Grice irony is a way blatantly to "flout" the second and most important maxim (tell the truth) without violating it: rather than believing a lie, the listener appreciates that a literally false utterance simply means something different.

This understanding of irony as saying something literally false and implying its opposite matches the classical definitions of εἰρωνεία and *ironia* by Anaximenes, Cicero and Quintilian;[17] but pragmatics help by explaining that one can violate the Cooperative Principle at the level of what is said but still respect it at the level of what is implied.[18] In particular, context and shared background allow one to decode irony through a twofold process: one takes an utterance literally, but upon realizing that it is at odds with its context,[19] rejects the literal in favour of non-literal meaning. Thus both Quintilian and Grice believe that irony is meant to be understood as such and both stress the importance of context: "delivery, character of the speaker and situation" ensure proper comprehension (*aut pronuntiatione intellegitur aut persona aut rei natura*, 8.6.54), or, as Grice has it, "context, linguistic or otherwise" (1975, 50) allows the hearer to appreciate "the conversational implicature" of an utterance, even if it literally flouts a maxim from the Cooperative Principle (48–50). This is a good reminder that classical insights on irony, being more nuanced and variegated than it is often recognized, have more to offer on irony than the single definition which became standard.

Similarly, for Grice irony, as a figure of rhetoric, belongs with metaphor, *meiōsis* (a sort of euphemistic understatement) and *hyperbolē*,[20] that is, with those figures which, being literally false, flout the second maxim but do not violate the Cooperative Principle, since they mean something else (52–53). This resembles the classification of the *Rhetorica ad Herennium*, which groups "irony" (*permutatio ex contrario*) with other "adornments of words," whereby words are

---

16 Grice (1975) 45–46.
17 *Rhet. Alex.* 1434b, 21; Cic. *De or.* 2.269 and 3.202; Quint. 9.2.44. In his analysis of εἰρωνεία in the *corpus Plutarcheum*, Opsomer concludes that the pragmatist approach with its focus on 'sincerity conditions' offers a more holistic model, able "to establish a comprehensive description for the various uses of the Greek εἰρωνεία" (1998) 3, cf. 19. Cf. Grice (1978) 124.
18 Grice (1975) 51–53. For a more detailed discussion about the contribution of Grice's pragmatics to the traditional understanding of irony, see Grillo (forthcoming, 2018).
19 Cf. Quintilian 8.6.54.
20 Grice (1975) 53 uses the following examples: irony is when A says "X is a fine friend", with both A and the audience knowing that X has just disappointed A; metaphor is saying "you are the cream in my coffee", and, like irony, involves two stages of interpretation; *meiōsis* is saying "he was a little intoxicated" of a man known to have broken all the furniture; and *hyperbolē* is saying "every nice girl loves a sailor".

transferred from their literal into a non-literal meaning (4.42). Metaphor is one of these adornments, is treated just before 'irony' and called with similar names: in 'irony' the "permutation" opposes literal and non-literal meaning, while in "metaphor" the permutation is based on a common denominator, thus being called *translatio* or *permutatio per similitudinem* (4.45–46).[21]

A few more examples can illustrate the use of this conversation between ancient and modern theories. In *De Provinciis Consularibus*, Cicero launches a harsh invective against Gabinius (against whom he held personal animosity): having listed his defeats, Cicero alleges that Roman provincials had to pay bribes "to that outstanding general of ours," *praeclaro nostro imperatori*.[22] The context of Gabinius' defeats demonstrates that both *praeclarus* and *imperator* are ironic. Later in the same speech Cicero reminds his audience that the senate exceptionally refused Gabinius' request for a supplication, but he and his friends "take this consolation, that the senate has refused a thanksgiving also to T. Albucius" (*hac consolatione utuntur, etiam T. Albucio supplicationem hunc ordinem denegasse, Prov. Cons.* 15). In fact the comparison with Albucius, rather than offering "consolation," provides Cicero with one more way to slander his target. He admits that there is a difference. Albucius defeated a bunch of unorganized thieves, while in the case of Gabinius,

> bellum cum maximis Syriae gentibus et tyrannis consulari exercitu imperioque confectum. (*Prov. Cons.* 15).
>
> "A war against the most powerful people and tyrants of Syria has been carried to completion under a consular army and authority."

Again, the context (of a refused thanksgiving) makes irony evident, and we can isolate some specific words saying one thing and meaning the opposite: e.g. *bellum*, or *maximis Syriae gentibus et tyrannis*, or *confectum*, since Cicero denies Gabinius the glory of a proper war, of fighting a proper enemy, and of carrying the "war" to completion. And yet in this case irony functions in more than one way, and a different model explains how.

---

[21] For *Ad Herennium*, *permutatio per similitudinem* differs from *translatio* in number, not in substance: when more than one metaphor (*translatio*) from the same realm occurs in the same sentence we have a *permutatio per similitudinem*. To use its example: "to what guard should we entrust our sheep, when dogs behave like wolves?" 4.46.

[22] *Ita gentes eae quae … vim argenti dederant praeclaro nostro imperatori*, "And so, the provincials who paid a large amount of money to our outstanding general …" *Prov. Cons.* 4, with Grillo (2015) 102.

Cicero's "Echoic Irony"

The superlatives and grandiose language of Cicero's false praise of Gabinius suggest that here irony operates also at another level. Indeed, I believe that with this phrasing Cicero imitates and mocks the language of the letter with which Gabinius had requested a supplication.[23] What especially generates irony, then, is Cicero's imitation of Gabinius' triumphalist claims, and noticeably, this type of irony does not immediately fit the definitions Cicero had available. We can better account for it by using a modern theory.

Between 1981 and 2012, four psychologists, Julia Jorgensen, George Miller, Dan Sperber and Deirdre Wilson, responded to Grice and put forth a new model, the so-called mention or echoic theory of irony.[24] This theory holds that, to use their own example, there is no doubt that a speaker saying "What lovely weather!" in the middle of pouring rain, speaks ironically; but there are two ways to account for it. As seen above, the traditional view, formulated by Cicero and Quintilian and tested by Grice, takes "the speaker to be using a figurative meaning opposite to the literal meaning of the utterance". The mention theory, instead, takes "the speaker to be mentioning the literal meaning of the utterance" and "identify[ing] the echoed material mentioned and the speaker's attitude toward it".[25] In other words, by saying "what lovely weather" in a storm the speakers are literally talking about lovely weather, the lovely weather they do not have, and by mentioning it they also voice disappointment at their expectation being cheated.

There are many instances of echoic irony in Cicero, as a few examples can demonstrate. In *Pro Sestio*, Cicero attacks Piso (against whom he also had personal animosity) for his look:

> Nam quid ego de supercilio dicam, quod tum hominibus non supercilium, sed pignus rei publicae videbatur? Tanta erat gravitas in oculo, tanta contractio frontis, ut illo supercilio annus ille niti tamquam videretur (*Sest.* 19).

> "And – my word! – what shall I say about that lofty brow of his, which struck people as not so much a brow, but a guarantee of the commonwealth: such seriousness was in his look, so furrowed in concentration was his brow – like a surety on deposit, it seemed to underwrite the full burden of his year as consul." (Trans. Kaster, Oxford 2006).

---

23 Cf. Grillo (2015) 160–161.
24 Sperber/Wilson (1981) 295–318; Jorgensen/Miller/Sperber (1984) 112–120; Wilson/Sperber (2012) 123–145.
25 Jorgensen/Miller/Sperber (1984) 115.

This statement must be taken literally, as it does not mean the opposite of what is says: Piso was renowned for his *gravitas*, he did have a prominent brow, and brows did signal character to Romans.[26] The irony, then, lies especially in its echoic force: it calls to mind Piso's look and specifically the expectation of *gravitas* that such a look elicited – an expectation (*pignus*) which was cheated, according to Cicero.

This model claims to replace the classical and Gricean theories of irony, but in my view it can coexist with them. For example, Cicero's ironically calling Gabinius "an outstanding general" can be seen as echoing the Romans' expectations of conquest and success and expressing disappointment at Gabinius' cheating them. In some cases, however, mention theory explains irony better than the traditional models.

In *Pro Caelio* Cicero cunningly picks up a quotation from the previous orator, Crassus, and uses it against Clodia:

> "Nam numquam era errans" hanc molestiam nobis exhiberet "Medea animo aegro, amore saevo saucia." Sic enim, iudices, reperietis quod, cum ad id loci venero, ostendam, hanc Palatinam Medeam ... (*Cael*. 18).

> "'for never would a wandering woman' have caused us all this trouble 'Medea, sick at heart, wounded by a wild passion.' For you will find out, gentlemen, what I shall show you when I come to that point – that this Medea of the Palatine ..." (Trans. Berry, Oxford 2008).

This quotation is filled with irony, and mention theory explains how: Cicero means the literal meaning of the utterance, which is about Medea; but we also easily identify the echoed material. *Palatina Medea* directly points to the unnamed Clodia, and Cicero manifests his attitude toward her, portraying her as a mad and dangerous woman.

Pro Plancio provides another passage which mention or echoic theory explains. In 54 Cicero defended Plancius, who had been elected curule aedile, against the prosecution of Laterensis, who had run for the same magistracy but had not been elected. Cicero allegedly declines to humiliate Laterensis: he was not elected – Cicero explains – only because, unlike Plancius, he relied on his noble birth and refused to canvass and please the people, who did not vote for him. To drive his point home, Cicero uses a *sermocinatio*, in which he imagines the people talking to Laterensis: the people complain that he was just not there when they needed him (*deinde sitientem me virtutis tuae deseruisti ac reliquisti*, 13) and that he did not please them in his campaign (*neglegenter petenti*, 13); then they

---

[26] Kaster (2006) 160–163.

beg him to beg them harder the next time (*condiscas censeo mihi paulo diligentius supplicare*, 13).

> ego tibi, Laterensis, Plancium non anteposui sed, cum essetis aeque boni viri, *meum beneficium ad eum potius detuli qui a me contenderat quam ad eum qui mihi non nimis submisse supplicarat.*
>
> Desiderarunt te, inquit, oculi mei, cum tu esses Cyrenis; me enim quam socios tua frui virtute malebam, et quo plus intererat, eo plus aberat a me, cum te non videbam. Deinde sitientem me virtutis tuae deseruisti ac reliquisti. *Coeperas enim petere tribunatum pl. temporibus eis quae istam eloquentiam et virtutem requirebant* ... pete *igitur eum magistratum in quo mihi magnae utilitati esse possis* ... qua re aut redde *mihi quod ostenderas, aut si, quod mea minus interest, id te magis forte delectat, reddam tibi istam aedilitatem etiam neglegenter petenti, sed amplissimos honores ut pro dignitate tua consequare, condiscas censeo mihi paulo diligentius supplicare* (*Planc.* 12–13).

> "I did not place Plancius above you, Laterensis, but since you are equally gentlemen, *I conceded my favor to the one who earnestly demanded it from me, rather than to one who did not beg too humbly for it.*
>
> My eyes missed you – it says – when you were in Cyrene; I had rather that I, instead of our allies, should enjoy your *virtus*, and the more I desired it the more it was far from me when I could not see you. Then when I was craving for your *virtus* you left and abandoned me. *You set out to stand for the plebeian tribunate at a time that demanded that eloquence and virtus of yours* ... Seek *then that office by which you can be of great use to me* ... Therefore either give me back *what you have promised or, if perhaps you care more for what pleases me less, I will give you this aedileship, even if you seek it without due care; but I believe that you can learn to beg me a bit more carefully to achieve the great honors which match your standing.*"

Clearly irony fills this comic *sermocinatio,* and yet the traditional model fails to explain how; indeed there is no contrast between words and their literal meaning. Irony is rather produced by an echo: in particular, Cicero evokes the form of a hymn of prayer. As the standard form of hymns demands,[27] the invocation of the addressee, Laterensis, is followed by a confession of preference, *Plancium non anteposui*; then *desiderarunt te* opens an aretalogy, or brief exposition of previous deeds, as usual stressing the relation linking suppliant and addressee, and the request, introduced by imperatives and formulaic language (*pete* and *redde*) follows; and lastly, the suppliant promises that, if the request is met with favour, Laterensis will be rewarded with what he desires – by being elected.[28] The echo of a prayer hymn highlights a pattern of ironic inversions: the people, in spite

---

27 Cf. La Bua (1998) 134–137.
28 I further explore this *sermocinatio* in relation to prayer-hymns in Grillo (2014) 220–221.

of having the power of granting election to Laterensis, act as suppliants, ironically playing up his distance from them, and suggesting that his noble birth and haughty posture worked against him; similarly, instead of reminding the addressee of a special relationship and previous favours, the people remind Laterensis of the lack thereof, pathetically recalling his withdrawal, which jeopardized their faith in his power and/or will to provide the needed help. Thus the echoic theory accounts for the irony of this passage, whereas the traditional model does not.

Classicists may enjoy spotting some classical antecedents to this theory.[29] For example, Anaximenes treats εἰρωνεία in the context of recapitulation, when one *mentions* something stated before, without needing to explain it (1434b, 21). Additionally, as Lausberg writes, often an orator ironically makes use "of the lexical range of values of his opponent and exposes its falsity by the linguistic or situational context" (§ 582). This use of irony consists of a sort of *sermocinatio* of the opponent's utterance, by means of echoing its "analytical terminology,[30] and thus expressing "an attitude toward it".

Classicists may also enjoy exploring the connection between mention theory and some literary approaches with which they are likely more familiar. According to mention theory there are two ways to produce irony: through a link to something specific, like Piso's look in *Pro Sestio* or Medea's character in *Pro Caelio*; and through a link to something general, like the *sermocinatio* in *Pro Plancio*, which does not call to mind a specific hymn, but rather the *type* of most prayer hymns. Equally, by saying "What lovely weather!" in a storm the speaker may ironically echo a specific weather forecast or "she might merely be echoing an expectation or hope that they have shared that the weather would be good".[31]

---

[29] Jorgensen/Miller/Sperber (1984) 112, perhaps too quickly, lump together the whole classical tradition, and, while giving it credit for "many well-described aspects of irony," they wrongly write that "classical accounts of irony assume a specialized mechanism of meaning inversion that does not seem to govern any other mental process". In fact, as seen above, the *Rhetorica ad Herennium* explains "irony" (*permutatio*) as a type of "allegory," or "a type of speech meaning one thing by the letter and one other by the meaning" (4.46) and groups allegory with other figures, including metaphor, explaining that they share as a defining feature the way that "language withdraws from the normal sense of words and is charmingly transferred into another meaning" (4.42). Similarly, an endless debate between lexica focuses on the mechanism and mental process by which tropes and figures (including εἰρωνεία) are shaped and on the differences between them. See West (1965) 230–231 on treaties *On Tropes*; other authors treat εἰρωνεία in their works *On Figures*, e.g. Alexander Sophist, Herodianus, Tiberius and Zonaios (Spengel 3.22.29; 3.91.20; 3.60.6; 3.164.12).
[30] § 902.3b; cf. 820; cf. Opsomer (1998) 17–18.
[31] Jorgensen/Miller/Sperber (1984) 115.

Mutatis mutandis, these two manners of references correspond to the dynamics of intertextuality: for instance, Virgil can activate an allusion to some specific words from Homer, who functions as "modello testuale", to borrow Conte's terminology, or he can call to mind broader modes or motifs, like elegiac, epic or Ennian. Such motifs then function as "modello codice", a *topos* that belongs to no one and to everybody and that as such is continuously revisited and reshaped.[32] Thus, the contemporary discourse about intertextuality, which remains very lively among classicists, mirrors the terms of the echoic model proposed by some psychologists. In either case, whether an author alludes to a specific passage or to a *topos*, all allusions are potentially ironic, as so many examples from Roman comedy or from Ovid or from Roman novels document.[33]

Cicero's Injudicious Statements

Just as the mention or echoic theory directly responds to Grice, in the attempt to disprove him, soon after the mention theory was formulated a new model was proposed to replace it. In 1984, Herbert Clark and Richard Gerrig put forth the pretence theory of irony,[34] explicitly responding to the mention or echoic model. According to pretence theory, the speaker using irony is "pretending to be an injudicious person speaking to an uninitiated audience; the speaker intends the addressee of the irony to discover the pretence and thereby see his or her attitude," and the audience "can take delight in being in on the pretence, in being a member of the inner circle".[35] This theory resembles Quintilian's understanding of *ironia* as a figure, which, as seen above (cf. n. 14), consists of pretence (*fictio*), as opposed to the trope, which results from the substitution of a few specific words and implies no pretence (*non aliud tamen simulat*, 9.2.45). Unsurprisingly then, this theory applies to certain passages better than the other two, as a few examples can demonstrate. In *De Provinciis Consularibus*, Cicero

---

[32] Conte (1986) 31; cf. Hinds (1998) 41.
[33] I intend to explore the interaction between mention theory and intertextuality further in a monograph on irony in Latin literature.
[34] (1984) 121–126.
[35] (1984) 121. As one can see, what drives these scholars is the quest for *the* model to explain irony *tout court*; what interests me, however, is whether any given model can help to explain classical texts; therefore, multiple models can coexist, and in certain cases that more than one model simultaneously applies even to the same passage, as I argue at the end of this paper.

recapitulates his tirade against the reappointment of his personal enemies, Piso and Gabinius, and says:

> Retinete igitur in provincia diutius eum, qui de sociis cum hostibus, de civibus cum sociis faciat pactiones ... (*Prov. Cons.* 12).[36]
>
> "Retain, then, in the province this one [Gabinius], who strikes private deals with the enemy at our allies' expense, and with the allies at our citizens' expense ..."

Noticeably, to explain this irony one could apply the first model and substitute *retinete in provincia* for *deducite* or *deripite de provinciis*, but the sustained irony can be better explained as a pretence to be an uninformed or ill-judged speaker, whose recommendation openly goes against common sense and state interests. Cicero gave this speech to the Roman senate, and no doubt his audience discovered "the pretence" and Cicero's attitude toward it as an absurdity. Arguably, one could apply the second model as well, and maintain that here Cicero echoes the proposal previously advanced by another senator; but the pretence theory accounts for this passage better than the other models. Later in the same speech, Cicero uses the same type of irony to support Caesar's reappointment in Gaul and asks the senators: *nam ipse Caesar quid est cur in provincia commorari velit* ("and what's the reason why Caesar wants to stay in the province?" 29). Then, to be sure, he responds to his own question:

> Amoenitas eum, credo, locorum, urbium pulchritudo, hominum nationumque illarum humanitas et lepos ... retinet (*Prov. Cons.* 29).
>
> "It is the pleasantness of these places, I believe, the beauty of their cities, these civilized and gentle men and people which keep him there ..."

This is no instance of *ironia ex contrario*. According to the precepts of ancient manuals of rhetoric, inserting "*non*" before *retinet* is not an option, since *ironia ex contrario* is produced by the *substitution* of a few specific words with their antonyms.[37] In this case, however, replacing either the subjects or the verb with their opposites (e.g. *amoenitas* with *barbaritas*, *pulchritudo* with *turpitudo*, etc. or *retinet* with *repellit*) would not reveal what Cicero means but simply produce another ironic statement ("barbarity keeps Caesar there" or "pleasantness drives him away"); and substituting both implies transforming the whole statement.

---

[36] There is no need to change the initial statement *retinete igitur* into a rhetorical question, as suggested by some editors, who miss the irony. Cf. Grillo (2015) 146.
[37] *Ut si quis hominem prodigum ... parcum ... appellet*, Rhet. Her. 4.46; *verba sint verbis diversa*, Quint. 9.2.45; cf. n. 14.

Quintilian would consider this a case of irony as a trope, which is not confined to one or two words and which implies *fictio*, pretence. This points into the right direction: given the chauvinistic attitude of Cicero's audience of Roman senators, there is no doubt that his sustained irony here consists of pretending to be another speaker, so grossly uninformed as to miss or overlook the difference between living in refined Rome and living in the middle of 'barbarity.'[38] In turn, irony signals Cicero's scorn toward such an uninformed speaker and utterance, thus pointing to his own sophistication, which he shares with the elite in-group of senators.

Similarly, in *Pro Caelio* Cicero famously accuses Clodia of incest with her brother:

> Quod quidem facerem vehementius, nisi intercederent mihi inimicitiae cum istius mulieris viro – fratrem volui dicere; semper hic erro. (*Cael.* 32; cf. 36).
>
> "I am restrained by my personal enmity with this woman's husband, I mean her brother – I'm always making this mistake!" (Trans. Berry, Oxford 2008).

The audience delights in the pretence, seeing through Cicero's 'slip' and self-correction (*reprehensio*), while the heavy accusation of incest, for which Cicero refuses to be accountable, lingers in our mind. In this example the pretence is immediately revealed as such, but in other cases there is some room for ambiguity; a potentially sincere statement seems meant to be taken literally, until another statement reveals the pretence. For instance, as seen above, in *Pro Plancio* Cicero has the people acknowledge his opponent Laterensis' eloquence: "You set out to stand for the plebeian tribunate at a time that demanded that eloquence and *virtus* of yours," *istam eloquentiam ... requirebant*. At first we may be inclined to take this utterance literally, especially after Cicero has treated his opponent mildly (cf. 2–7). Later in the same speech, however, Cicero portrays Laterensis as a rather poor speaker, who screams (*clamitas, Laterensis*) and who seems to have been educated not in Rhodes, like Cicero, but among the barbarian Vaccaei (84). Thus, his 'compliment' for "that eloquence of yours" is revealed for what it is, ironic pretence. To be sure, the first two models also provide an explanation for this use of irony: according to the first, *virtus* and *eloquentia* stand for their opposite, while according to the second, Cicero is talking about the *virtus* and *eloquentia* Laterensis does not have, thus voicing his disenchantment. The pretence model, however, explains this instance better, in at least two ways: it takes into account that the audience may be taken in by the pretence and hence find

---

38 For more evidence of this attitude, see Grillo (2015) 219.

pleasure in discovering it as such;[39] and it explains how, once the pretence is clear, those who appreciate it become part of an in-group, which exists by virtue of leaving someone else out. In other words, this theory contemplates more than one level of audience.[40] Indeed this type of irony is subtle, and not everyone gets it: for instance, the Bobian scholiast writes that "Laterensis was equally eloquent and noble" (*nec minore facundia quam generis nobilitate praedito, argumentum Planc.*) thus proving that he missed it.[41]

Clark and Gerrig dutifully acknowledge that irony comes from εἰρωνεία, which involved some pretence from the start. The main difference is that, according to their model, irony is meant to be understood, at least by some, while in Greek εἰρωνεία often indicates cunning dishonesty or mischievous deception.[42] The pretence model thus comes closer to Latin *ironia* than to Greek εἰρωνεία. In particular, Latin manuals of rhetoric included pretence, *fictio*, in their understanding of irony, and, as seen above, for[43] Quintilian *fictio* is the mark of irony as a figure of speech (as opposed to the trope). Modern psychology confirms this understanding, but the pretence model exalts *fictio* to the defining feature of irony as such. Other than helping to explain specific passages, there is much value in this model, which contemplates different levels of audience. In particular, the notion that by understanding irony at someone else's expense one becomes "a member of the inner circle" resembles the dynamics of Roman invective, as some recent studies have explained it.[44] This is one more way in which the interdisciplinary cross-fertilization which volumes like this promote promises to be particularly productive.

It will be clear by now that I am more interested in the relation between these modern models and ancient theories and texts than in the debate about which of these models is 'right' at the expense of the other ones. In my view, different ways to decode irony can coexist and prove alternatively more or less fitting to explain various passages. Indeed, as a way to summarize before drawing some conclusions, we can take a look at an instance from another *post reditum* speech and

---

39 Clark/Gerrig (1984) 123 persuasively use Swift's *Modest Proposal* to exemplify this type of ongoing pretence.
40 "Speakers are not just ironic: They are ironic only to certain listeners," Clark/Gerrig (1984) 124.
41 Cf. Grillo (2014) 222–223.
42 Cf. e.g. Aristophanes *Clouds* 449; Plato *Soph.* 268a; Theophrastus *Char.* 1; cf. Ribbeck (1876), Büchner (1941), Bergson (1971).
43 Quint. 6.3.90 and 9.2.46; *TLL* 6.1.648.35–44.
44 E.g. Corbeill (2002).

see how each of these theories provides a different explanation and how each explanation helps to make sense of Cicero's sophisticated use of irony.

During the trial of Sestius, in 56, Cicero abused Vatinius, a witness, who had deposed against his client. The next day, Vatinius tried to rebuke Cicero, who responded with the *Interrogatio in Vatinium*. This *interrogatio* is a document of full invective, based on Cicero's comparison between himself and Vatinius, a typical *dignitatis contentio*. Among other things, Vatinius alleged that during his exile Cicero was not as missed and loved as he thought (*Vat.* 6–7). Vatinius must have especially dwelt on this point, since his own fame for being unusually funny and good-humoured (cf. Elder Seneca, *Contr.* 7.4.6 and Younger Seneca, *Dial.* 2.17) may have gained him points in the *contentio*. As childish as it may seem, Cicero decides not to let this allegation go unchallenged and replies:

> Scilicet aspera mea natura, difficilis aditus, gravis vultus, superba responsa, insolens vita; nemo consuetudinem meam, nemo humanitatem, nemo consilium, nemo auxilium requirebat (*In Vat.* 8).

> "No doubt I am a prickly sort of person, difficult to approach, heavy of countenance! I answer people arrogantly, rudeness is my habit! No one missed my society, my good nature, my advice, my assistance!" (Trans. Shackleton Bailey, Atlanta 1991).

Cicero was so known for being easy-going and approachable, that everybody must have appreciated the joke. In one way, this joke certainly responds to the 'traditional' or Gricean understanding of irony since the context demonstrates that words like *aspera natura, difficilis aditus, superba responsa* or *insolens vita* are not to be taken literally, but simply mean the opposite of what they say. The Cooperative Principle is 'flouted' at the literal level but not at the level of the implicature. But these words also specifically respond to the allegation by Vatinius, an allegation which Cicero echoes. "What lovely weather!" ironically uttered in pouring rain can target a specific forecast still fresh in the audience's mind. Similarly, Cicero's utterance targets Vatinius' recent allegation, exposing its absurdity. The mention theory therefore explains how Cicero, by calling to mind Vatinius' words in a reworked context, makes him the butt of his irony. Lastly, Vatinius' contention looks absurd, and the pretence theory explains that Cicero achieves irony also by pretending to be an uninformed speaker talking to an uniformed audience; in this case the audience is allowed to see the pretence, thus joining Cicero's in-group, at the expense of the pretended uninformed speaker who, of course, is Vatinius himself. Thus each model is not only applicable, but in fact necessary to do justice to Cicero's cunning use of irony, an irony which transforms a theoretically frightening comparison into a joke.

In conclusion, Cicero's *post reditum* speeches demonstrate that a dialogue between disciplines like Classics and Psychology has much to contribute to our understanding of irony. Classicists can borrow refined models, which account for so many ironic utterances found in classical texts and which, at times, help to decode some classical passages better than the classical theories themselves. But Classicists can also enjoy discovering the classical roots of the modern theories they borrow. And in turn, Psychologists can value the historical depth of such a rich tradition, which can provide further foundation for their research. Indeed, Greek and Latin texts offer a sophisticated understanding of irony, which is less monolithic and uniform than is often believed.

Paul Earlie
2 Psychoanalysis and the Rhetorical Tradition: Theory and Technique

I

For all the richness of his classical culture, Freud has curiously little to say about the rhetorical tradition. For some, this ellipsis is simply constitutional. According to his faithful biographer Ernest Jones, Freud never really went in for "oratory" when addressing an audience,[1] a view endorsed by his English translator and editor James Strachey, for whom "[Freud's lecturing style] was never rhetorical [...] his tone was always one of quiet and even intimate conversation (SE, XV, 5–6).[2] That Freud's prose *is* rhetorical and is so in a way that is unusually persuasive seems scarcely objectionable today. What is more striking is that the relationship between psychoanalysis and the rhetorical tradition never seemed of much interest either to Freud himself, who appears to have studiously avoided mention of the topic, or to scholars of classical antiquity, who have preferred to devote the principal part of their attention to psychoanalysis's therapeutic retrieval of ancient myth and tragedy.[3]

In one sense, this situation is understandable. Parallels between psychoanalytic therapy and ancient tragedy are as numerous as they are diverse, from the importance placed on dialogue and *katharsis* to the necessity of formal constraints on space and time. These affinities explain why Freud, particularly in the early stage of his career, nourished such an abiding interest in the writings of the tragic poets. And yet, resemblances between the analyst and the rhetor are just as prominent: both are committed theorists, teachers, and practitioners of the *logos*; both are concerned with *pathos*, or affect, and its relationship to the spoken utterance; both emphasise the plasticity of character (*ethos*) in achieving persuasive results. The question, then, remains: why, given the force of such affinities, did

---

[1] Jones (1953) 375.
[2] "SE", henceforth in the text, refers to Freud (1953–74).
[3] For a concise history of the latter, see Bowlby (2009). Rhetoric, the *technē* par excellence for inhabitants of the supremely verbal *polis*, is mostly absent from more recent studies of Freud and classical antiquity (e.g., Armstrong (2005); Oliensis (2009)), though Le Rider (2002) provides important examples of the place of rhetoric in Freud's gymnasium curriculum.

Paul Earlie, University of Bristol

https://doi.org/10.1515/9783110482201-015

Freud circumvent classical rhetoric with such an impressive degree of insouciance? To attribute this lacuna to personal disposition alone is to evade the many wider-reaching questions it raises, chief among which are the role of language in the "analytic situation"[4] and Freud's complex relationship to the latter vis-à-vis the scientific ambitions of psychoanalysis.

As George Makari has shown, Freud's model of the mind was rooted in the new aspirational sciences of the nineteenth century (biological Darwinism, psychophysics, neuroanatomy), tempered as this model was by typical Victorian frustrations regarding the limitations of scientific capability. As a consequence, Freud never relinquished his desire "to furnish a psychology that shall be a natural science" (SE, I, 295), as he phrases it in his incomplete 1895 manuscript, "Project for a Scientific Psychology". He merely replaced the anatomizing vocation of his early career with the spatialized, psychical models of psychoanalysis, what he called "structures" or "topographies". These fictive models were only ever intended as an expedient if temporary step on the road to eventual scientific legitimacy since the deficiencies in our description would probably vanish if we were already in a position to replace the psychological terms by physiological or chemical ones" (SE, XVIII, 60). Nonetheless, Freud's decision to abandon a research career in neurology and train as a physician was a momentous one, for it very quickly led him to the aetiology of hysteria, the logic of dreams, and the universality of the Oedipus complex. The direct necessity of treating patients untreatable by existing methods led Freud not only to the "speculative" models he so vaunts in *Beyond the Pleasure Principle* but also to the experimental *bricolage* by which he sharpened his therapeutic technique. This early search for a method led Freud to methods as distinctive, and controversial, as hypnosis and cocaine, before he stumbled on two techniques which became the cornerstone of analytic therapy for the remainder of his life: the interpretation of the patient's free associations and the manipulation of the patient's transference.

This discovery was, of course, also a rediscovery. But while the scientific, philosophical, and literary roots of Freud's breakthrough have been well documented, psychoanalysis inheritance of the rhetorical tradition has been subject to less scrutiny, perhaps partly due to Freud's own indifference to the subject. I will try and show here how the principle technical innovations of psychoanalytic therapy – free association and the transference – both draw on a long Western tradition of reflection on the persuasive power of language (*logos*), character

---

[4] Freud's indifference to rhetoric may stem from an excessively restricted view of rhetorical "context", i.e. limiting it to judicial or political situations of urgency. What Freud calls the "analytic situation" nonetheless fulfils each of Bitzer's three criteria for a "rhetorical situation" (1968) 6.

(*ethos*), and emotional appeal (*pathos*). Free association and the transference reproduce the two key modes of rhetoric as *technē*: rhetoric as persuasion and rhetoric as interpretative tool. With respect to the latter, the necessity of a rhetorical approach to the interpretation of the unconscious is required because the unconscious employs a wealth of rhetorical displacements (e.g., ellipsis: omission of a key term; metonymy: part for whole; periphrasis: talking around) in order to slip past what Freud calls psychical "censorship" (SE, XXII, 15) and into conscious life. The unconscious metaphorises its message through the symptom, requiring an analyst well-versed in the distinction between tenor and vehicle: "as soon as writing, which entails a liquid flow out of a tube on to a piece of white paper, assumes the significance of copulation, or as soon as walking becomes a symbolic substitute for treading upon the body of mother earth, both writing and walking are stopped because they represent the performance of a forbidden sexual act" (SE, XX, 90). But the analyst must also employ rhetorical persuasion as a means of galvanising the progress of the treatment. The analyst's handling of the transference clearly draws on the old rhetorical proofs of *pathos* (the arousal or abreaction of the patient's affective responses) and *ethos* (the analyst's "mirroring" of a particularly important character in the patient's life).

Although psychoanalysis draws on the resources of the rhetorical tradition, it is by no means reducible to a simple process of persuasion.[5] For, to use a distinction that has long played a role in rhetorical theory, if psychoanalysis seeks to persuade, it must also convince.[6] By influencing the transference, the analyst can persuade and thereby alter the structure of the patient's unconscious. Yet for the analysis to achieve any measure of success, the patient must be consciously convinced that they grasped the truth of their condition. Such conviction can only be brought about by the dialectical process of analysis, that is, by rational argumentation. Only reasoned argument can appeal to the logical domains of consciousness and the preconscious, while, conversely, only the analyst's rhetorical technique can appeal to and thus persuade the non-logical domain of the unconscious.

Psychoanalytic therapy also relies on a third type of discourse, however: the discourse of science. Psychoanalysis has always depended on scientific principles which, irrespective of their number or mutability, play a determined and determining role in structuring the dialectical-rhetorical encounter. This does not

---

5 To claim that psychoanalytic therapy is sustained by "rhetorical analysis" alone (Van den Zwaal (1988)) is to miss both the dynamic dialectic of the analytic encounter and the scientific principles which supposedly underpin it.
6 See Perelman (1991) 26–31.

mean that these discursive modes (scientific, dialectical, rhetorical) are always in harmony with each other. In Freud's case, there is a clear desire to understate the rhetorical mode and accentuate the scientific credentials of analysis, for reasons which are no doubt historically strategic. A key argument of the current article, however, is that the specificity of psychoanalytic therapy lies not in its prioritising of any single mode but in its attempt to offer a coherent synthesis of all three. Recent controversies surrounding the burgeoning field of "neuro-psychoanalysis"[7] remind us that such synthesis has always been controversial, and that the relations between each mode have always been unequal, dynamic, and evolving.

II

To investigate psychoanalysis' integration of these three discursive modes, it is useful to return to a thinker whose work already provides such a model. Throughout his writings, but principally in the *Rhetoric* and the *Topics*, Aristotle stresses the complementary nature of dialectical, rhetorical, and scientific (i.e. demonstrative) proofs.[8] This complementarity can be stated succinctly: scientific knowledge (*epistēmē*) is produced when syllogistic demonstration (*apodeixis*) is made from certain necessary principles (*archai*).[9] When the premises are not necessary, but disputed or merely probable opinions (*endoxa*), what is required is dialectical syllogistic (the subject of Aristotle's *Topics*) or, in certain contexts, the rhetorical *enthymeme* (the subject of the *Rhetoric*).

We have already seen how Freud aspired towards a psychoanalysis founded on the model of the natural sciences (SE, XXII, 187–8), but that precise empirical knowledge of the electro-chemical mechanisms underpinning psychical life frustrated such ambitions. To fend off accusations of "suggestion", Freud borrowed a number of principles from biology and physics, where deductions from fundamental axioms had already produced an impressive and broadening body of knowledge (*epistēmē*).[10] Inspired by Gustav Fechner, for instance, what Freud called the "principle of constancy" referred to the psychical apparatus's tendency to keep the internal quantity of excitation as low or as constant as possible, thus explaining the mechanism of repression and the partial discharge of drive energy

---

[7] See, paradigmatically, Solms/Turnbull (2011); Malabou (2012).
[8] See, for example, *Rhetoric* 1 1, 1355a4–18 (references are to the Barnes edition unless stated otherwise).
[9] *Posterior Analytics* 1 6, 74b5–12.
[10] On Freud's borrowing from contemporary sciences, see Sulloway (1979); Makari (2008).

in the "symptom". But while physicists could test the validity of their principles through the observation of moving bodies, limitations in neurobiology meant that Freud's *Konstanzprinzip* could be tested only indirectly, through the dialectical exchange of analyst and analysand and what it revealed about the relative intensity of the patient's drives.

The dialectic interaction of analysis played a pivotal in testing the foundational axioms of psychoanalytic therapy. Unlike Socratic dialectic, Aristotle's dialectic does not aim at the timeless truth of a universal Form but serves a critical role in scrutinising the foundations of "the philosophical sciences".[11] At its most concrete, Aristotle's dialectic involves an "exchange between participants acting in some way as opponents".[12] In a dialectical debate, the "answerer" typically poses a thesis or proposition which the "questioner" tries to refute by bringing out a latent contradiction in the premises. In the analytic situation, dialectic is useful for the same reason it is in Aristotle: it allows the questioner to test a proposition put forward by the patient without having knowledge of the truth or falsity of the premise in question. In this way, analysis aims, as dialectic does in Aristotle, at "securing premises"[13] since it only by means of the latter that the patient's conviction can be attained and the cure effected.

The road to conviction is not, however, straightforward. Following interpretation of the patient's free associations, the analyst confronts him or her with a thesis (what Freud calls a "construction") concerning the structure of the patient's unconscious. As these constructions are accepted or rejected by the patient, consciously or unconsciously, they are progressively refined by the analyst until a "recollection" emerges and the analysand has reached a state of conviction. This, at least, is the basic structure outlined by Freud in his final paper on technique, "Constructions in Analysis" (1937). Here Freud repeatedly emphasises the dialectical nature of analysis: it "involves two people, to each of whom a distinct task is assigned" (SE, XXIII, 258). He aims to refute the commonly held view that psychoanalysis is a dogmatic mode of interpretation, that it is founded on a sophistical logic of "Heads I win, tails you lose" (SE, XXIII, 257). In other words, if the patient agrees with the analyst's interpretation, the interpretation is correct; if he or she rejects it, this is a sign of his or her resistance to it. In rejecting this view, Freud argues that progress in the treatment is only ever achieved through equal exchange between patient and analyst. "We do not pretend," he writes, "that an

---

11 *Topics* 1 2, 101a25–27. For a detailed treatment of the relationship between dialectic and scientific demonstration, see Evans (1977).
12 Smith (1999) 58.
13 Smith (1999) 60.

individual construction is anything more than a conjecture which awaits examination, confirmation or rejection" (SE, XXIII, 265).

While an "interpretation" concerns a fragment of distorted material (a symptom or dream-image, for example), an analyst's "construction" is a consistent argument drawing on a number of interpretations which providing a picture of the patient's unconscious (SE, XXIII, 261). The dialectical structure of analysis proceeds, ideally, as follows: "the analyst finishes a piece of construction and communicates it to the subject of the analysis so that it may work upon him; he then constructs a further piece out of the fresh material [including, crucially, the patient's openness or hostility to the original construction] pouring in upon him, deals with it in the same way and proceeds in this alternating fashion until the end" (SE, XXIII, 260–1). In this way, the patient's responses – which may or may not be "resistances", which may or may not be conscious – feed back into the reciprocal spiral of meaning-making that is the analytic situation. The danger of the unjustified "imposition" of a construction is guarded against by the very dialecticity of this process. In the case of a false construction, the patient's reaction will be tepid and no fresh material will follow, allowing the analyst to discern whether he or she was on the right path or has somehow gone astray. The alternating structure of falsehood and truth is thus actively dialecticized (or, in Hegelian language, "sublated") by the hermeneutic rules of analytic technique (SE, XXIII, 162). This movement continues until the analyst attains a "construction", i.e. an internally consistent picture of the patient "forgotten years", that is both "trustworthy" and "in all essential respects complete".

The subtlety of Freud's phrasing here ("in all essential respects") takes us to the core of the distinction between Socratic and Aristotelean types of dialectic. In Plato's dialogues, most famously the *Meno*, Socratic questioning seeks to bring forth a forgotten truth that is both eternal and external, on the model of the truths of geometry. In the dialectical encounter of analysis, however, what is in question is not a necessary timeless truth but a truth which is internal and historical. If Socratic dialectic terminates in the intuition of an ideal Form, psychoanalytic dialectic is undertaken in a spirit of provisionality or, to use Freud's own language, "interminability".[14] For Aristotle, dialectic is not a positive science but a method of negative critique which is always in some sense incomplete, or rather, to-be-completed. For Freud, similarly, the very notion of a "complete" construction is, like the Borgesian map which covers the entirety of territory it purports to

---

[14] SE, XXIII, 209–53. Freud himself rejects the "approximation" of psychoanalytic therapy and the Socratic method (SE, XVI, 280).

represent, a theoretical fiction. Every construction "is an incomplete one, since it covers only a small fragment of the forgotten events" (SE, XXIII, 263). In psychoanalysis, this structural incompleteness takes several forms – the uninterpretable "navel" of the dream (SE, V, 525), the retroactive revision of the meaning of the past (*Nachträglichkeit*),[15] Freud's late conclusion that analysis is always to some extent "interminable" – but in each case it refers to a structural axiom with which analytic therapy must contend. The therapeutic consequences of this are considerable, for if every construction is incomplete, then the "cure" cannot be triggered by a complete correspondence of the construction (the reasoned argument concerning the structure of the patient's unconscious) with the historical truth of what has been repressed.

From where, then, does the analytic cure arise? Several clues are provided in the closing pages of Freud's paper. If the patient's reactions to a construction are "rarely unambiguous", then "only the further course of the analysis enables us to decide whether our constructions are serviceable or unserviceable". This language of functionality points again to the fact that a construction need not present a complete picture of a state of affairs in order to be "serviceable", i.e. effective in bringing about a cure. What is important, we are told, is that the analyst's "conjecture" is eventually replaced by the patient's "conviction" (SE, XXIII, 265). If there is congruence between the two, this does not always entail a "recollection" on the patient's part of the repressed material. Indeed, it is sometimes the case that "an assured conviction of the truth of the construction achieves the same therapeutic result as a recaptured memory" (SE, XXIII, 266). This concession is particularly striking because it suggests that the real aim of analytic therapy is not the Platonic *anamnesis* of recollection per se, but the patient's reasoned conviction that what he or she has grasped is the truth of their illness. In both cases, i.e. cure by recollection and cure by belief in the construction, the common element is not the reawakening of a memory; it is the patient's "conviction" of having grasped a truth that has emerged through the dialectical process of analysis.

This emphasis on convincing/conviction, however, brings psychoanalytic therapy into dangerous alignment with rhetorical persuasion. Freud indeed acknowledges the "danger of our leading a patient astray by suggesting, by persuading him to accept things which we ourselves believe but which he ought not to" (SE, XXIII, 262). But here, as in Plato and Aristotle, the dangerous incursion of sophistic rhetoric ("Heads I win, tails you lose") calls for the scrupulous observation of technique: only correct adherence to the dialectical method of analysis can

---

[15] See Laplanche/Pontalis (1988) 11–114.

guard against unjustified persuasive suggestion (SE, XXIII, 263). It is my contention, however, following Mikkel Borch-Jacobsen's forceful account of the return of "suggestion" in Freud's later work,[16] that the type of rhetorical (i.e., non-rational) persuasion that Freud seeks in this passage to expel from psychoanalytic treatment is in fact a fundamental component of analytic treatment. This is because, as Freud was all too aware, however dynamic the dialectical exchange between analyst and analysand, every analysis eventually encounters an impasse: the patient's "resistance" to the cure (SE, XVI, 286–302). Since rational constructions alone cannot induce the patient to give up these resistances, the analyst must adopt classical techniques of persuasion in order to dynamize a treatment that will otherwise founder in inertia.[17]

The necessity of adopting different approaches – one based on rational argument (dialectic), the other on rhetorical persuasion – is explained by Freud's topographical distinction between the *logical* domains of consciousness (perception, thought) and the preconscious (stored memories and experiences), and the essentially *non-logical* domain of the unconscious (repressed wishes, traumas, and libidinal urges).[18] Reasoned argument is insufficient to bring about the cure; it must be supplemented by personal influence, that is, the analyst's handling of the patient's transference-resistance through the arousal of emotions by means of an appropriate presentation of the analyst's character. In other words, only the proofs of *pathos* and *ethos* can bring about conditions in which the analysand will engage openly with the analyst's reasoned constructions (*logos*).

It is striking that Freud, who so vaunts the systematising potential of psychoanalytic theory, seems unaware that the power of both the words and character of the speaker to engage the emotions was already the subject of systematic investigation in antiquity. Indeed, several of Freud's technical recommendations regarding conscious and unconscious influence are the subject of commentary in Aristotle's *Rhetoric*. An example of this rich crossover can be found by comparing Aristotle's text with a short technical paper by Freud, "Wild Psychoanalysis"

---

16 Borch-Jacobsen (1990).

17 Freud distinguishes between conscious and unconscious resistance. The former is "an *intellectual* resistance", in that "it fights by means of argument" (SE, XVI, 289); the latter, "the id's resistance", is more recalcitrant but nonetheless more susceptible to rhetorical persuasion. For a detailed discussion of this distinction, see SE, XX, 224–5.

18 The unconscious's transgression of logical categories is exemplified in the absurdity of the dreamscape: "dreams are disconnected, they accept the most violent contradictions without the least objection, they admit impossibilities [...]. Anyone who when he was awake behaved in the sort of way that is shown in situations in dreams would be considered insane" (SE, IV, 54; see also SE, V, 543).

(SE, XI, 221–7). In this paper, Freud discusses the dangers of treatment practiced by those insufficiently versed in the theory and technique of psychoanalysis. He recounts the case of a newly divorced woman who was advised by her physician – on the basis of a minimal familiarity with psychoanalytic therapy – that her anxiety was caused by a lack of sexual satisfaction. Since her religious background obliged her to reject his prescribed course of treatment (remarrying her husband or taking a new lover), her anxiety worsened. As the woman remained unconvinced by the physician's "construction", he referred her case to a personality (*ethos*) of some authority in the field of psychoanalysis: Sigmund Freud – not to *treat* her condition but merely to *confirm* the doctor's original hypothesis.

On the one hand, the physician's lack of success stems from an ignorance of the dialectical method of analysis: he attempts to impose his conjectured construction on the patient without applying the appropriate dialectical techniques of interpretation. But he also misunderstands the rhetorical dimension of analysis, believing that Freud's reputation alone will suffice to persuade the patient to accept the initial construction. These difficulties are only compounded by his ignorance of the scientific principles underpinning the dialectical and rhetorical techniques of analysis, in this case the principle of constancy: the idea that "blocked" internal excitation can be abreacted through simple sexual satisfaction is a gross mischaracterization of analytic theory.

Given the woman's obvious "hostile feelings" towards him, Freud is most critical of the physician's innocence of the transference (SE, XI, 221), which means that he is essentially powerless against the patient's resistances. For Freud, the latter can only be overcome by bypassing the patient's conscious resistances (which will eventually become susceptible to rational argument) and by altering those resistances which remain unconscious (and are thus susceptible only to rhetorical persuasion). The only "means of persuasion" available to the analyst is the manipulation of the positive or negative affective charges of the patient's transference. It is not the case, as the physician believed, that the authority or reputation of a particular analyst is decisive in analytic treatment; rather it is the analyst's ability to reflect, unobtrusively, the character or *ethos* of a figure of personal importance to the patient which enables the resolution of the transference-resistance. For Aristotle, if rhetoric is to function as a *technē* appropriate to a maximal variety of situations, the confidence the speaker inspires must "be due to the speech itself, not to any reestablished reputation by the speaker".[19] If *ethos* as proof were based on the speaker's actual character or personality, the inflexibility of the latter would in fact inhibit, in the majority of cases, the

---

[19] *Rhetoric*, 1356a9–10. On this point, see Brunschwig (1996), 46.

persuasive power of the orator. It would hamper the orator's ability to influence the audience's emotional responses (*pathos*) since appeals to affect are often built on the orator's *ethos*. The analyst influences the patient's affective responses by presenting him- or herself as a "blank slate" on which the patient can project a pre-existing (most often, but not always, parental) model. Like the ideal orator of Aristotle's *Rhetoric*, who attunes his self-presentation to the character (*ethos*) or characters (*ethoi*) of a given audience,[20] Freud argues that "the doctor should be opaque to his patients and, like a mirror, should show them nothing but what is shown to him" (SE, XII, 118).[21] Only later, once the patient has "formed a sufficient attachment (transference) to the physician for his emotional relationship to him to make a fresh flight impossible" (SE, XI, 226), should the analyst offer the patient a reasoned account of the workings of his or her unconscious.

III

In his classic text on analytic technique, "Variations on the Standard Treatment" (1953), Jacques Lacan ridiculous those analysts who use the "stylish" notion of counter-transference (the analyst's affective investment in the patient) as a means of shirking "the action that it is incumbent upon him to take in the production of truth" (2006: 276). While Freud's mirror metaphor suggests an ideal of non-intervention on the part of the analyst, Lacan insists that the analyst must play an active role in all parts of the analytic treatment. Indeed, the very idea that the analyst enjoys a kind of splendid isolation is a fiction, since even the analyst's "silence implies (*comporte*) speech" (2006: 291).

What type of speech is Lacan referring to here? His text makes a sharp distinction between the truth of discourse (*discours*) and the truth of speech (*parole*), the former referring to language's "correspondence to the thing" (2006: 291) and thus with scientific "knowledge of reality", the latter referring to the truth of the unconscious articulated in and through the patient's speech. Despite their fundamental incommensurability, each mode of truth – *discours* and *parole* – is "altered when it crosses the path of the other truth" and therefore each plays complementary roles in the subject's experience of the world. The precise nature

---

[20] Aristotle (2006) 148–56. For Grimaldi "[the aim of Aristotle's] study of the major character types is to show the speaker how his *ethos* must attend and *adjust* to the *ethos* of varied types of auditor if he is to address them successfully" (1998, 2: 186).

[21] In this way, in Mahony's elegant formulation, "the analyst does not so much persuade as effect a persuasion" (1974) 417.

of this complementarity is developed in a second distinction made by Lacan: between convincing (*con-vaincre*) and persuading (*per-suader*).²²

For Lacan, "discourse (*discours*) proceeds to con-vince, a word that involves in the process of reaching an agreement" (2006: 292). Discourse refers to the agreement of two or more interlocutors concerning a given state of affairs, i.e. the "correspondence" between a verbal picture and the reality it represents. It is analogous to Aristotle's notion of dialectic in so far as the agreement concerns a particular construction of reality (or thesis). At the same time, reaching agreement on a particular construction of reality (*discours*) is hampered by the continual interruption of the truth of the unconscious (*parole*): "this process [of convincing] is carried out while the subject manifests bad faith, steering his discourse between trickery, ambiguity, and error. But this struggle to assure so precarious a peace would not offer itself as the most common field of intersubjectivity if man were not already completely per-suaded by speech". In this passage, Lacan, like Freud, holds the unconscious to be the organ of persuasion and the ego that of conviction, even if his somewhat negative (structuralist) assessment of the latter marks a clear divergence from Freud ("the subject loses himself in the discourse of conviction, due to the narcissistic mirages that dominate his ego's relation to the other").

On the other hand, as in Freud, it is because the subject is "completed persuaded by speech" that the analyst must draw on the rich resources of the rhetorical tradition: "we can see, in the most unexpected manner, in the elaboration of the unconscious's most original phenomena – dreams and symptoms – the very figures of outdated rhetoric, which prove in practice to provide the most subtle specifications of those phenomena" (2006: 299). Such comparisons between unconscious phenomena and rhetorical figures and tropes were a common intellectual *topos* in the postwar period, originating in the work of Roman Jakobson but perhaps most authoritatively articulated in Lacan's "linguistic" unconscious.²³ Unlike many of his contemporaries, however, who preserved an essential distinction between psychoanalysis and rhetoric through the figure of analogy, for Lacan the unconscious is not "like" rhetoric: it *is* rhetoric. And if the psychoanalyst is not "like" a rhetor, it is because the psychoanalyst "*is*

---

22 The role of this distinction in Lacan may be traceable to his engagement with contemporary theorists of rhetoric such as Chaïm Perelman, to whose work Lacan responds in "Metaphor of the Subject" (2006) 755–8. For Perelman, "the term *persuasive* [applies] to argumentation that only claims validity for a particular audience, and the term *convincing* to argumentation that presumes to gain the adherence of every rational being", (1969) 28–9.
23 Jakobson (1956); Todorov (1982); Benveniste (1971).

a rhetor (*rhéteur*), [...] he *rhetifies* (*rhétifie*), which implies that he rectifies".[24] The rectification that the patient seeks in analysis, then, is intrinsically linked to the analyst's status as a *rhetor*, a word we must take not only in its traditional sense – as *teacher* of persuasion through the study of tropes – but also in the sense of a committed *practitioner* of persuasion, as orator.

Existing scholarship on Lacan's use of rhetoric has examined the importance of tropes and the textbooks of Cicero and Quintilian in understanding the rhetorical turns of the patient's speech (*parole*).[25] Lacan, for instance, famously identifies the mechanisms of unconscious defence with the figures of classical rhetoric:

> This is why an exhaustion of the defense mechanisms [...] turns out to be the other side of unconscious mechanisms [...]. Periphrasis, hyperbaton, ellipsis, suspension, anticipation, retraction, negation, digression, and irony, these are the figures of style (Quintilian's *figurae sententiarum*), just as catachresis, litotes, autonomasia, and hypotyposis are the tropes, whose names strike me as the most appropriate ones with which to label these mechanisms. Can one see here mere manners of speaking, when it is the figures themselves that are at work in the rhetoric of the discourse the analysand actually utters?" (Lacan 2006: 433).

Part of the role of the analyst-rhetor is to interpret such mechanisms rhetorically. The role of the analyst is never simply one of interpretation, however; he or she must also induce or persuade the patient to reflect on the latent meaning of such "turns" of speech and to give up the resistances which motivate it. My focus here will be on precisely this dimension of the analytic equation: the means by which the analyst intervenes actively and rhetorically in the progress of the cure. While Lacan's relationship to classical rhetoric may not be all-determining, it clearly goes beyond the mechanical application of rhetorical reading to the distorting ruses of the patient's unconscious (free association). To paraphrase Marx, the goal of psychoanalysis is not simply to interpret the unconscious, the point is also to change it. In examining how the analyst sets about to alter the structure of the analysand's unconscious, I will draw on a much underexploited corpus of texts: the written testimony of Lacan's own patients. More specifically, I will make

---

[24] Lacan (1977) 7.
[25] Chaitin (1996); Mahony (1974); Fink (2004) 72–5. This reading is summed up by Mahony (425): "in resisting free association or "pure" referential discourse, the patient thereby tries to influence, convince the analyst. The analysand's resistances are rhetorical, being greatly involved in maintaining his superego or *ethos* before his auditor". For contemporary rhetorical studies" embrace of Lacan, see Lundberg (2012).

reference to George Haddad's detailed account of his analysis with Lacan, though a wealth of competing material is also available.²⁶

What the detailed examination of such texts reveals is that, for Lacan at least, the analyst's handling of the transference functions at both the concrete, micro-logical level of trope (Lacan deploys irony to intensify the transference and thereby dynamize the cure) and at the larger macro-logical level of persuasion (Lacan employs the rhetorical proofs of *pathos* and *ethos* to induce the patient to give up his or her resistances). In this way, the analytic situation offers an organic synthesis of two dimensions of rhetoric that are sometimes seen to be in conflict: rhetoric as the study of tropes and rhetoric as a process of persuasion.

One of the most significant yet controversial ways in which the Lacanian analyst intervenes in the session is through the technique of "scanding" (*scanner*). Scanding refers to the analyst's attempt to structure the patient's free associations by means of "punctuation" or "interruption". In free associative speech, we have seen, the analysand employs of a series of "spontaneous" rhetorical figures to keep him or her from confronting certain unconscious ideas. The role of the analyst is not only to interpret such speech (and formulate a more or less likely "construction"); it is also to persuade the patient to reflect on its latent meaning and, eventually, to abandon the resistances which underpin it. In Lacanian psychoanalysis, this is achieved through "scanding" the patient's associations, a technique that can be as simple as a well-timed exclamation ("Huh!") or the repetition of a phrase that the patient has just uttered.²⁷ The most extreme, and contentious, method of punctuating the session in this manner is to terminate it without warning, a technical innovation of Lacan that is sometimes called the "short session".

Scanding in fact falls into a very technical rhetorical category: paralipsis, a subset of irony which consists in "drawing attention to something in the very act of pretending to pass it over".²⁸ In Haddad's account of his treatment, for example, he recalls Lacan's punctuation of his free association with a series of inscrutable sniggers (*ricanement*) or seemingly indifferent sighs: "once my statement had described a closed loop, Lacan interrupted me, leaving in the statement's hollow a mysterious significance".²⁹ At face value such dismissals underline the

---

26 See Roudinesco (1999) 504, n.7 for a (now somewhat dated) bibliography of such testimony; more recently, Gérard Miller (2012) has filmed a series of documentary-interviews with Lacan's former patients.
27 Fink (1999) 15.
28 http://rhetoric.byu.edu.
29 Haddad (2002) 102 (all translations my own).

insignificance of what has just been said, but in the charged meaning-laden situation of analysis they can have the opposite, paraliptic effect. The power of this technique lies in the fact that it is not immediately determinable if such dismissals do in fact signify their opposite, that is to say, whether such speech acts have a literal value ("what you have just said has no bearing on your analysis") or a metaphorical one ("what you have just said is rich with unconscious significance"). The problem of irony, and perhaps the very source of effectiveness as trope, has always been one of uncertainty: how can we know if our interlocutor is being sincere or not? This uncertainty tends to be written out of heavily formalized rhetoric manuals, though its efficacy has resurfaced in recent decades in a postmodern turn from the constative aspect of irony (this is what I *really* meant) to its performative, persuasive function (this is what my proposition does: inspire questioning).[30]

In the analytic situation, the analyst's irony is an open-ended problem, one which constantly stimulates the patient to question the truth of his or her repressions. As Lacan puts it in an early seminar, irony is "far from being an aggressive reaction, irony is primarily a means of questioning, a mode of question. If it has an aggressive element, it is structurally secondary in relation to the question element".[31] This reference to aggression raises a second and no less important dimension of irony: its relationship to affect. For Hutcheon, "there is an affective "charge" to irony that cannot be ignored and that cannot be separated from its politics of use if it is to account for the range of emotional response (from anger to delight) and the various degrees of motivation and proximity (from distanced detachment to passionate engagement)".[32] Irony may indeed signal the withdrawal of affect, but it also engages emotion in a powerful way through the recursive self-questioning it throws back on the audience. This dimension is a crucial element of Socrates' use of *eironeia*. Plato's Socrates deploys irony to biting rhetorical effect in his ceaseless questioning of the citizens of Athens, deliberately blurring the boundaries between his own ignorance and knowledge in a way which arouses the hostility or anger of his interlocutors. In a cognate way, the psychoanalyst feigns ignorance (through the punctuation of a "huh" or the repetition of a phrase) in order to arouse the analysand's positive or negative emotions and ultimately encourage reflection on the sources of resistance.

As a trope, irony never occurs in isolation but is always deployed within the context of a larger process of persuasion. While it can stimulate the interlocutor to self-reflection, it also plays a wider role in the patient's experience of

---

[30] For Linda Hutcheon, this uncertainty is the very source of "irony's edge" (1994) 11.
[31] Lacan (1994).
[32] Hutcheon (1994) 15.

the transference. Haddad's account is useful here because it shows, at a concrete technical level, how Lacan's use of scanding aims at stimulating a crisis of *pathos* that will eventually lead to the working-through of the neurosis. The title of Haddad's narrative, *The Day Lacan Adopted Me*, is an (ironic?) allusion to the highly transferential nature of what would become a nine-year analysis with Lacan. By projecting his tense relationship with his father onto his relationship with Lacan, Haddad is able to accept the futility of his craving for paternal approval and become, against the wishes of his biological father but with those of his "adopted" father, an analyst in his own right. Haddad's memoir is as an immensely rich source of insight into the practical dynamics of the transference, but I can only comment briefly here on how Lacan makes use of scanding to influence Haddad's transferential *pathos* and eventually effect a cure.

The book's narrative clarifies the degree to which Lacan's therapeutic practice was predicated on the plasticity of the analyst's self-presentation (*ethos*). Where Freud cautioned analysts to practice "abstinence" or "privation" (SE, XVII, 162) in relating to patients, to act as an impassive "receptive organ" or "telephone receiver" for the discourse of their analysands (SE, XII, 115), Lacan's technical procedure consisted in direct intercession between the patient and his or her unconscious affective state. Haddad's text thus portrays an analyst who "did not hesitate to offer a paternal gesture in taking the hand of his patient, often on the verge of tears, speaking to him or her with words of affection, "*mon petit, ma bien chère*"". Such techniques aim at intensifying the transference through the use of gestures, verbal and non-verbal, which appeal to the patient's unconscious projections:

> He reacted to some of my remarks [...] with sighs full of anxiety and emotion, with handshakes which were some days more insistent than others. While accompanying me in a friendly manner to the door of his consulting room, or while opening the corridor window over the courtyard I had to pass through when leaving the "clinic", he would shout "See you tomorrow! See you tomorrow!" as if I was somehow in danger of forgetting our next meeting. I felt this agitation, whose sincerity I never doubted, like the spur of a rider pushing me beyond my limits of possibility [..]. In this way an entire series of small satisfactions or privations, so important to the intense transference relationship he encouraged, came to dynamise the cure.[33]

It is only when Lacan intensifies the frequency and shortness of their sessions, however, that a crisis is provoked which enables Haddad to grasp the meaning of his analysis. Confronting Lacan over his apparent callousness, Haddad's aetiological epiphany is described in the following terms: "it was precisely this ques-

---

33 Haddad (2002) 100.

tion of the father, of his hoped for yet unbearable death, which formed the hard bone of my relationship to Lacan, of my quasi-delirious transference".[34] My argument here, and throughout this article, has been that Haddad's realization, based as it is on his reasoned conviction regarding a given construction, could not have occurred without the transference relationship, i.e. without the analyst's use of rhetorical persuasion to appeal indirectly to unconscious affective charges. If psychoanalysis is by no means reducible to such *techne rhetorike*, it cannot entirely do without them either.

A final question: if Lacan has done more than any other theorist to reacquaint psychoanalysis with its rhetorical roots, how can we explain his later devotion to the *matheme*, the diagrammatic representation of the structure of the unconscious which seems to run so counter to the contingencies of rhetorical persuasion? The point of the latter is that it represents not content as such, but rather the purity of a timeless "structure" – what Freud would call a "principle" – from which the theoretical and technical practice of psychoanalysis can proceed. Lacan, like Freud, bases the dialectical structure of the analytic situation on scientific principles (*archai*), such as the structures of linguistics or geometry or set theory. But scientific principles alone, as Freud himself concedes, are incapable of leading to a cure. If knowledge of the structure of the unconscious were enough to rid the patient of a particular pathology, then, as Freud notes, "listening to lectures or reading books would be enough to cure him" (SE, XI, 225), just as staring at, or wrangling meaning from, one of Lacan's *mathemes* will not in and of itself effect a cure. Scientific principles alone are not enough to ensure the success of the treatment. The power of psychoanalysis lies in its integration of dialectical and rhetorical modes which, while they can never be entirely assimilated to scientific principles, are continually informed and shaped by them.

---

34 Haddad (2002) 166.

Aaron Turner
3 Thucydides, Groupthink, and the Sicilian Expedition Fiasco

Introduction

Decision-making is the foundation of Thucydides' narrative of the Peloponnesian War. Through his use of speeches and his characterization of particular individuals and states Thucydides demonstrates the decision-making processes that determine the war's origin, its development, and, implicitly, its outcome. It strikes me that the *History* could essentially be read as a series of decisions that drive the historical events of the narrative and that in order to understand these events we must first understand the decisions that instigate them. For Thucydides, the Athenian decision to invade Sicily is a bad one. Not only do the Athenians totally miscalculate the strength and divisiveness of the numerous Sicilian states but they absolutely fail to consider any contingency plans in case the expedition is unsuccessful.[1] Blinded by greed (*pleonexia*) and compelled by desire (*erōs*) the Athenians throw everything they have at Sicily and the result is an unmitigated disaster. The unprecedented loss of military personnel and resources suffered in this fiasco contributes enormously to the final defeat of Athens in the Peloponnesian War. In this paper, I argue that in making this decision the Athenians exhibit the same symptoms that Irving Janis identified in 1972 as conducive to his theory of Groupthink. I argue that Thucydides implicitly demonstrates conditions highly comparable to those Janis explicitly formulates in his theory of Groupthink.

---

[1] Lest we forget what Rhodes (1988) 245 calls "the most serious inconsistency in the *History*", referring to Thucydides' statement in 2.65.11 that the failure of the expedition was "not so much" (*ou tosouten*) on account of the Athenians "miscalculating their enemy's power" but was rather more facilitated by internal affairs which hampered the expedition. This statement is particularly puzzling considering how much the miscalculation of Sicilian forces is borne out in Books 6 and 7, especially in the text surrounding the speeches of Alcibiades and Nicias. Hornblower (1991) 347–349 argues against Thucydides' claim that the expedition was not well supported: "On the contrary it was well supported with reinforcements". Of course, Westlake (1969) 166–167 is quite correct when he asserts that the use of *ou tosouten* (not so much) does not completely invalidate the efficacy of the Athenians' miscalculation, Cf. Rood (1999) 161; Cawkwell (1997) 76.

Aaron Turner, Royal Holloway, London

The Concept of Groupthink

Irving Janis' model of Groupthink derives from his analysis of twentieth century fiascos and the decision-making processes that led to their occurrence. Groupthink is "a mode of thinking that people engage in when they are deeply involved in a cohesive in-group, when the members' strivings for unanimity override their motivation to realistically appraise alternative courses of actions".[2] Janis pioneered the concept of Groupthink when he struggled to understand the decision-making process of President John F Kennedy's EXCOMM committee that was responsible for the Bay of Pigs fiasco. During this process, important information was withheld if it upset the conformity of the group and deeply flawed assumptions went unquestioned. The spectacular failure of this incident prompted Janis to consider whether broader more generalized conditions conducive to bad decision-making might be at fault here. He identified similar errors of judgement in numerous other events, including the Watergate Scandal, the escalation of the Korean War, and the apathy of the American military concerning warnings about an impending Japanese attack on Pearl Harbor. Following his analysis, Janis concluded that the decision-making groups involved in all these incidents suffered from Groupthink. Such a flaw in decision-making is symptomatic of certain antecedent conditions and a high degree of group cohesiveness among members. Initially, two types of antecedent factors that contribute to the materialization of Groupthink were established: structural faults of the organization and provocative situational contexts. Together with a high degree of group cohesiveness these factors, according to Janis, produce several symptoms of Groupthink which in turn cause several defects in decision-making.[3]

---

[2] Janis (1982) 9. The Merriam-Webster Online Dictionary (2010) defines groupthink as "pattern of thought characterised by self-deception, forced manufacture of consent, and conformity to group values and ethics".

[3] Groupthink is not without its critics. Park (2000) 873 writes that there is "very little consensus among researchers on the validity of the Groupthink model". See also, Aldag/Fuller (1993) 533–552; Longley/Pruitt (1980) 74–93; 't Hart (1990). Despite its controversy the Groupthink theory has been widely accepted (Cf. Mitchell/Eckstein (2009) 164). Baron (2005) 219 has found that the syndrome occurs in a far greater number of group settings than initially conceived. For some excellent recent discussions of the Groupthink model, see: Wilcox (2010); Forsyth (2009) 336–350; Kowert (2002) 97–124.

Origin, Function, and Agency of Groups

Janis' analysis of bad decision-making in groups was not without precedent. Before such a model of Groupthink could exist some basic understanding of the concept of a group and how it functions would first need to be established. It is generally acknowledged in the study of groups that there must be a significant degree of cohesion among group members, i.e. they must share the same values and goals. Without shared ambitions to unite the group constituents might simply be considered individuals rather than group members. A group may be defined in different ways. For instance, "a group is a collection of individuals who have relations to one another".[4] Or a group is "a bounded set of patterned relations among members".[5] Or "a group is a social unit which consists of a number of individuals who stand in (more or less) definite status and role relationships to one another".[6] In all these instances, people in a group are understood to be linked by their membership.[7]

How might we understand social group membership in Thucydides? In the *Archaeology,* Thucydides begins his narrative by presenting the human condition devoid of all social properties: the removal of *nomos* to isolate the purest *phusis*. At 1.2, Thucydides describes a Hobbesian 'state of nature' in which individuals live out nomadic existences in isolated groups. A constant fear of invasion prohibits the safe pursuit of wealth facilitated by commerce and agriculture. In order to escape from this state of nature individuals are compelled to form groups under the sovereign rule of strong individuals. At the core of this process is the idea that "the love of gain made the weaker willing to serve the stronger" (1.8.3). The social group in Thucydides then, at least in its initial capacity, was formed to enable the safe pursuit of natural and material wealth.

What is apparent from this passage is that, for Thucydides, human beings are fundamentally homogenous in nature. The antithetical construction of Athenian daring (*tolma*) and quickness against Spartan moderation (*sōphrosunē*) and slowness are not innate characteristics but rather social properties that develop as a result of the group's original collectivising. Thucydides explains the development of social groups in relation to their environmental

---

4 Cartwright/Zander (1968) 46.
5 Arrow/McGrath/Berdahl (2000) 34.
6 Sherif/Sherif (1956) 144.
7 Forsyth (2009) 4.

conditions.⁸ Sparta, he writes, was established in region of Greece blessed with the most fertile soil which meant there was constant competition for the land. In Attica, the soil was of a much lower quality and so contention among those inhabiting it was not so intense (1.2.3–6).⁹ For Thucydides, the development of the social and political infrastructures of Sparta and Athens were grounded in these situational conditions. Due to the intense competition for resources, stringent laws were introduced in Sparta to constrain contention and foster cohesion among group members. Given the relative poverty of natural resources in Attica, the lack of competition encouraged a much more liberal attitude among group members.

For Thucydides, it is evident that social properties are symptomatic of the group striving for cohesion in order to satisfy the primary purpose of the group: ensuring the safe pursuit of wealth. Rational and prudent decision-making processes must be seen as facilitating this purpose. For instance, the formation of state alliances after the Persian invasion follows the exact same formula as that which motivated the original collectivization of individuals. Thucydides employs the same model he uses to explain the collectivization process in order to explain the emergence of the Delian and Peloponnesian Leagues following the Persian invasion. He writes:

> "The Barbarian was repelled by a common effort; but soon the Greeks, as well those who had revolted from the King as those who formed the original confederacy, took different sides and became the allies either of the Athenians or of the Lacedaemonians; for these were now the two leading powers, the one strong by land and the other by sea" (1.18.2).

Like the nomadic individuals seeking to escape the state of nature, the weaker Greek states subjected themselves to the rule of the strong, in this case, Athens or Sparta. For Thucydides, the Persians represent the same external threat that motivated the original collectivization process. The fear of a future Persian invasion compels the weaker states to subsume under a sovereign ruler. Even Thucydides' presentation of the Peloponnesian War can be seen as a product of this paradigm. He identifies Spartan fear of the growth of Athenian power as the "truest cause" (*alēthestatē prophasis*) of the war, and the "least avowed in speech" (1.23.6). However, Athens' motivation for going to war against Sparta can be viewed in precisely the same way. Pericles' instigation of war is not predicated on imperial

---

8 I agree with Lebow (2003) 146–147 when he states that Thucydides modelled his analysis on the contemporary theories of the Hippocratic physicians, who argued that social characteristics of peoples are attributed to their physical environment. Cf. Jouanna (2000) 657; Lloyd (1979) 23.
9 On this 'soil paradox', see Marshall (1975) 26–40. Cf. Foster (2010) 14.

aggression but on the view that any concession to Spartan arbitration would be detrimental to the Athenians' expected standard of living:

> "You are not really going to war for a trifle. If you yield to them in a small matter, they will think that you are afraid, and will immediately dictate some more oppressive condition; but if you are firm, you will prove to them that they must treat you as their equals" (1.140.4–5).

Pericles fosters fear within the *dēmos* in order to encourage war. Balot is critical of Pericles' rhetoric in this speech: "Unlike the hortatory vision of his funeral oration, these arguments are designed to control the Athenians by stimulating their anger, aggressiveness, and indignation".[10] Indeed, Pericles is often criticized for his 'warmongering' on the basis of this reluctance to repeal the Megarian Decree.[11] But Pericles does not invoke fear to encourage an aggressive and indignant *dēmos*. He does encourage war and uses fear as its catalyst but this fear is substantiated by his understanding of historical processes and the role of emotions that drive them. The Peloponnesian War, then, is a product of the same rational decision-making on the parts of both the Athenians and the Spartans. The function of the *Archaeology* is to contextualize these decisions within a historical precedent. In doing so, Thucydides demonstrates the constant and unchanging purpose of the social group: the safe pursuit of wealth. This paradigm is the foundation of rational choice within Thucydides' understanding of social phenomena. Group membership, either within societies or state-alliances, is thus predicated on maintaining the pursuit of wealth that the purpose of the group itself entails.

An issue that might be conceived in attributing the Groupthink syndrome to Thucydides' explanation of the decision-making process leading to the Sicilian Expedition is that Janis identified the symptoms of Groupthink in small groups whereas comparatively Thucydides is dealing with an Athenian assembly that could often consist of as many as 5,000 citizens.[12]. One solution, I would argue, is evident in Thucydides' textual characterization of the Athenian *dēmos*. Throughout the narrative crowds of people are often defined as a single homogenous entity exhibiting singular emotions. Consider, for instance, the uniform anger (*orgē*) that the Athenian masses (*homilos*) direct toward Pericles when the effects of the war begin to impinge on their lifestyle. Their temper is only

---

10 Balot (2014) 118. Cf. Konstan (2010) 190.
11 Adcock (1927) 186–187; Andrewes (1959) 225.
12 Thucydides himself states that the Athenians were rarely able to assemble more than 5,000 at the Pnyx (8.72.1). Further literary and archaeological evidence suggests that attendance would unlikely surpass 6,000 citizens: cf. Hansen (1991) 128–132.

pacified when Pericles is fined and "with the usual fickleness of a crowd" he is re-elected and his position restored (2.65.3). In rhetorical contests, the crowd is often divided into two opposing camps whose views represent the particular argument of one of the speakers. In the Mytilenean Debate, public opinion is almost split right down the middle (3.49.1). In the debate concerning the Sicilian Expedition the ratio is far more one-sided (6.15.1; 6.24.4). The reason why such political consonance exists is because debates and their subsequent decisions are almost always reduced to the possibility of two outcomes. It generally boils down to whether something *should* or *shouldn't* be done and so it doesn't matter if six or six thousand people are voting as long as there are only two plausible results there will only be two modes of thought. Or in the case of the Sicilian Expedition: one.

Another solution we might consider is the rudimentary characteristics of individuals that Thucydides identifies in his state of nature (1.2). Human beings are presented as entirely homogenous and function only according to fear and self-interest. The formation of the social group serves to suppress fear in order to enable the safe pursuit of self-interest. Social properties that are symptomatic of this collectivization process, such as national character (*tropos*), honour (*timē*), and justice (*dikē*), are transient properties that lose their meaning or dissipate entirely when circumstances such as plague and revolution induce a breakdown of social norms. The psychological drives of human nature– fear (*phobos*) and self-interest (*ōphelia*) – are constant and universal. These drives share an ubiquitous presence throughout the *History* and, I would argue, form a foundational symbiosis in Thucydides' explanation of historical processes. Throughout the narrative human action is entirely dictated by this fear/self-interest paradigm, and so for Thucydides the homogenous nature of the crowd is in fact predicated on their adherence to these universal symbiotic psychological drives. In their decision to invade Sicily the fear that traditionally regulates self-interest is compromised by the Groupthink syndrome, which diminishes the crowd's ability to recognize the dangers of the expedition.

Concerning the theory of Groupthink itself and its applicability to groups much larger than those Janis' initial foray examined, we might consider alternative psychological theories that support the plausibility of Groupthink manifesting in large groups. Sluiter, following Sunstein, has argued that good decision-making in large groups relies on an efficient and comprehensive dispersal of information and that in such circumstances "groups spectacularly out-perform individuals".[13] Good decision-making in large groups is thus contingent upon each group

---

13 Sluiter (2011) 35. Cf. Sunstein (2006).

member possessing a sufficient amount of knowledge in order to fully understand the ramifications and potential outcomes of the proposed decision. The absence of such an important factor in the decision-making process is precisely the definition of Groupthink. Therefore, we could well argue that the risk of Groupthink contaminating decision-making processes increases according to the size of the group making the decision. In large decision-making groups, the ability to disseminate information efficiently becomes more difficult. Furthermore, it could also be argued that conformity rather than Groupthink might be a more appropriate determinant to attach to poor decision-making in large groups. Conformity "refers to the act of changing one's behaviour to match the responses of others".[14] As I will demonstrate in this chapter, however, conformity is in fact a product of Groupthink rather than an alternative explanation. The homogenous crowd that Thucydides presents does not simply imply conformation among members of the assembly. Good decisions, such as the reversal of Cleon's ruthless decree against the Mytileneans, are made because the rhetorical structure of the Athenian democracy allows deliberation and reconsideration. Even the Athenian decision to go to war against Sparta is considered by Thucydides to be a good decision, regardless of his retrospective knowledge of their eventual defeat in 404. It was a good decision because Pericles' informed appraisal of Spartan military strength and resources convinced the *dēmos* to vote for a conflict they realistically should have won. The paradigmatic force of fear and self-interest, not conformity, drives their decision.

The Emergence of Groupthink

The Athenians break the mould when they choose to invade Sicily. This decision is not grounded in the same paradigm that drives both the Athenians and the Spartans to war against each other in 431. Only self-interest (*ōphelia*), propelled by lust (*erōs*) and greed (*pleonexia*), motivates the expedition. The reason, I suggest, is implicit in Thucydides' presentation of the debate preceding the invasion and in the events leading up to the debate. It is my argument that within his explanation Thucydides reveals an understanding of decision-making that Irving Janis would much later formalize in his theoretical framework of Groupthink.

Janis identifies seven symptoms of Groupthink and delineates these symptoms into three main types.

---

[14] Cialdini/Goldstein (2004) 606.

Type 1 – Overestimation of the group
1) *Illusions of invulnerability shared by most or all members, which creates excessive optimism and encourages taking extreme risks.*
2) *An unquestioned belief in the group's inherent morality, inclining members to ignore the ethical and moral consequences of their decisions.*

Groups exhibiting symptoms of Groupthink generally assume that their choices are prudent and that everything is working perfectly. This degree of unwarranted optimism was understood by Janis to stem from "illusions of invulnerability." Thucydides himself perceived an illusion of invulnerability among the Athenians following their unexpected successes against the Spartans in the Peloponnesian War. He writes:

> In their present prosperity they were indignant at the idea of a reverse; they expected to accomplish everything, possible or impossible, with any force, great or small. The truth was that they were elated by the unexpected success of most of their enterprises, which inspired them with the liveliest hope (*elpidos*) (4.65.4).

While this attitude existed prior to Brasidas' extremely damaging campaigns in Thrace, which eventually brought about the Peace of Nicias, it does betray a growing optimism within Athens concerning their supreme self-perception. In fact, during his speech condemning the launching of the Sicilian Expedition Nicias himself elucidates this excessive confidence:

> There was a time when you feared the Spartans and their allies, but now you have got the better of them, and because your first fears have not been realized you despise them, and even hope to conquer Sicily. (6.11.5)

Diodotus previously warned against the prevalence of unchecked hope in the Mytilenean Debate, arguing that blind obedience to desire is more ruinous than even the most obvious dangers (3.45.5). Diodotus' prophetic remarks concerning hope are picked up by the Athenian envoy at Melos, who implore the Melians to act prudently and not to rely on the hope that justice, the Spartans, or even the gods, will save them (5.103). That such an admonishment of blind hope immediately precedes the Athenian decision to invade Sicily has not been lost on modern commentators.[15] The Melian Dialogue is itself saturated with Athenian self-conceptions of their pre-eminence across Greece. Even their alleged motive

---

15 On this juxtaposition, see Finley (1942) 323; Liebeschuetz (1968); Parry (1981) 199–200; Macleod (1983), 59–60; Connor (1984) 158; Orwin (1994) 97–141; Kallet (2001) 12; Marincola (2001) 70; Rengakos (2006b) 297.

for attacking Melos – that the smaller, autonomous Greek states represent the real danger to them because their independence undermines the Athenians' imperial integrity (5.99) – is founded on the idea of Athenian supremacy.[16]

The Athenian argument in the debate at Melos is perhaps most indicative of what Janis called "an unquestioned belief in the group's inherent morality, inclining members to ignore the ethical and moral consequences of their decisions." The Melian Dialogue exemplifies one of the major underlying themes of the entire narrative: the concept of 'might is right'. What is particularly evident in this exchange is the contrasting attitude toward the 'inherent morality' of imperialism expressed here and in the speech of the Athenians at Sparta before the war.[17] In their opening gambit, the Athenians immediately dismiss from their own argument any ideas about the legitimacy of their rule based on their heroic conduct during the Persian War (5.89). In comparison, the Athenian justification of empire at Sparta was practically founded on emphasising the role of the Athenians against the Persians and their subsequent liberation of the smaller states (1.73.1–3). Such justifications are considered superfluous by the Athenians at Melos. Indeed, they have no reason to justify their actions and no cause to convince the Melians that their dominion is legitimate. Their doctrine is simple: "the powerful exact what they can, and the weak grant what they must" (5.89). Invocations of honour by the Melians are similarly dismissed by the Athenians, who assert that "the question is not one of honour but of prudence" (5.101. Cf. 5.107). By discarding honour as an incentive for human action, the Athenians distance themselves more from their pre-war predecessors, who identify honour, along with fear and self-interest, as one of three all-powerful motives (1.76.3). By exhibiting a 'might is right' attitude and ignoring the historical validity of their rule the Athenians demonstrate a significant departure from their pre-war speech at Sparta. One of the main purposes of that element of the speech at Sparta was to emphasize the volition of the allies in incorporating themselves in the Delian League. This is significant because it reconciles the nature of alliances with that of societies and creates an understanding of how groups form. The elimination of this process in the Athenians' attempted subjugation of the Melians represents a shift in the relationship between strong and weak entities. No longer do the weak attach themselves to the strong for "the love of gain" (1.8.3). Instead they are presented with an ultimatum: join

---

16 Cf. "For we are masters of the sea, and you who are islanders, and insignificant islanders too, must not be allowed to escape us" (5.97).

17 Strauss (1964) 192 notes a uniformity between the Athenian speech at Sparta, Pericles' speeches, and the speech at Melos, even stating that "[Pericles'] political principle did not differ from that of those Athenians [at Melos]". Cf. Palmer (1992) 64.

or die. This attitude is precisely what led the Athenians to invade Sicily. Their inherent belief in their own legitimate ambition to dominate and rule – in their own *dunamis* – impelled them toward their own destruction.

Type 2 – Close-mindedness
3) *Collective Rationalization – collective efforts to rationalize in order to discount warnings or other information that might lead the members to reconsider their assumptions before they recommit themselves to past policy decisions.*
4) *Stereotypes of out-groups – stereotyped views of enemy leaders as too evil to warrant genuine attempts to negotiate, or as too weak and stupid to counter whatever risky attempts are made to defeat their purpose.*

The speech of Alcibiades encouraging the Athenian *dēmos* to persevere in their decision to invade Sicily is entirely representative of Janis' idea of 'close-mindedness'. Much like Pericles' assessment of Sparta's economic and military capacity, Alcibiades attempts to push forward his policy of war by providing the *dēmos* with an account of Sicilian resources and military strength. Thucydides is in total agreement with Pericles' assessment of Spartan resources and his foresight that the Athenians would win the war. Pericles himself later confirms his prediction of Spartan strategy and thus proves that his assessment was accurate. Thucydides' demonstration of Alcibiades' assessment of Sicilian resources lacks the same conviction. The majority of the assembly were "reluctant to rescind the vote" (6.15.1) following Nicias' first speech and Alcibiades was quick to snuff out their hesitance when he argues:

> Having determined to sail, do not change your minds under the impression that Sicily is a great power ... They are a motley crew, who are never of one mind in counsel, and are incapable of any concert in action. Every man is for himself, and will readily come over to anyone who makes an attractive offer; the more readily if, as report says, they are in a state of internal discord (6.17.2).

At this point, Thucydides has already invalidated Alcibiades' assessment of Sicily by remarking how "most of them knew nothing" (6.1.1) about the size and strength of the island's inhabitants.[18] His narrative of the expedition itself reinforces Alcibiades' baseless and misguided appraisal. As Nicias warned, an Athenian invasion might inspire the Sicilian cities "to unite against [Athens] in fear" (6.21.1). Athenagoras and Hermocrates also predict such an outcome (6.33.5; 37.2). Indeed, both Messene and Catana refused to aid the Athenians (6.50.1–4). Camarina

---

18 Yunis (1996) 106 writes: "Alcibiades recycles a paltry myth of Sicily as consisting of poorly armed, disorganised, primitive poleis and full of useless barbarians". Cf. Stahl (1973) 70–71.

was equally disposed against supporting the Athenian expedition (6.52.1–2).[19] The Athenians failed to obtain support from Carthage and Etruria (6.88.6). As Hornblower suggests, "the Athenian failure to win over non-Syracusan Sicily was absolutely crucial".[20] Alcibiades, wittingly or unwittingly, misunderstood one of the most fundamental characteristics of human action – that individuals and states unite in fear of a common enemy – to the detriment of the *polis*.

Type 3 – Pressures towards Uniformity
5) *Self-censorship of deviations from the apparent group consensus, reflecting each member's inclination to minimize to himself the importance of his doubts and counter-arguments.*
6) *A shared of illusion of unanimity concerning judgements conforming to the majority view.*
7) *Direct pressure on any member who expresses strong arguments against any of the group's stereotypes, illusions, or commitments, making clear that this type of dissent is contrary to what is expected of all loyal members.*
8) *The emergence of self-appointed mindguards – members who protect the group from adverse information that might shatter their shared complacency about the effectiveness and morality of their decisions.*

This particular 'type' is slightly more difficult to reconcile with Thucydides' text on account of the more specialized and precise language employed. Broadly speaking Janis is identifying several elements that signify in-group pressures towards uniformity meaning members are discouraged from expressing their reservations about the group decision. Nicias is clearly the expedition's biggest naysayer but his support is limited, as Thucydides says that only "a few took the side of Nicias" (6.15.1). Against Alcibiades' speech which showcased only the glory and profits to be made from the expedition, as well as its apparent simplicity, Nicias labours to convince the *dēmos* that such a task would be much harder than they imagine and proceeds to demonstrate "the magnitude of the force that would be required" (6.19.2). His effort to dissuade the *dēmos* produces the opposite effect:

> Far from losing their enthusiasm at the disagreeable prospect, they were more determined than ever; they approved of his advice, and were confident that every chance of danger was now removed. All alike were seized with a passionate desire to sail ... the enthusiasm of the

---

[19] Camarina is later the subject of debate between Euphemus and Hermocrates who both seek its alliance but the Camarinaens, fearing the Athenians more, offer moderate aid to Syracuse (6.88.1).
[20] Hornblower (2008) 357. Cf. Rood (1998) 165: "Nicias' warning that the cities might unite in fear is fulfilled".

> majority was so overwhelming that, although some disapproved, they were afraid of being thought unpatriotic if they voted on the other side, and therefore held their peace. (6.24.2–4)

This reaction is a product of the initial "reluctance" of the *dēmos* "to rescind the vote" (6.15.1) and exposes the Athenians' absolute unwillingness to be led astray from their desire to invade Sicily. Alcibiades almost certainly embodies Janis' idea of a "self-appointed mindguard," single-handedly allaying any fears or concerns the group might have regarding the capability of the Athenians in occupying the island and the legitimacy they have in doing so. Even the few doubters that remained feared "being thought unpatriotic" and withheld their reservations about the dangers of the expedition, thus fulfilling Janis' seventh symptom concerning pressured conformity.

Groupthink in Full Swing

With the Groupthink syndrome evidently manifested in the Athenians' collective psyche we might now consider the defects of decision-making that Janis understood to be symptomatic of Groupthink. The seven defects are as follows:
1) *Incomplete survey of alternatives* – *limiting the discussion to only a few alternatives without a survey of all possible alternatives.*
2) *Incomplete survey of objectives* – *limiting discussion to only a few objectives without a survey of all possible objectives.*
3) *Failure to examine risks of preferred choices.*
4) *Failure to reappraise initial rejected alternatives* – *failure to re-evaluate initially discarded alternatives for non-obvious gains that may have been overlooked.*
5) *Poor information search* – *not seeking the advice of experts in specific fields.*
6) *Selective bias in processing information at hand* – *selective bias so that the group uses information that supports their preferences but ignores information that counters it.*
7) *Failure to work out contingency plans* – *failure to consider how other groups might react, or to develop contingency plans for possible failures and setbacks.*

Athens' inability to consider alternative courses of action or alternative objectives once the Peace of Nicias had been established was perhaps contingent upon Alcibiades' assessment of what makes Athens Athens: continuous expansion. In his opposing speech advocating the launching of the expedition, Alcibiades attempts to inspire fear in the *dēmos* by emphasising the dangers of inactivity. He states that "a state used to activity will quickly be ruined by the change to inaction" (6.18.6–7). Modern scholars tend to equate Alcibiades' insistence on constant expansion with the conduct of Athenian imperialism before the war and with the Corinthians' portrayal of Athenian dynamism in their speech at Sparta (1.70.2–3).[21] But Alcibiades' vision of Athens is not consistent with that of Thucydides. In Nicias' corresponding speech warning the Athenians against the invasion of Sicily one of Nicias' primary arguments is the lack of threat that the Sicilians pose to Athens at the current time (6.11.2). Thucydides perceives Syracuse to be another Athens in-the-making and Nicias dispels the fear that a united Sicily would threaten Athens.[22] He remarks that Syracuse and her allies would not attack Athens for the exact same reason that Athens should not attack Sicily – because empires "should not be likely to make war against another empire" (6.11.3). Forde dismisses Nicias' suggestion that "empires, once established, become fundamentally defensive or conservative".[23] But this is precisely how Thucydides characterizes the Athenian Empire at its inception. By assimilating the nature of the empire with that of a tyrant (cf. 1.40.1; 1.122.3; 1.124.4; 2.63.2) it allows Thucydides to minimize to his readers the aggression that Athens displays in its pursuit of empire. In the *Archaeology*, tyrants are defined by their reclusivity and lack of enterprise (1.17.1). I would argue that the degree of imperial aggression exhibited by Athens in the *Pentekontaitia* is suppressed by Thucydides in order to differentiate their initial pursuit of empire from their more destructive behaviour during the war, specifically the decision to invade Sicily.

It is this alleged suppression of Athenian aggression that has divided Thucydidean scholars concerned with this period of expansion. Such suppression is evident from the numerous omissions made by Thucydides in the Pentecontaetia.[24] Hornblower argues that "Thucydides systematically understated Athenian aggressiveness in the run up to war".[25] Badian is similarly disposed, claiming

---

[21] Palmer (1992) 96; Mills (1997) 68; Ober (1998) 107–110. Connor (1984) 166 writes: "The significance of Alcibiades' speech, then, lies not in the force of its arguments for action against Sicily, but in its understanding and illumination of Athenian character".

[22] As Rawlings (1981) 162 points out, Thucydides makes clear that Syracuse was a potential Athens. Cf. Saxonhouse (2006) 172; Ober (1996) 78–80; Hawthorn (2014) 175.

[23] Forde (1989) 62. Hornblower (2008) 330 is equally dismissive of this "dubious" claim.

[24] As de Romilly (1963) 91 notes: "... he makes no mention of the transference, in 454, of the treasury from Delos to Athens; he makes no mention of the triumph, in 443, of a policy which consisted in using the money contributed by the allies for other purposes than waging war; he makes no mention of the division of the allies into five districts, which took place at the same time and marked the beginning of an imperial mode of organization, or of the fusion of Athena's treasury with the federal treasury. Yet these different measures both marked and brought about the transformation of the allies into subjects". Cf. Tsakmakis (1995), 85–87.

[25] Hornblower (1994) 131–166. Cf. Shanske (2006) 158–159.

that Thucydides' treatment of the Samian Revolt (1.115–117) is "tellingly philo-Athenian".²⁶ For Thucydides, the expansion of the empire after the Persian War was predicated on necessity. This process is given historical precedence in the *Archaeology* when sovereign rulers of groups would expand their rule in order to "increase their wealth and provide for their poorer followers" (1.5.2). As we saw earlier, it was "the love of gain" (1.4.1) that motivated weak individuals to subordinate themselves to a strong leader. The same process is observed in the alliance of states, who rally behind either Athens or Sparta in order to protect themselves from future Persian invasions (1.18.2). The greedy and aggressive Athens that Thucydides depicts in the events of the Melian Dialogue and the Sicilian Expedition is far removed from the Athens depicted here, whose ambition and expansion is propelled by necessity alone. So, then, when Nicias debunks Alcibiades' assertion that Syracuse might one day pose a threat to Athens (6.11.3) he is in fact demonstrating a consistent logic with Thucydides and his own interpretation of events. His proposal, too, that the Athenians should "expend our new resources upon ourselves at home, and not upon begging exiles who have an interest in successful lies" (6.12.1), is consistent with the logic of the tyrant who refused to "extend their thoughts beyond their own interest, that is, the security of their persons, and the aggrandisement of themselves and their families" (1.17.1). Nicias' alternative course of action is discarded by Alcibiades on account of his misunderstanding of imperial expansion. Instead he advocates policies grounded in self-interest in order to secure the support of the *dēmos* who see the expedition as an opportunity to improve their own fortunes while disregarding the inherent risk that such an endeavour holds. An incomplete survey of objectives and alternatives occurs precisely because of the lack of financial gain that these entail.

The total failure of the Athenians to fully examine the risks of the expedition (Janis' third defect in decision-making) has already been partially covered in the analysis of the Groupthink syndrome. Another such risk that requires attention was how the Sicilians, and indeed the Spartans, might react to the impending expedition. This relates specifically to Janis' seventh defect: "failure to consider how other groups might react". The Athenians evidently considered the Syracusans "too weak and stupid to counter" their purpose and failed to entertain the possibility that envoys would be sent to Sparta to appeal for aid. Sparta itself was eager to help the Syracusans. Athenian defeat would undoubtedly benefit

---

26 Badian (1993) 138–140. Pelling (2000) 98 argues against such a viewpoint and suggests that "it is hard to think that Thucydides' concern is really to maximise Spartan and minimise Athenian aggression" in the build-up to the Peloponnesian War. Cf. Foster (2010) 62–64; Stahl (2006) 331; Stadter (1993) 37–38; Powell (1988) 442–444.

the Spartans when the tenuous peace treaty inevitably expires. Alcibiades dismisses Nicias' argument that by invading Sicily they "leave many enemies behind" (6.10.1) by proclaiming that "nothing [at home] ... need interfere with the expedition" (6.17.7) to the detriment of the city. The Spartan general Gylippus was sent to Sicily and transformed the fighting capability of the Syracusan army. Gylippus' superior tactical and leadership abilities ensured naval victory in the Great Harbour of Syracuse (7.69–72) and the final victory over the fleeing Athenian infantry forces (7.74–85).

Janis' seventh defect also refers to the failure of the group to "develop contingency plans for possible failures and setbacks." Such an oversight on the part of the Athenians is made poignant when, having been defeated in Sicily, their insecurities at home cultivates further discord against them: "The states which had been neutral determined that the time had come when, invited or not, they could no longer stand aloof from the war; they must of their own accord attack the Athenians" (8.2.1). Furthermore, given that absolute victory was allegedly assured, such a vast armament was deployed to Sicily that it was difficult for those in Athens to comprehend the significance of the defeat, for "they had lost a host of cavalry and hoplites and the flower of their youth, and there were none to replace them" (8.1.2). While the Athenians did manage to reconstruct their navy and hold out in the war for a further seven years their failure in Sicily, at least in Thucydides' estimation, was ultimately responsible for their defeat against Sparta and the subsequent loss of their empire. This conclusion is evident at 2.65 where Thucydides laments the demagogic nature of Pericles' successors, whose "private ambitions and private interests ... had disastrous effects in respect both of themselves and of their allies" (2.65.7). The Sicilian Expedition was the culmination of these private ambitions and thus the misguided decision to invade Sicily ultimately decided the fate of Athens both in terms of her defeat in the Peloponnesian War and the loss of her imperial hold over Greece.

Conclusion

For Thucydides, it is clear that the Sicilian Expedition was the result of bad decision-making. I have shown throughout this chapter that the conditions Irving Janis explicitly formulated and categorized into his theory of Groupthink are themselves implicit in Thucydides explanation of the Athenian decision to invade Sicily. Given the significance of the failure of the expedition we might suggest that the entire narrative itself is teleologically inclined toward explaining how and why the Athenians threw caution to the wind and embarked on an expedition that promised excessive wealth and glory but delivered unmitigated disaster. Groupthink, according to Janis, occurs when the group is in a state of extremely high cohesion. For the Athenians this degree of cohesion was reached under the administration of Pericles' successors. They were "more on an equality with one another, and, each one struggling to be first himself, they were ready to sacrifice the whole conduct of affairs to the whims of the people" (2.65.10). Pericles, on the other hand, was able to produce prudent policies based on his control of the masses – he "led them rather than was led by them" (2.65.8). Under Pericles decision-making was good because Pericles combined wisdom (*gnōmē*) and foresight (*pronoia*) to dictate Athenian affairs. The assimilation of his successors' political ambitions with the short-sighted and indulgent whims of the masses creates a dangerous cohesiveness between the two entities that results in the onset of Groupthink. Therefore, Thucydides not only perceives a pressured social conformity among the Athenian masses (i.e., Janis' seventh symptom) but also a psychological conformity. Without the guidance of wisdom and foresight to dictate policy-making Alcibiades becomes a demagogue, converting the short-term ambitions of the masses into principles of foreign policy. This development is compounded by the intense stress the Athenians feel under the pressure of the war and the plague; what Janis might call a "provocative situational context". Under such conditions the Athenians no longer see the long-term benefits of the social group and the established role differentiation between strong and weak – leader and led – becomes blurred. Such a breakdown of social norms is elucidated by Thucydides in his explanations of the plague that sweeps Athens in 430/29 (2.47–54) and of the Corcyraen Revolution (3.82–84), which denotes broader implications for the rest of Greece suffering from *stasis*. Groupthink, or rather the conditions that Janis defined in his formulation of Groupthink, is the product of such *stasis*. Social unrest in Athens destabilizes and cripples the traditional structure of the social group. Had Janis read the *History* he may well have been struck by how similar Thucydides' approach to understanding group dynamics and bad decision-making was to his own. And while Janis can posthumously add another example of an historical event exhibiting the groupthink syndrome to his catalogue, Thucydides can rest assured that his "possession for all time" is confirmed once again to be a possession for our time.

Richard Seaford
4 Mystic Initiation and the Near-Death Experience

The Near-Death Experience (NDE) has been the object of much modern research. The first scholar to argue for its relevance to ancient Greek texts was – so far as I know – Jan Bremmer (2002), who considered "five descriptions which could be possibly be considered as NDEs", but without mentioning mystic initiation. Mystic initiation was an ancient ritual that can best be described as a rehearsal for death that was meant to overcome the fear of actual death. Its elimination by Christianity left a large gap in the western religious imagination.

In two papers (2005 and 2010) I suggested the (direct or indirect) influence of NDEs on further ancient texts and on the ritual of mystic initiation by which the texts were influenced. Recently Yulia Ustinova (2013) has produced what is now the best, the most detailed, and the most comprehensive account of the topic. What I propose here is to (1) reproduce two important ancient texts, and briefly reiterate my argument of 2010, (2) situate these two texts in their context, (3) add two substantial points to my earlier argument, and (4) indicate the difficulties confronting modern psychology in its attempt to understand NDEs. The overall aim is to bring not only NDEs to the attention of those studying the ancient world but also ancient texts to the attention of those studying NDEs.

(1) I reproduce below the two texts most important to my argument of 2010. The fragment of Plutarch is perhaps our most important account of the *experience* of being initiated into the mysteries. Significantly, it compares this experience to the experience of dying. The other text is one of the numerous passages of Euripides' *Bacchae* that reflects the ritual of mystic initiation.[1] The underlinings in both passages make it clear that there are significant similarities between mystic initiation and the (otherwise inexplicably odd) experience of Pentheus. It is because the passage of *Bacchae* reflects and evokes initiation, rather than because of some inexplicable delusion or psychosis, that Pentheus acts in the way he does.

It is true that Plutarch seems to refer to the Eleusinian mysteries, whereas *Bacchae* concerns the mysteries of Dionysos. But Dionysos was present (as

---
1 Seaford (1996).

Richard Seaford, University of Exeter

Iakchos) in the Eleusinian mysteries, and both Aristophanes' *Frogs* and Plato's *Phaedrus* conflate Eleusinian with Dionysiac mysteries.² I must also note that at *Bacchae* 630 the editors have universally and erroneously replaced the manuscript *lectio difficilior* φῶς (light) with the conjecture φάσμ' (apparition), because none of them had any inkling of the considerations that I present in this paper and in my commentary on the play (1996).

Plutarch fragment 178

> In this world the soul is ignorant, except when it is already in the teleutan [to end or die]. Then it has an experience like that of those being initiated into the great mysteries. And so teleutan and teleisthai [to be initiated] are similar as verbs and in the actions they denote. At first wanderings and tiring runnings around, and anxious uncompleted journeys, then before the completion itself all the terrors, shuddering and trembling and sweat and awe. But after this a wonderful light met (the initiand) and pure places and meadows received him, with voices and choral dances and solemnities of sacred sounds and holy visions. Among these now he – made complete and initiated and free – moves around at large, crowned, celebrating the rituals, and is with holy and pure men, looking on the uninitiated and impure mob of the living trampled by itself [i.e. on the ground] in much mud and mist, in fear of death clinging to sufferings through not believing in the blessings there [in the hereafter].

Euripides Bacchae *604–635*

> Dionysos: ... Have you astounded by fear fallen to the ground? ... But raise up your bodies and take courage, putting trembling from your flesh.
>
> Chorus: O greatest light for us of the joyful-crying bacchanal, how gladly I looked on you in my isolated desolation.
>
> Dionysos: Did you come to faintheartedness when I was being sent in, thinking that I would fall into the dark enclosures of Pentheus?
>
> Chorus: How could I not? ... But how were you freed, having fallen in with an impure man?
>
> Dionysos: ... [Pentheus tied up a bull], panting out his wrath, dripping sweat from his body, biting his lips. But I calmly sat close by and watched. During this time Bakchos came and shook up the house and on the tomb of his mother ignited fire. And Pentheus when he saw it, thinking that the house was on fire, rushed this way and then that way, telling the servants to bring water; and every slave was hard at work, toiling in vain. And having abandoned this toil, on the assumption that I had fled, he rushes, having seized a sword, inside the dark³ house. And then Bromios – I say what seemed to me – made a light in the court-

---

2 Riedweg (1987) 30–69.
3 This translates the tiny emendation κελαινῶν (Verrall) for ms. κελαινὸν for argument see Seaford (1996) 201–202.

yard. And Pentheus charging against it rushed and stabbed at the shining < > as if slaughtering me ... through <u>exhaustion</u> he dropped the sword and <u>collapsed</u>.

The modern literature on the NDE is immense.[4] Suffice it here to say that generally agreed features of the 'core experience' are departing from the body, entry into darkness (often in a tunnel); movement towards a light, which is also somehow a person (the Being of Light); a beautiful place, such as a meadow; a feeling of peace and well-being; life review; seeing (deceased) relatives and friends; receiving knowledge about the nature of the universe; a sense of ineffable reality and of unity; permanent removal of the fear of death.

There is for ancient mystic initiation (and in texts that reflect it) evidence for all these features (except perhaps life review and seeing dead relatives). I refer readers to Ustinova (2013). In my two earlier papers I focused especially on the Being of Light, and cited – besides the two passages above – a large number of ancient Greek passages that are associated with mystic initiation and identify a deity with a light. It is also worth recalling here the influence (direct or indirect) of the initiatory role of light on divine epiphanies in the Acts of the Apostles.[5]

(2) The Plutarch fragment combines phraseology influenced by a famous passage of Plato's *Phaedrus* (248–250) with elements derived from Eleusinian initiation ritual.[6] The *Phaedrus* passage is a description of a heavenly vision that Plato describes as a mystic initiation.[7] Plato, who was a contemporary of Euripides, in various works evokes or alludes to mystic initiation,[8] and had surely been himself initiated. Plutarch's account of Eleusinian initiation is a synthesis of his own experience (for he too had very likely been initiated) with Plato's sublimated version.

As for the *Bacchae* passage, it is one of numerous passages in the play that reflect and evoke the ritual of mystic initiation. The strange (and otherwise inexplicable) experiences of Pentheus – not only his behaviour in the passage quoted but also, for instance, his 'fluttering anxiety' (*ptoēsis*), and seeing two suns and two cities of Thebes – can be related to the experience of the mystic initiand. The theme of the play was the introduction of Dionysiac mystic initiation to Thebes (20–25, 39–40). That is to say, the play dramatized an aetiological myth of mystic

---

[4] For a recent survey, see Greyson (2014a).
[5] Seaford (1997).
[6] Riedweg (1987) 65–66; Graf (1974) 132–138. Graf underestimates what could be enacted (or evoked) in the Eleusinian ritual.
[7] 248b1–5, 249c7, 250b–c; Riedweg (1987) 30–69.
[8] e.g. *Symp.* 210a1, *Phaedo* 108a, *Republic* 560e, *Cratylus* 400, *Meno* 81a–b.

initation, and so – like other aetiological myths of ritual (e.g. the *Homeric Hymn to Demeter*) – prefigured details of the ritual to be established. I have argued all this in detail in my Commentary on the play (1996).

Nor is the *Bacchae* the only Athenian tragedy that evokes ritual. A number of rituals – notably mystic initiation, the wedding, the funeral, the procession, animal sacrifice, and supplication – were more central to the life of society, and more familiar to people in general, than is any religious ritual of our era. And because these rituals were also both dramatic and highly emotional, they were frequently evoked by tragedy for emotional effect, in a manner and to an extent that have been unfamiliar to European theatre audiences ever since.[9]

(3) In this section I add two points to my earlier argument.

(a) Evidence has been presented by Kevin Clinton for the presence during Eleusinian initiation of statues illuminated from within. It consists of a number of ancient texts[10] together with a votive plaque from the sanctuary showing Demeter with rays of light emerging from her head.[11] To this evidence I would add the numerous passages identifying deities with light in a mystic context: for instance, in the *Homeric Hymn to Demeter*, which is in various respects aetiological of the Eleusinian mysteries, 'a light shone far out from the immortal skin of the goddess ... the compact house was filled with radiance like lightning' (278–280). The creation of statues illuminated from within shows how concretely the NDE (specifically the Being of Light) might be represented in mystic ritual.

(b) In the *Bacchae* passage the chorus – after anxiety, individual isolation, and falling to the ground – welcome the epiphany of Dionysos, whom they call "greatest light". This represents the mystic transition – attested e.g. in the Plutarch passage – from isolated anxiety to communal joy (a transition with profound political potential),[12] a transition effected by light in the darkness. Pentheus too undergoes the preliminary phase of isolated anxiety (again, for detail compare Plutarch), but when the light appears to him in the darkness and he recognizes it as Dionysos (just as the chorus have called Dionysos in his epiphany "greatest light"), he *attacks* it. The myth of Pentheus represents the *persistence* of the phase of anxious resistance, what Plutarch calls "clinging to sufferings", that in the ritual is eventually abandoned. Pentheus

---

9 From the copious scholarship, see e.g. Foley (1985); Seaford (1994).
10 Notably Plato, *Phaedrus* 249e–250c, 254b. With the latter passage I suggest we compare *Bacchae* 647 (and my commentary *ad loc.*).
11 IG II² 4639.
12 For this political potential, see Seaford (2012) 274–278 and (2013).

too is, much later in the drama, eventually made to abandon it by Dionysos, but only so as to be sent to Hades (in contrast to the imagined Hades temporarily inhabited by the initiates). Myth can express as a reality what in the ritual is merely imagined, and the mystic transition will not be effective unless the uninitiated are made fearful (by the myth as well as by the ritual).

In general, the NDE passes from a phase of anxious isolated resistance to a phase of profound well-being that is often associated with the Being of Light. But there are cases (a minority) that resemble the normal NDE except that the dying person *rejects* his new environment, feels *isolated*, and has to struggle for his continued existence: the transition to well-being does not occur. These may be called Negative Near-Death Experiences (NNDEs). A study[13] based on over 100 interviews with NNDE experiencers found that the same kind of experience can be viewed positively in a normal NDE but negatively in a NNDE. For instance, 'a Being composed entirely of light can seem to be a trick of the devil or a punishment of some kind'. It has been suggested that the unpleasantness of some NDEs derives "from the resistance to the experience, not from the experience itself".[14] What might have become a NNDE can turn pleasant "once the person relaxes into the experience". I suggest that the NNDE is a source for Pentheus' persistently anxious resistance, his isolated clinging to sufferings, and specifically for his hostility to the light that he recognizes as a person (Being of Light) but nevertheless attacks.

The *Bacchae* passage is not the only ancient Greek text that was probably influenced by the NNDE. Plato in the *Phaedo* (108) infers from certain rituals (surely mystic rituals) that the way to the underworld has many forks and windings, and then contrasts the *pure* soul, which finds gods as companions and guides to the underworld, with the *impure* soul, which resists, suffers, and is dragged to the underworld where it is shunned by all and *wanders around bewildered and alone*. For Plato this distinction had implications for how we should lead our lives. And so the question should be raised of whether Euripides too represents Pentheus as the *kind of person* who, like the impure soul described by Plato, is imagined as likely to experience death entirely negatively. That is to say, does Pentheus have characteristics – over and above his mere rejection of Dionysos – that make him that kind of person? This then leads to a further question: do modern NNDE experiencers tend to

---

13 Atwater (1992).
14 Greyson (2014b).

be a certain kind of person? The current answer to this last question seems to be no (see below), but research in this area may still have a long way to go.

(4) How do we explain the NDE *physiologically* and *psychologically*? A useful recent survey of this issue, with extensive bibliography, is by Greyson (2014a). I conclude by indicating two problems for explanations hitherto proposed, and a suggestion for future, interdisciplinary progress.

A common kind of psychological explanation is provided by the expectancy model: the NDE, it is sometimes claimed, is a fantasy constructed – as a defense mechanism – out of personal and cultural expectations. The problem is that NDEs apparently often conflict with such expectations. My impression from looking at some of the numerous studies is that the typicality of the NDE generally prevails over pre-existing variations in the NDE experiencers – variations in religion, in knowledge or ignorance of NDEs, in culture, and in psychological make-up. An instance of this prevailing is provided by the representation – in a very different culture of two and half millennia ago, ancient Greece – of what we can merely from modern experience clearly identify as the NDE.

The other problem is this. Besides various physiological processes, there are also various anomalous or abnormal states that have been adduced to explain the NDE, such as hallucination, dissociation, depersonalization, and derealization. But the NDE generally enters a phase that is lucid, ordered, pleasant, peaceful, and typical. A sense of personal identity is not lost (but may be detached from bodily sensation, and may combine with a sense of unity with others). And a sense of reality is not lost: in fact the experience may seem especially real, albeit ineffable. This remarkable combination of features was – I suggest – a factor in the Greek desire to enact in their rehearsal for death (mystic ritual) the reports of NDE experiencers. But the combination also seems very different from the anomalous or abnormal psychological states that have been adduced to explain the NDE. This objection also presents a problem for the physiological explanations, for which moreover we still lack the necessary experimental data. Indeed it is significant that in his survey, Greyson finds serious problems with each of the explanations for the NDE that have been proposed (psychological, physiological, or the separation of mind from body), and concludes with a far-reaching aporia: "Controversy persists over whether that invariance [of NDEs through the centuries and around the globe] is a reflection of universal psychological defenses, neurophysiological processes, or actual experience of a transcendent or mystic domain".[15]

---

15 Greyson (2014) 358.

Modern researchers study the NDE as an entirely *individual* experience. Perhaps therefore there is a lesson for them from the ancient manifestations of the NDE. On the one hand the ancient NDE is strikingly similar to ours. On the other hand there is a world of difference between the *location* of the NDE in the individual consciousness then and now. In the ancient material that we have examined the NDE is represented in the communal enactment of myth (in drama) and of ritual, enactment that might even have political significance. But the modern NDE remains an experience of discrete individuals. Moreover, fifty years ago (at least in the West) nobody, or almost nobody, spoke of NDEs (let alone considering them worthy of study). The phenomenon had to be gradually extracted by researchers from the privacy of certain individuals.

And so the NDE can be communally present on the one hand or on the other hand intensely private and generally unknown. The question then arises of *why* the NDE was communally present in Greek antiquity, and yet generally unknown – or internally repressed? – in (say) the first half of the twentieth century. This important question has never been asked. An answer would probably require the introduction of anthropological and socio-historical factors, which accordingly cannot ultimately be excluded from our current attempts to understand the relation of the NDE to the individual mind.

Jennifer Radden
5 Burton's *Anatomy* as Classical, and Present-Day, Mind Science

Introduction

Scientists and philosophers were ushering in the modern world when Robert Burton finished the first edition of his great *Anatomy of Melancholy* (1621), and brought out the ever-expanding editions that followed in 1624, 1628, 1632, 1638. (A posthumous one followed in 1651.) His Oxford colleague Harvey had in the 1620s described the circulation of the blood; by 1620 Bacon's *Novum Organum* had inaugurated experimental and empirical method as we have come to understand them; Descartes was redirecting epistemology with the *Meditations* (1641), and ideas about affective states in *The Passions of the Soul* (1649). Yet Burton resolutely turned backwards. His writer's persona Democritus Junior was a reincarnation of the pre-Socratic atomist. Some of his strongest influences, like those of the Renaissance humanists, trace to ancient philosophy and medicine: particularly, Galenic humoral medicine, Aristotelian faculty psychology, and Hellenistic ideas about curbing the passions. With these classical underpinnings, the *Anatomy* has usually been seen as the last, late-flowering product of Renaissance thought – and it was. As such, Burton's debt to classical thinking, much of it interwoven with Christian theology, is powerful and compelling. Yet from the perspective of the early twenty-first century sciences of mind, I think it can be shown, this work is also noteworthy. It demonstrates an embodied mind, a model of mental functioning, and notions of affect regulation, that are each strikingly resonant with contemporary cognitivism and brain science, and contains implications of philosophical, psychological and psychiatric significance.

After introducing Burton's life and work in Part 1, and summarizing some of the particular elements of his ideas about mental processes and the remedies and preventatives he recommends for melancholy, I'll focus in Part 2 on the three particular classical elements noted above: the Aristotelian faculty psychology, Galenic humoral medicine, and Stoic ideas about regulating the passions. These classical underpinnings of the *Anatomy*, I want to illustrate in Part 3, allow us to see Burton's efforts as surprisingly consonant with today's mind sciences. As such, they are potentially useful in contemporary efforts to treat the affective disorder of depression, with its strong parallels to Burtonian Melancholy.

Jennifer Radden, University of Massachusetts, Boston

https://doi.org/10.1515/9783110482201-018

1. The Man and his Anatomy

Robert Burton (1577–1640) was an English bibliophile and Oxford don, a Protestant clergyman, and a prodigious scholar. In each subsequent edition after the 900-page First Edition of 1621, his book grew larger. His time was spent quietly at Christ Church College. He never married, and took on few pastoral duties. Instead, his lifetime's work involved revising, embellishing and augmenting his massive book – offering a further explanation, example, or correction here, an engraved frontispiece or scholarly digression there.[1] Rather than seeking originality, his aim was to assemble a compendium of all human knowledge about melancholy. The *Anatomy* touches on every imaginable topic: as well as an encyclopaedia, it is also health advice, medical text, consolatory and pastoral literature, and medical, philosophical and psychological analysis. Central to the work were Burton's references to the long canon of writing about melancholy or *melancholia* (the two were, and are here, used interchangeably), that begins with Hippocratic aphorisms, is elaborated extensively by Galen and the great medical thinkers of the Middle East, such as Avicenna, and restored to Western scholarship through the Renaissance. In addition to this canon of writing, the extent of his intellectual curiosity apparently unlimited, Burton read the Greek and Roman philosophers, orators, tragedians and historians.

These classical influences came in two forms. The Renaissance humanists' revival and translation of, and commentaries on, classical texts had left more than a hundred years of such scholarship on which Burton could, and did, draw.[2] In addition, the scholar could avail himself of copies of the original Greek and Latin texts, as Burton also did, often providing his own translations. My particular emphasis here is the classical influences on the *Anatomy*, but it should be added that inheritances from the Church Fathers, medieval and Early Modern theology and the writings of the Renaissance medical men, including his countryman Timothy Bright, are equally central to the work understood as a whole.

They are all there, in the *Anatomy*, and we might be pardoned for supposing that nothing original at all can be drawn from Burton's welter of quotations, paraphrases, descriptions of learned debates, and lists of eminent thinkers. However,

---

[1] All page references in what follows are to the Fourth Edition (1632), edited by Faulkner/Kiessling/Blair (1989–2000).

[2] By the early seventeenth century, there were also the rich pictorial traditions, and elaborate iconography, surrounding depictions of the four humours, and the figure of Melancholy. And there were the literary and dramatic traditions, in works such as those by Shakespeare, and Milton.

that would be mistaken. Burton's aim was to produce something like an encyclopaedia, it is true, not an original treatise.[3] If not original ideas, however, the *Anatomy* contains original arrangements, inferences and emphases, as Burton himself recognizes. ("'Tis all mine, tis none mine" he says, of his book.) Moreover, interspersed with neutral descriptions, where no judgment is passed, we find places where the author is clear in siding with one view or another, or adamant (as he is when he disagrees with his beloved Stoics over their deterministic materialism), that some scholars are mistaken.

2. Three Classical Elements

Aristotle and Aristotelianism

The *Anatomy*'s faculty psychology is Aristotelian. The separate faculties or units of the psyche or soul are assigned according to function: the Rational soul has as its instruments understanding and will; the Sensitive or Sensible soul encompasses the five outward senses together with the Common Sense,[4] memory and imagination; and the Vegetative soul controls processes of growth, nutrition and reproduction. The workings of the faculty of Imagination, in the Sensitive soul, have a special place in the *Anatomy* account. Following the classical canon on melancholy that traces to Hippocratic and Galenic medicine, together with the emphasis of the Renaissance doctors, the condition known as Melancholy or Melancholia is depicted as a deficiency or weakness afflicting the Imagination, which is at the same time too intense, and prodigious, and unruly. That deficiency engenders disorder or imbalance of the Passions, typified by unwarranted, and excessive, fear and sadness. This condition arises as the result of a failure to curb an imagination that is overly fecund, or intense, and engages in unproductive and dangerously idle – although appealing and enjoyable – "opinions" and "fancies". The Imagination is rebellious, and disinclined to submit to Will or the dictates of Reason. And it dominates through its power to arouse and

---

[3] On the intentions behind Burton's efforts, including this one, see Gowland (2007). Other important scholarly work on the *Anatomy* includes Jackson (1986); Lund (2010); Schmidt (2007); Tilmouth (2005); Bamborough (1989–2000).
[4] The Common Sense (in the Aristotelian usage) was a sensory capacity serving to coordinate the data introduced through the five outward senses, and to apprehend the "common sensible" qualities (such as size, shape, duration, etc.) that are known through more than one sense.

stabilize the Passions. Since we are all possessed of an imagination and drawn to the pleasures of day-dreaming and other forms of idle speculation, Burton thinks, we are all at risk of succumbing to melancholy. He repeatedly insists that rather than any humoral temperature, an unruly Imagination is responsible for melancholy symptoms. "I may certainly conclude," he asserts

> [that] this strong conceit or imagination, is *astrum hominis*, the rudder of this our ship, which reason should steire, but overborne by phantasie, cannot manage, and so suffers it selfe and this whole vessel of ours to be overruled, and often overturned (I,2,3,2).

As the rudder of our vessel, Imagination and imagining join thought, feeling and humoral states in the hectic, multi-causal and multi-directional interactionism that characterizes the *Anatomy* model of mental processing.

> To our imagination commeth, by the outward sense or memory, some object to be knowne … which he mis-conceiving or amplifying, forthwith communicates to the Heart, the seat of all affections. The pure spirits flocke from the Braine to the Heart, by certaine secret channels, and signifie what good or bad object was presented; which immediately bends it selfe to persecute, or avoid it; and withal, draweth with it other humours to helpe it: so in pleasure, concurre great store of purer spirits; in sadnesse, much melancholy blood; in ire, choler. If Imagination be very apprehensive, intent, and violent, it sends great store of spirits to, or from the heart, and makes a deeper impression, and greater tumult, as the humours in the Body be likewise prepared, and the temperature it selfe ill or well disposed, the passions are longer and stronger. So that the first steppe and fountaine of all our grievances in this kinde, is … Imaginatio, which misinforming the Heart, causeth all these distemperatures, alteration and confusion of spirits and humours. (I,2,3,1).

Whether stimulated by memory, imagination, or some immediate perception, a thought or representation occurs and is registered, but also interpreted with accompanying evaluative appraisal. The stronger the imagination the more intense and disruptive are the person's affective attitudes about the thought, with their accompanying humoral and other bodily changes, and action tendencies. Notable here is the role of Imagination in triggering the sequence (the "first steppe and fountaine"). But the part played by the humoral constitution or temperature is shown equally important in affecting the outcome ("makes … greater tumult, *as the humours in the Body be likewise prepared, and the temperature it selfe ill or well disposed*"). Although the mind is more often the instigator of one of these sequences resulting in disturbed passions, the humoral disposition of the body (its temperature, in this instance), also plays a part. Remembering, dreaming, fantasizing, and speculating, as well as more imagistic forms are all functions of the Imagination. Moreover, as part of the Sensitive Soul, imagining partakes of the bodily as well as the intellectual, somehow straddling the two.

Because of its special power to ignite and destabilize Passions that in turn bring about further bodily changes, the Imagination apparently initiates these sequences. Burton sometimes asserts that this makes the Imagination, rather than any "distemperature of the body" the *cause* of Melancholy. Yet other passages in the *Anatomy* make clear that humoral states and tendencies, temporary and inborn, as well as other bodily conditions, will also often affect the Passions and the Imagination. So this is a multi-causal analysis, reflecting multi-directional sequences or loops uniting the bodily with the cognitive through affective states. In fact, the *Anatomy* describes at least three different forms taken by the causal interactions resulting from melancholy. In one, the initial mental state alters the humoral arrangement (which in turn affects the Passions, again changing further mental states such as thoughts). Then, sometimes the body is the initiating source of these changes, as happens when we fail to adhere to an appropriate diet, over-exercise, or lack sleep. And last, as is hinted at in the above passage, bodily states act as a diathesis, combining with some additional mental state to produce affective disturbance. Burton summarizes this array of multi-directional causal sequences:

> the body works upon the mind ... disturbing the soul and all the faculties of it ... so, on the other side, the mind most effectually works upon the body (I,2).

As this mixture of proximate causes suggests, melancholy has an illimitable number of origins. Behavioral and mental habits; passing humoral fluctuations as well as more fixed states arising from individual temperament, tendencies and bodily changes, but also all manner of experiences, even astrological signs – these all initiate symptoms of melancholy.[5] In the plethora of causes cited, the *Anatomy* conception of disease matches that of other Early Modern thinkers such as the influential disease classifier Thomas Sydenham (1624–1689). In contrast to the nineteenth century model derived from the discovery of bacterial infections, the earlier approach was focused not on underlying causes but on signs and symptoms observed through the course of the disease's natural history. This conception was also tied to a notion of "cure", or remedy. Not a single treatment matching an underlying specific, morbid state would effect improvement, it was emphasized. Rather, what was required was a whole host of interventions, most of them preventive, that together, in the manner of holistic healing, brought about balance within the broader bodily and psychic systems.

---

[5] Burton scholars disagree over whether demonic influences should be included in this enumeration, or whether, like his more enlightened contemporary, the Renaissance doctor Johann Weyer, Burton avoids supernatural causes. For a discussion of these disagreements, see Gowland (2007).

Galenic Medicine

The canon of writing on melancholy that Burton so extensively cites is imbued with Galenic humoral medicine. As one of the several diseases of the black bile (alongside haemorrhoids, dysentery and skin eruptions), the condition known as Melancholy (or sometimes translated 'Melancholia') is extensively discussed in Galenic writing.[6] And the influence of that tradition left Galen's analysis, and approach to treatment, largely unchanged throughout the medieval era. By the Renaissance, some had begun to question and challenge Galenic assumptions – Paracelsus for example, who rejected the humoral basis of medicine. And more empirical approaches and discoveries were gradually taking hold by the time Burton wrote, when adherence to orthodox Galenic medical lore was giving way to attitudes and practices closer to those we associate with modern science. The effect of these changes on the *Anatomy* are not entirely agreed-upon. It has often been read as a work of humoral orthodoxy, and certainly Burton's references to contemporaries like Paracelsus suggest polite indifference towards any wholesale rejection of Galenic medicine. Nonetheless, although reliance on particular explanations employing humoral substances and the animal spirits was slowly being eclipsed by more accurate causal hypotheses, humoral ideas, categories and distinctions lingered as metaphors long after the seventeenth century. (Indeed, they are with us still.) And although they have rarely been taken this way, Burton's references to the humors in explaining Melancholy should perhaps be read in these looser and less literal terms.

Regardless of this issue, however, the *Anatomy* does adhere to Galenic traditions in its overarching definition of melancholy and in proposals for treating, and averting melancholy symptoms. Melancholy is distinguished from other conditions along classical medical lines. It is without fever. (On Burton's definition, Melancholy is: "a kind of dotage without feaver, having his ordinary companions feare, and sadnesse, without any apparent occasion" (I,1,3,1).) It is distinguished from madness, moreover, by appeal to the characteristic subjectivity of melancholy (in the states of unwarranted fear and sadness or sorrow), as well as by its relative lack of severity and violence. Madness is more "vehement, raving, and violent" than melancholy, and

> *without all feare and sorrow*, with such impetuous force and boldnesse, that sometimes three or foure men cannot hold [patients] (I,1,1,4, emphasis added).

With regard to remedies for Melancholy, Burton shared the humanists' skepticism of contemporary medical practices, but his attitude towards classical medical

---

[6] The primary source here is Galen's *On the Affected Parts*.

lore was unfailingly respectful. Like many other works from Renaissance and Early Modern times, the *Anatomy* is a kind of self-help manual based on Galenic humoral lore framing a *regimen sanitatis* through adherence to the six "non-naturals" which were the elements affecting our bodily constitutions: exercise, fresh air, sleep, diet, evacuation, and perturbations provoked by the passions).

The "cures" (or we would perhaps more safely say "remedies") enumerated and explained in the *Anatomy* are shaped by other influences as well, including Medieval Christianity, and the vaunted place of the imagination in Renaissance and Early Modern times, especially the role assigned to aberrant imagining by Renaissance medical thinkers like André Du Laurens (1558–1609), Felix Plater (1535–1614) and Johann Weyer (1515–1588). But these remedies are largely classical, reflecting their ancient origins in two ways. They are based loosely on Galenic humoral medicine, and they also exhibit Hellenistic philosophy and the Stoic's unparalleled attention to regulating the passions.

Following Galenic medicine Burton lays out his primary remedial principles, which emphasize preventative self-help. From the Patient himself, as he says

> the first and chiefest remedy must be had ... if he be willing, at least, gentle, tractable, and desire his owne good (II,2,6,1, page 101).

The person can and should become his own physician, by following the regimen for maintaining healthy humoral balance, prescribed through the six non-naturals of Galenic medicine.[7] The body's constituents were natural, and included its qualities of heat, cold, warmth and dryness, for example, and the humors themselves, along with the animal spirits that transported humoral substances around the body. The non-naturals each altered the individual's humoral balance.[8] As everyday mental and behavioral habits, the six non-naturals could be acquired and exercised, at home, and alone. They demanded no more than regular practice, close attention and self-control. With this emphasis on daily self care, Galenic medicine had ascribed significant value to self-mastery – an attitude with which Burton entirely concurred. Failure to adhere to the regimen, he deems a "want of [self] government." And by such failure, he warns, we not only engender Melancholy, but risk moral depravity. We

> degenerate into beasts, [and] transforme our selves (I,1,1,1).

---

[7] The Galenic regimen adhered to by Burton was one of several put forward by medical authorities at the time. See Tilmouth (2005) 532–534.
[8] For a thorough discussion of these aspects of humoral medicine, see Arikha (2007); Foucault (1988).

These elements of classical medicine demonstrate not only the specific measures required to prevent the humoral imbalance associated with melancholy, and the importance of self care. They also illustrate the way in which, in classical thinking, health and unhealth were attributes of the non-bodily soul, or psyche, as well as of the body. It is true that the body brought about psychic changes and the psyche, bodily ones; illness, disease, and imbalance were attributed to souls and minds, as well as to bodies. These ideas had been adopted and reinforced by Medieval Christianity, and are integral to Burton's understanding of disease from both sources.

Stoic Regulation of the Passions

The valuing of self-mastery and self-control runs through Stoic doctrine, where identifying and taking charge of what is within our control, and practicing serene acceptance of things lying outside it constitute a key element of how to live well.[9] Burton diverges from the Stoics on several matters, including their failure to acknowledge the freedom of the will, but he thoroughly agreed with them about self control. And, it was the Stoics who most thoroughly and carefully wrote of what Burton sees as the central challenge posed by melancholy: adhering to the sixth of the non-naturals. To prevent melancholy, the person must curb and regulate his Passions, utilizing his Imagination to do so. And the distinctive ideas about the passions, the self and its powers, values and ends, associated with the Stoicism of Chrysippus, Seneca, Epictetus and Marcus Aurelius are an obvious source for these ideas.

With the Stoics, Burton accepts that Passions such as fear, anger, and love are tied to erroneous judgements. (This analysis was closely related to today's cognitivist theories of emotion. On those theories, cognitive states are essential accompaniments, or even constituents, of affective states.[10]) Thoughts and beliefs are open to adjustment, and will in turn curb, and alter, the Passions that contain, and are a consequence, of them. The Stoic sage who had attained moral and intellectual perfection would achieve a state of tranquillity (*ataraxia*), untroubled by feelings of any kind. Although scholars would disagree with his interpretation, for Burton (along with much of the neo-Stoic writing of the Renaissance), the entirely apathetic state in which the person

---

9 For an explication of these Stoic ideas, see Gill (2009); Sorabji (2000); Nussbaum (2003); Robertson (2010).
10 See Nussbaum (2003); Goldie (2010).

is without Passions is the one sought by the Stoics. And with that goal, he disagrees.[11] The approach and methods proposed for curbing the Passions associated with Stoic exercises are acceptable, including regular critical analysis of one's cognitive states of belief and imagination. But, seeking to be "without all manner of passions and perturbations whatsoever," he insists, would be mistaken, since such a state of tranquility would be an impossible one to achieve. No Stoic, Burton insists, nor any

> so wise, none so happy, none so patient, so generous, so godly, so divine, that vindicate himself, so well composed, but *more or less some time or other*, he feeles the smarte of it [Melancholy].

Rather than seeking to entirely expunge the Passions, Burton wants to regulate and change them through habits of self-analysis. Seeking balance (or *krasis*) between the Passions, Imagination and Reason is a goal that seems to place Burton closer to the Aristotelianism that promoted moderate, rather than extreme, passions, achieved through their careful, habituated regulation. Feelings were central to the moral life and the achievement of *eudaimonia,* for Aristotle, and Burton agreed. However, they must be of the right kind: at the right time, about the right things, towards the right people, for the right end, and in the right way.[12]

The exercises involved in regulating the Passions, attributed to Chrysippus, Epictetus, Seneca and Marcus Aurelius, are found in no single treatise, but they were well known.[13] And Burton demonstrates familiarity with them in his recommendations concerning the sixth non-natural, although he dispenses with the details of the Stoic epistemic process of belief acceptance. Understood by him, the Stoic exercises involve careful and rigorous assessment of evidence and inductive reasoning patterns. Thus, in one passage Burton instructs a person who claims to see signs of demonic influence (a not uncommon situation in those times). He addresses the person directly, and requests that he reconsider his suspicions:

> Thou thinkest thou hearest and seest divells …' tis not so, 'tis they corrupt phantasy, settle thyne imagination, though art well. Thou thinkest thou has a great nose, thou art sicke, every man observes thee, laughes thee to scorne, *perswade thy selfe* 'tis no such matter: this is feare only, and vaine suspition.

---

11 The Stoic sage "is not entirely impassive, *contrary to the popular conception of a Stoic*" (Long (1986) 206–207, emphasis added). It was a popular misconception even in their own time, it should be added, when the Stoics were also ridiculed for their views on the passions.
12 Aristotle, *Nichomachean Ethics*.
13 The texts from which they are drawn are Seneca's *Letters*, Epictetus's *Handbook* and the *Meditations* of Marcus Aurelius, as well as from descriptions of Stoicism by later classical writers.

At moments of discontent, sadness and heaviness, he advises

> we must ask *why*, and *upon what ground*? Consider of it, he admonishes, "*examine it thoroughly*" (II,2,6,1, page 103 emphases added).

By paying attention to our beliefs, assumptions and inferences, and subjecting them to critical assessment and skeptical review, we can dissuade ourselves from accepting them. Attentively employed, these practices will serve to avert, dispel, and heal melancholy symptoms, Burton implies. And these daily cognitive exercises aimed to eliminate unwarranted belief and ill-formed judgement must particularly be directed towards flights of the Imagination. The unfettered play of the Imagination, although enjoyable, is dangerous, it is stressed. This is because imaginings and feelings are an endless goad to one another. Imaginings and errant beliefs prompt feelings, feelings in turn foster misleading imaginings. To curb unruly and overweening passions and avert melancholy or dispel its passing presence, we must monitor and correct the conceits, fantasies and wilful blindness that result from the solitary, careless, self-indulgent ruminating he calls "melancholizing". The lure of these "phantastical and bewitching thoughts ..." is a constant danger. They

> so urgently, so continually set upon, creep in, insinuate, possess, overcome, distract and detain ... [some people] they cannot go about their more necessary business, stave off or extricate themselves, but are ever musing, melancholizing, and carried along (I,2,2,6).

His attention on quelling excessive, or the wrong kind of, imagining, Burton may also derive his emphasis on these imaginary objects from the Stoic stress on the here and now (*hic et nunc*). Attention to the present moment in Stoic thought, it has been pointed out, frees us from the passions, "always caused by the past or the future".[14] The characteristic symptoms of melancholy, whether passing or habitual, are unwarranted fears and sorrows. The here and now is also the actual rather than hypothetical, and a passage from Epictetus seems to capture exactly the apprehensions that run through much of the *Anatomy*,

> we always exaggerate, and represent things greater than the reality. In a voyage, for instance, casting my eyes down upon the ocean below, and looking around me, and seeing no land, I am beside myself, and imagine that, if I should be shipwrecked, I must swallow all that ocean; nor does it occur to me, that three pints are enough for me (*Discourses* II,16,111).

---

[14] Hadot (1995) 84–85. Contemporary cognitive therapy has developed this emphasis on the here and now and integrated it into mindfulness practices. See Robertson (2010).

Danger lies in all these objects for Burton as well: those that are unchangeably past, or hypothetically future are *not now*; and those that are merely imaginary are *not here*. Worries and fears such as Epictetus's all disturb the Passions. Whether Burton knew such troubling concerns from personal experience, as is often suggested, from his observation of others, or from descriptions like this by the ancients, he does seem to entirely concur with this depiction of the inner life of imagination-fostered worry and unwarranted distress.

The Stoic-inspired cognitive exercises addressing the sixth of the non-naturals, together with the elaborate daily regimen called for in avoiding, averting and "curing" melancholy, share certain characteristics. They are self-help, as we saw: homely, personal remedies requiring self-control, and attentive daily practice. Burton did not think all melancholy was amenable to such remedies, he acknowledges that there are states so entrenched and "chronic" as to constitute an untreatable disease. This, he described as Melancholy in Habit, the chronic condition that is, he believes, disease properly so-called. In contrast, were the passing states of sadness and worry that he regards as inescapable aspects of being human and calls Melancholy in Disposition. Thus

> Melancholy ... is either in Disposition, or Habit. In Disposition, is that transitory Melancholy, which goes & comes upon every small occasion of sorrow, need, sickness, trouble, fear, grief, passion, or perturbation of the Mind ... from these Melancholy Dispositions, no man living is free .... This Melancholy of which we are to treat, as in Habit ... a Chronic or continuate disease, a settled humor ... not errant but fixed, and as it was long increasing, so now being (pleasant, or painful) grown to an habit, it will hardly be removed (I,1,1,5).

The confusion of naming as forms of melancholy both the severe, chronic condition, and passing states of sadness and worry, is warranted on Burton's account because they can be seen as later and earlier stages of the same disorder. His analysis is longitudinal, so the disposition might through time become the more severe, entrenched state.

As well as beyond self-help, the person afflicted with chronic melancholy is in some cases also beyond the help of friends and medical authorities, and effectively incurable. The conception of melancholy in the *Anatomy* is focused on habituation. The chronic, incurable condition (Melancholy in Habit) is one resulting from neglect of the simple measures that initially could have prevented it. And melancholy stubbornly resists treatment once it becomes habituated ("it can hardly be removed"). Remedy then, is seen as based on prevention, and on this matter also, Burton turns to the ancient medical authorities for support. Of the good rules and precepts we learn from ancient physicians, he says, the first is to "withstand the beginning". This, Burton insists, quoting Ovid, is a precept "which all concurre upon" (III,2,5,2, page 208) For,

> he that will but resist at first may easily bee a conquerer at the last (III,2,5,2).

These "good rules and precepts" about early prevention stemmed from a time when little was known about specific causes, and remedies were for the most part ineffectual, making early prevention the safest and surest approach. And the same remained true in Burton's own era. Melancholy may be treated or at least mitigated, as he says,

> if it be withstood in the beginning, maturely resisted, and as those ancients hold, *the nayles of it be pared befor they grow too long.* (III,3,4,1).

'Prevention' can mean entirely averting or reducing the severity of initial symptoms; reducing the length of initial or subsequent phases; or reducing the likelihood of developing melancholy-inducing habits. With his emphasis on *"paring the nails before they grow too long"*, Burton apparently accommodates each of these interpretations. Even in those whose inherent temperament strongly predisposes them towards Melancholy, with greater effort, applied early, chronic Melancholy may be able to be averted.

3. The Anatomy and the Mind Sciences of the Twenty-first Century

Our era has seen a remarkable opening up and exchange between the related sciences of psychology, medicine (including medical psychiatry) and philosophy, as well as the new hybrid fields like cognitive neuroscience, and cognitive psychiatry. The 'silos' around these different disciplines that earlier prevented such productive interdisciplinary work have been eliminated in part due to advances in understanding both mind and brain. The widespread adoption of cognitivist theories of mind, such as Fodorian functionalism, or the presuppositions of cognitive science, is an example of the first; and the new technologies affording observation of the brain and its workings to establish links with behavioural and subjective states, illustrates the second. The expression "mind sciences" best covers this broad research domain, and it is a domain that nicely fits the *Anatomy*. Burton turned his back on most of the new science emerging during his times. Yet separated from the humoralism through which it is expressed, his encyclopaedic summation of all that had come before, in classical, Renaissance, and Medieval psychology, deserves our respectful attention. In the last part of this chapter, I want to note some aspects of the *Anatomy* that make it such an agreeable fit.

First, the model of mind employed by Burton is strikingly consonant with the cognitivist presuppositions that form the prevailing paradigm of twenty-first century psychology. In this respect, it is better matched to contemporary thinking than the psychology associated with Cartesianism that held sway for the several hundred years between Burton's seventeenth century and the new paradigms coming with cognitivist psychology in the twentieth century. In France, Descartes was at work on his *Discourse* (1637) and *Meditations* (1641) at the same time as, in England, Burton laboured over revising the *Anatomy*. (Neither thinker knew of the other, as far as we can determine.) Both, as faithful Christians, were dualists. But they adhered to very different conceptions of the mind to body relationship. For Descartes in his early work from the 1630s, the mind was essentially and by explicit definition a thinking substance, and the body an extended and unthinking one. By contrast representations and ideas are attributed to both mind and body in the *Anatomy*, and the Sensitive or Sensible faculty containing the Common Sense and Imagination somehow straddles the intellectualistic and corporeal. (Representations move from the mind to the body, and through the body, transported by the animal spirits, as we saw. This was a position that Descartes also reached, but only with later writing on the passions from the 1640s.) As a consequence, consciousness and self-awareness are not awarded the special place in Burton's scheme of things that they are in Descartes' early work where they are identified with thinking substance. Self-knowledge is not privileged, nor, indeed, is the self identified with the conscious mind. In each of these characteristics, Burton's model corresponds to the assumptions of modern day cognitivism, and with its spare, "cognitive" unconscious mechanisms. There are other similarities as well. Burton's system recognizes the centrality of those affective states that contemporary neuroscience has shown to be embedded in all higher cognition. And he acknowledges the pain/pleasure systems and the relation now understood to exist between the emotion and reward systems. Although Burton's quaint anatomy and physiology remain of only historical interest, the substance of what he says conforms with what is known about the role of the amygdala, insular cortex, and ventromedial prefrontal cortex from work like that of Joseph LeDoux, and Antonio Damasio. Burton's multi-directional causal loops also correspond to the mechanics of mental functioning identified by contemporary neuroscience. Damasio portrays emotions and feelings as emerging out of an elaborate, looping exchange between different systems, which begin with a stimulus (from outside the mind or – as in a memory, or entirely imaginary objects – within it) that is processed in the visual cortices, and ends with a felt state accompanied by "the representation of the object that caused the emotion in the first place". In more recent work (2012), Damasio has also made room for multi-directional causal sequences in his references to the way, once an emotion has been triggered, it is altered not merely by the neurobiology that makes it possible, but by attitudes towards it that take place in the conscious mind, thus forming feedback loops along Burtonian lines. And LeDoux has similarly adapted his account to accommodate the way emotions may arise from cognitive processes in a top-down fashion (LeDoux 2015).

Second, Burton's emphasis on the imagination and its functioning in inciting, and controlling, the Passions also finds parallels in contemporary psychology and brain science. Its importance corresponds to findings about the "resting" or "task negative" system has been identified within attentional networks as the brain's default mode of operation (the Default System Network).[15] This operation has been shown to be common, normal, and an indispensable part of cognitive functioning. Its capabilities include speculating, conceiving, imagining, day-dreaming and imaging – which are the characteristic functions of the Burtonian Imagination. Separate findings on cognitive states involving "mind wandering" or "time travel" similarly confirm these parallels.[16]

Most of these findings about the Default System Network and mind wandering involve normal mental processes. Yet they can readily accommodate the imbalanced and dysfunctionally habituated frames of mind that Burton wants to emphasize in depicting how disordered Imagination and feeling, and careless and self-indulgent cognitive habits, together yield the recalcitrant moods and fears afflicting the melancholic. More particularly, the activity Burton calls "melancholizing", seems to correspond to the ruminating, idle, repetitive ideas and default mode "mind wandering" that have been linked to depression. Rumination on negative thoughts engenders negative moods, and the interaction between the thoughts and moods creates a vicious cycle.[17] From this body of research it has been concluded that depressed individuals are more likely to be in the default state and once engaged, are more likely to stay there – thus invoking the tendency towards a habituated condition stressed by Burton.

These parallels and echoes are of considerable interest. But Burton's remedies seem to have more immediate implications for the treatment of and approach to affective conditions like depression which, while not to be equated with melancholy, resemble it.[18] The illimitable number of causes of melancholy cited in

---

15 See Buckner/Vincent (2007); Andrews-Hanna/Smallwood/Spreng (2014); Schacter (2012); Gerrans (2014).
16 See Killingsworth/Gilbert (2010); Kam/Handy (2013).
17 Nolen-Hocksema (1991, 2000); Nolen-Hocksema et al. (2008); Huffziger/Reinhard/Kuehner (2009).
18 See Radden (2003).

the *Anatomy* correspond to present day recognition that much, if not all, depression is brought about by a comparable range of exogenous and endogenous risk factors and triggers.[19] And Burton's emphasis on the range of remedies that must be applied together, has parallels in contemporary questioning about the applicability of the common cause and single (magic bullet) remedies associated with much biological psychiatry and psychopharmacology.[20] Rather than a single, endogenous cause that will respond to a particular remedy on the model of bacteriological infections and their treatment, it is increasingly speculated that affective disorders such as depression should be subject to a range of therapeutic responses.[21] Thus, Alternative, Complementary, and Integrated Medicine are increasingly appealed to not only in other areas of medicine, but in mental health care.[22] For depression, Burton's emphasis on prevention has also been increasingly recognized, the almost exclusive earlier attention to treatment increasingly seen to be too little, too late.[23]

The most obvious parallel with contemporary treatments for affective disorder is, of course, cognitive therapy. The Stoic-inspired therapy for regulating the passions that Burton recommends in relation to the sixth non-natural, has been widely, and apparently successfully employed with affective disorder. (The link between these Stoic ideas and current forms of cognitive behavioural (CBT) and mindfulness therapy has been thoroughly explored.[24]) Closest to the program of *self*-help that Burton recommends, may be forms of mindfulness practice, and very recent trends including the use of the Internet for guidance, and apps for phones that address the individual directly.[25]

There are differences of interpretation and assumption still dividing Burton's recommendations from those applied to today's disorders. Thus, he portrays melancholy as a danger we must all fight against with vigilance and unfailing

---

[19] These generalizations are complicated by classificatory distinctions. Some argue, for example, that there are true endogenous depressions, whose causes are likely more limited in number. For a review of the history of these classificatory issues see Shorter (2011).
[20] On these network models, see Cramer/Borsboom/Aggen/Kendler (2011); Kendler/Zachar/Craver (2011); Wichers (2014); Zachar (2014).
[21] For the historical shift to conceptions of disease causation postulating a single, endogenous cause, see Thagard (1997).
[22] Dobos/Tao (2011); Eardley/Bishop/Prescott (2012); Frass/Strassl/Friehs (2012); Pampallona et al. (2004); Rhead (2014).
[23] See Walsh (2011); McLaughlin (2011); Mrazek (1994); O'Connell/Boat/Warner (2009).
[24] See Beck/Alford (2009); Biegler (2011); Dobson (2010).
[25] Van Straten/Cuijpers/Smits (2008); Van Voorhees (2011); Hollandare/Johnsson/Randestad/Tilfors (2011).

attention to the *régime sanitaire*. Some people will be by temperament or experience more prone to succumb to the habit of melancholy. Nonetheless, we are all at risk. If we neglect our health until it is too late, any of us might find himself the victim of chronic, untreatable disorder. This attitude towards preventive self-help runs rather contrary to many contemporary attitudes about affective disorder, when the sufferer is depicted as a victim, and one whose very condition robs her of the self-control and motivation to engage in such a daily regimen. Burton's analysis does not challenge this picture. He acknowledges that there are those whose condition leaves them beyond self-help, or even the help of friends and doctors. But his conception of disease, as we saw, is a longitudinal one, emphasizing disease course. So this state of disorder is understood within a temporal context, where degrees of habituation are acknowledged. According to his habituation model of melancholy, in those cases the sufferer must have neglected the daily practice of preventive self-help while such a response was within her power. The model whereby as the result of our genetic disposition, or earlier experience, Depressive Disorder will be for some an immovable fate, is not entirely contrary to Burton's idea, however. True, it omits the significance of early prevention and attentive self care: caught early, the habit may have been averted. But Burton has no illusions about how difficult such prevention can prove, especially in those whose natural tendencies incline them towards melancholy and towards the pleasures and comforts of idle, solitary "melancholizing".

Conclusion

Although Burton ignored the evidence of modern science around him, and turned instead towards the great legacy of classical medical and philosophical writing from the ancients, I have tried to show, what he has left us finds many convergences with post-Cartesian cognitive psychology as well as other contemporary mind sciences. His anatomy and physiology can have little to teach those sciences. But as we confront the challenge imposed by widespread and apparently increasing depression in our own time, the remedial principles of self-help, prevention, and complementary healing cannot be easily dismissed.

Christopher Gill
6 The Psychology of Psychotherapy: Ancient and Modern Perspectives

The aim of this discussion is to explore the relationship between the ancient philosophical therapy of emotions, developed between the third century BC and second century AD, and modern psychotherapy, especially CBT (cognitive and behavioural psychotherapy). The main focus will be on psychology, in line with the overall theme of this volume, but, as will become clear, the psychological dimension is closely connected with other aspects, such as ethics and modes of communication. Why is this topic of special interest for the study of ancient psychology, and why is it especially worth considering now? The second question is addressed first, and the explanation may also help to answer the first question.

The key point is that recent developments in modern psychotherapeutic practice have made it much more plausible than before to take the ancient philosophical therapy seriously *as a mode of psychotherapy*, conceived in modern terms. For much of the twentieth century the dominant mode of psychotherapy was Freudian, or Jungian, psychoanalysis, which was centred on bringing to consciousness the unconscious sources of psychological disorders (often taken to be located in infant traumas) and by that process working towards psychological maturity and health. Freud and Jung are, of course, key figures in the history of modern psychotherapy, and Freudian influence remains very powerful in modern Western culture and thought. However, as I understand the position, Freudian-style psychoanalysis has become a relatively minor strand in modern psychotherapeutic treatment, at least in the UK and USA, and most current practice is based on some version of CBT. The evidence base for the effectiveness of CBT, it is claimed, is very strong, whereas the evidence base for the effectiveness of Freudian-style psychoanalysis is much weaker.[1] Although there are significant

---

[1] See Eysenck (1952) for an early and influential challenge to the therapeutic effectiveness of psychoanalysis; see also Gregory (2004) 777–779.

Note: I appreciate the invitation to present this paper at the Leuven conference and the helpful and thoughtful comments on the paper and stimulating discussion at the conference more generally. I am also grateful to the Leverhulme Trust for awarding a Leverhulme Emeritus Fellowship, which enabled me to carry out the research and composition of this paper.

Christopher Gill, University of Exeter

https://doi.org/10.1515/9783110482201-019

differences between CBT and ancient philosophical therapy, discussed shortly, the ancient approach is much more comparable with CBT than with Freudian psychoanalysis. In particular, CBT shares with ancient philosophical therapy a focus on conscious beliefs and on deliberate efforts that the client can make for herself to understand and to improve her psychological state and to change her behaviour or situation. In this respect, there is much more basis for comparison between ancient and modern psychotherapy than before,[2] and perhaps too an opportunity for ancient approaches to inform modern practice (a suggestion developed at the end of this discussion).

To provide the basis for this comparison, I outline the history and main characteristics of these ancient and modern approaches. The ancient approach is found in a genre of writing which was widely practised between the third century BC and the second century AD, and which had a reasonably distinct and consistent character. The genre emerged in the Stoic and Epicurean schools of philosophy, though it was adopted later by some thinkers writing in a Platonic-Aristotelian or eclectic mode, such as Plutarch and Galen.[3] The genre reflects salient features of Stoic and Epicurean ethics, which were partly, though not wholly, shared by the Platonic and Aristotelian traditions in that period. The core idea is that human beings have an in-built capacity to create, or to undermine, their own happiness. Happiness (*eudaimonia*) is conceived in objective terms, as 'flourishing', we might say, though it carries with it the subjective sense of well-being which is what 'happiness' normally means today. Happiness, in this philosophical tradition, consists in, or at least depends on, developing virtue (*aretē*), or the virtues, conceived as those qualities of understanding, character and mode of action and relationship which are fundamental to a good human

---

[2] In Gill (1985), I took Freudian or Jungian psychoanalysis as the assumed modern approach (especially as presented by Storr 1979), and so reached a more negative conclusion about the extent to which ancient methods of psychotherapy, including philosophical ones, prefigured modern ones. See also, on ancient, esp. Stoic, and modern psychotherapy, Gill (2010) 354–360.

[3] A brief overview of the genre of philosophical therapy of emotions: Chrysippus (3rd cent. BC Stoic), 'therapeutic book' (Book 4 of *On Passions*); Philodemus (1st cent. BC Epicurean), many works including those on avoiding fear of death and anger; Lucretius, *On the Nature of the Universe (De Rerum Natura)* Book 3 on confronting fear of death; Cicero (1st cent BC Academic Sceptic), *Tusculan Disputations*; Seneca (1st cent AD Stoic) *On Anger (De Ira)*, *On Peace of Mind (De Tranquillitate Animi)*; Plutarch (1st cent. AD Platonist), various works including *Avoiding Anger (peri aorgēsias)*, *On Contentment (peri euthumias)*; Galen (2nd cent AD, medical and philosophical writer), *Avoiding Distress (peri alupias = de Indolentia)*, *The Diagnosis and Cure of Psychological Affections (and Errors) (Aff. Dig.,* and *Pecc.)*; Stoic writings combining protreptic, therapy and advice: Epictetus (1st cent. AD Stoic teacher), *Discourses, Handbook*; Marcus Aurelius (2nd cent. AD emperor influenced by Stoicism), *Meditations*.

life. Two other crucial Stoic and Epicurean ideas, which are, however, *not* shared with the Platonic-Aristotelian approach, are these. One is that all human beings as such are naturally capable of developing in a way that leads towards virtue and happiness, as these notions conceived in the relevant theory. The other is that emotions depend directly on beliefs, and that the quality of our emotions is radically changed by ethical development. In Stoic theory, for instance, ethical development brings with it the loss of ill-judged, negative and destructive emotions or passions (*pathē*), such as anger and hatred, and the formation of well-judged, positive and beneficial emotions (*eupatheiai*) such as good will and joy. The 'therapy of emotions', then, in Stoic-Epicurean and, to some extent, other writings in this genre, centres on promoting the kind of ethical development, in understanding, character, mode of action and relationship, that carries with it this type of emotional transformation. If we accept the Stoic-Epicurean assumptions on this point, change of belief by itself carries with it change in emotion and state of mind without the need for separate, habituative, modification of non-rational parts of the personality. This is, arguably, a strength of the Stoic-Epicurean therapeutic strategy – though, again, one that depends on accepting their psychological views.[4]

What about the other side in this comparison – the history and main features of CBT? There are a number of strands in this approach, and the methodology seems to be one that is open to change and modification. Key common features, indicated already, include a rejection of the backward-looking focus of Freudian psychoanalysis, centred on unearthing from unconsciousness the buried roots of current psychological states. The focus is on the present and future, and on steps that the person concerned can take, as a conscious agent, to address his or her problem and bring about change. Another key feature is the use of short interventions (typically, eight one-hour weekly sessions), designed to support the client's own efforts at change in this period, in sharp contrast with the extended, sometimes life-long, process of Freudian psychoanalysis. A third feature is a commitment to on-going assessment of the effectiveness of the specific method used, which is often appraised in comparison with other psychotherapeutic methods

---

[4] See, on ancient philosophical therapy and its theoretical presuppositions, Gill (2010), ch. 5, esp. 246–251, 280–300, Gill (2013b); also, on Stoic and Epicurean thinking on ethical development, Gill (2006) 129–145, 177–186, and on Stoic emotions, Gill (2006) 244–266. On Stoic emotions and development, see also Graver (2007), chs. 4 and 7. On Chrysippus' (Stoic) therapy, see Tieleman (2003), ch. 4; on Philodemus and therapy, see Tsouna (2007), chs. 4–5; on philosophical therapeutic strategies, see Sorabji (2000), chs. 15–16. For important earlier studies of the genre, see Hadot (1969), Nussbaum (1994).

and also, of course, with the other, most widely used, method of modern treatment for psychological disorders of all kinds, namely drug therapy.[5]

How far can we compare modern CBT, or indeed modern psychotherapeutic practice of any kind, with the ancient philosophical therapy of the emotions? I think there are some genuine similarities in the underlying project of both types of practice, as explained shortly. But there are also some important differences, or at least complications involved in undertaking the comparison. Modern psychotherapy forms a distinct and well-recognized procedure, centring on pre-arranged one-to-one dialogues between therapist and client with (largely) agreed objectives. The main modern sources used for this discussion are academic textbooks about this procedure, written for psychotherapeutic researchers and practitioners (n. 5). Our evidence for ancient philosophical therapy consists of a much more diverse collection of essays, literary letters or dialogues, reports of informal lectures, quotations and discussions of lost works and so on.[6] Can we identify, embedded in this ancient material or underlying it, anything like the one-one psychotherapeutic dialogues we now take as standard? Well – perhaps and to some extent.[7] But it is clear we are dealing with a process that was much less formalized and distinct than modern psychotherapeutic meetings. Also, we need to recognize that these various literary works, as well as the kinds of oral communication they represent, constitute an important vehicle of the therapy being offered. Actually, in the modern world too, where there are so many kinds of communicative vehicles for ideas and methods (oral, written, technological), this feature of ancient psychotherapy is a highly suggestive one; but we need to note the difference from the standard modern pattern.

A second question to be faced is this. Modern psychotherapeutic treatment is offered to those who present themselves as distressed or disturbed, and who believe that they could be helped by the therapeutic process and its effect on their lives. Is that also true of ancient philosophical therapy? The answer is, again: perhaps and to some extent. Here are two passages that point in this direction.

---

[5] See Hawton/Salovskis/Kirk/Clark (1989); Hayes/Strosahl/Wilson (1999); Herbert/Forman (2011).

[6] See refs. in nn. 3–4.

[7] As far as I am aware, there has not been a sustained attempt to reconstruct therapy as a social practice on the basis of the literary evidence; nor is it clear how far the evidence allows us to do this. For some suggestive moves in this direction, see (on Epicurean therapeutic discourse), Nussbaum (1994) 117–136; Tsouna (2007) chs. 4–5; also (on Epictetus' Stoic discourses to students and visitors to his school), Long (2002) 43–64. See also passages cited in next paragraph.

> (Serenus talking to Seneca) I ask you, therefore, if you possess any cure (*remedium*) by which you can check this fluctuation (*fluctuationem*) of mine, to consider me being worthy of being indebted to you for tranquillity. I am aware that these mental disturbances (*motus animi*) I suffer from are not dangerous and bring no threat of a storm; to express to you in a true analogy the source of my complaint, it is not a storm I labour under but seasickness: relieve me, then, of this malady (*mali*), whatever it may be, and hurry to aid one who struggles with land in his sight.[8]
>
> One of the young men in my circle, who used to suffer grief (*aniasthai*) over trivial matters, realized the fact one evening; and he came to me first thing in the morning, admitting that he had been awake all night over this, and that at some point it had occurred to him that I did not suffer grief in the same way, even in response to great matters, as he did in response to trivial ones. He desired to learn how this had come about – whether it was the result of training, of particular doctrines, or simply because I had been born like that. I told him the truth. In all cases, I said, nature has great power in childhood: so too does emulation of those amongst whom one lives. Then, at a later stage, the important factors are doctrines and training.[9]

However, it must be acknowledged that much ancient philosophical therapy was rather differently conceived and presented. Philosophical therapy was understood, especially in the Stoic and Epicurean schools which originated this genre, as part of a programme for 'cleansing' or 'curing' misguided and destructive emotions. This process was seen as one that would, if carried through successfully, free people from psychological disturbance and distress. But the message and the therapeutic programme were disseminated widely and not only to those who presented themselves as distressed or as looking for support of a specific kind.[10]

Thirdly, there are significant differences between ancient and modern modes of therapeutic dialogue. Modern psychotherapeutic dialogue aims to be supportive and collaborative; it is also, at least in principle, non-judgemental and non-moralistic. The pre-arranged, private session between therapist and client offers a kind of protected space and time in which the client is not subject to the kind of judgements and reactive attitudes she might experience at other times. The characteristic mode of ancient philosophical dialogue or communication is more asymmetrical in the relationship established between teacher and listener and is more like lecturing or instructing. Also, the therapeutic process is not, even

---

[8] Seneca, *De Tranquillitate Animi* 1.1–2, trans. Davie (2007) 115. On this dialogue as a whole, see Griffin (1976), 321–327.
[9] Galen, *Psychological Affections* (*Aff. Dig.*) V.37 (Kühn) (=25 De Boer), trans. Singer in Singer (2013) 270. On Galenic therapy and the form of this work, see Singer (2013) 205–232, including discussion of the use of addressees (218–219); also Gill (2010) 252–262.
[10] For stress on this dimension of philosophical (at least Stoic and Epicurean) therapy, see Nussbaum (1994), chs. 4, 9; Tieleman (2003) ch. 4; Gill (2010) 280–315.

in principle, ethically neutral or non-judgemental; nor does it offer a protected space like the modern therapeutic session. On the other hand, the Stoic and Epicurean versions of this practice, in particular, do offer a new vantage point on the core principles of ethical life and on human psychology. While this new standpoint, in some ways, *extends* the scope of what is subject to ethical judgement, compared with conventional social frameworks, it also *revises and enlarges* the perspective within which someone may make judgements on himself and it does not simply reinforce existing moral frameworks.[11]

Despite these differences between ancient philosophical therapy and modern psychotherapy, there are certain important underlying similarities in the underlying aim of the therapy offered in each case. These similarities apply rather generally; for instance, they apply, to some degree, to Freudian psychoanalysis. However, there are also more specific points of contact between CBT, in its various versions, and ancient philosophical therapy, especially Stoic, which are explored more closely later.

Both ancient and modern versions of psychotherapy address problems that (it is supposed) can be resolved or improved through a psychological change that the client or patient can, in whole or in part, bring about herself. That is, the client is regarded as a psychological agent. The agency or action involved is reflexive or self-related; it presupposes the capacity to affect and change the way one thinks or feels or relates to others in a way that resolves or mitigates the original problem. A second common feature is this. The therapeutic process is often conceived as a two-stage or two-aspect method. The first stage or aspect consists in a critical exploration of the client's mind-set or belief-system (or the totality of influences on the problem), with a view to clarifying for the client the salient factors that seem to be causally effective in producing the sense of distress or disturbance. The second stage or aspect consists in helping the client to bring about the change (which is at least partly internal or self-related) needed to remove or mitigate this sense of distress or disturbance and to do by her own efforts. Despite the differences noted earlier between ancient and modern approaches, and between different versions of ancient and modern psychotherapy, I think this broad pattern holds good and justifies us in saying that ancient philosophical therapy constitutes psychotherapy *in a modern sense*.

It was suggested earlier that ancient philosophical therapy is much closer to CBT than to Freudian or Jungian psychoanalysis, both as regards psychological

---

[11] For instance, Stoic and Epicurean therapy promote the adoption of revisionist views about what count as good or justified emotions, and about the best form of interpersonal or social relations; see refs. in nn. 4, 10.

assumptions and therapeutic methods. To see how far this resemblance goes, it is useful to look more closely at the history and main features of CBT. Researchers tend to identify three main, partly overlapping, phases or 'waves' of CBT.[12] The first phase, in the 1950s and 1960s, was centred on behaviour and behaviour-change. It was informed by the psychological movement of 'behaviourism', which focused on behaviour rather than the supposed psychological causes of behaviour. It was also influenced by experiments on animals which were successful in changing behaviour by stimulus-response methods. The psychotherapeutic process was centred on finding motivational rewards which would lead the client to make changes in behaviour, which, it was supposed, which would carry with them changes in emotional state. The second phase in the late 1960s, 1970s and 1980s – on the face of it, rather sharply different in approach – saw a shift towards cognition as the key theme, and marked the influence of cognitive psychology and cognitive theories of emotion. 'Cognitions', in this type of theory, are not necessarily conscious processes, such as beliefs, reasoning or knowledge. They are, rather, units of 'information' of various kinds, which can be embedded in perceptions, memories, thoughts, and which underlie conscious belief-patterns or 'belief schemas', as they have been called. Crucially, however, they are seen as key causal factors in producing behaviour and emotion. A central theme of the cognitive approach is that we are disturbed not so much by events as by our reactions to these events; the cognitive basis underlying these reactions is seen as the crucial factor. Hence, the psychotherapeutic process focuses on helping people to examine critically their beliefs, to challenge 'cognitive errors' of different kinds in their beliefs (exaggerated fears and anxieties, for instance) and to work towards a cognitive framework that they and others find credible and workable, and which enables them to cope with life and relationships. Behaviour-change is seen as an important part of this process; however, in this approach it is viewed as a means of bringing about, and consolidating, the cognitive change that is the crucial factor.[13] CBT, cognitive-behavioural therapy, then, is an amalgam of these two strands, in which different therapists may place greater weight on the behavioural or the cognitive dimension of the process.

Since the 1990s, there have been further additions or developments in what is sometimes called 'third-wave' CBT. One, termed 'Mindfulness', uses relaxation exercizes, such as breathing and yoga, and meditation, to encourage clients to

---

[12] See Hawton/Salovskis/Kirk/Clark (1989) ch. 1; Herbert/Forman (2011) ch. 1.
[13] On cognitive therapy, see Robertson (2010) chs. 1–2; Herbert/Forman (2011) chs. 2, 11. On therapeutic modification of cognitive 'errors', see Hawton/Salovskis/Kirk/Clark (1989) ch. 3 (on anxiety), ch. 6 (on depression).

focus on the present rather than dwelling unhelpfully on the past or worrying about the future. The main influence here has been Buddhism (at least, secular, Westernized Buddhism). 'Mindfulness' techniques, it seems, are sometimes used on their own and sometimes in conjunction with other variants of CBT. The appeal of this approach is, perhaps, that it counteracts what might seem to be the rather mechanical or intellectualist character of therapy which is centred solely on behaviour-change or cognitive change.[14] A further, rather more complex, development is the emergence of Acceptance and Commitment Therapy (ACT). There are two, relatively distinct stages in this therapeutic process (ACT), both of them incorporating some salient differences from other types of CBT. The first stage is an attempt to explore the various factors in the current problematic situation, in an honest and open, but also unpressured and fairly gradual, way. This is characterized as 'Acceptance'; however, this does not signify accepting the validity of the way things currently appear, but rather exploring, examining or 'entertaining' how things appear without necessarily endorsing their validity. The factors are not limited to behaviour or cognitions; they can include any factors – actions, beliefs, emotions and facts in a person's situation – which have a direct bearing on the person's current state of mind. (This approach is characterized as 'functional contextualism' – identifying factors that, in functional terms, *make a difference* (negatively) to one's state of mind and well-being.)[15] The second stage, building on the first, centres on commitment to taking action of some kind to change the factors that are now recognized as being the source of the problem. This stage has a number of possible components; but three are of special interest because they are similar to recommendations made in ancient, especially Stoic, psychotherapeutic guidance, as brought out later. One is identifying in your situation factors that can or cannot be changed by actions you can take. Another is 'values-clarification', that is examining your underlying value-system and seeing how far your current life and actions match this. A third is making a firm and decisive 'commitment' to make the changes on which you have decided.[16] ACT, then, forms a distinct and coherent version of CBT, though it seems that elements of the ACT approach can also be applied eclectically within other types of CBT treatment.[17]

---

[14] See Herbert/Forman (2011) chs. 3, 6, 11–13.
[15] See Hayes/Strosahl/Wilson (1999) 18; Herbert/Forman (2011) 38.
[16] For these three elements in ACT, see Hayes/Strosahl/Wilson (1999) 78–79, 221–228, 243–249 respectively.
[17] On ACT, see Herbert/Forman (2011) ch. 10, also chs. 11–13 (compared with other CBT approaches). For the two main stages in ACT, see Hayes/Strosahl/Wilson (1999) chs. 4–6, 7–9 respectively; for an outline of stages or processes in ACT, see Herbert/Forman (2011) 237–238.

This outline of features of CBT may indicate points of contact with ancient philosophical therapy, at least with its underlying project, if not its typical procedures; and these connections are explored further now, with special reference to Stoic therapy. Epictetus' *Discourses* provide the main parallels, though the similarities identified apply to the Stoic approach more generally. On the face of it, Stoic therapy is closest to the 'cognitive' strand in CBT, as developed by Aaron Beck and Albert Ellis. However, the links may be closer still to the rather more complex therapeutic pattern offered by ACT, despite some initial differences from the Stoic approach.

The most obvious similarity between cognitive therapy and Stoicism is one that Beck and Ellis themselves recognized: they repeatedly quoted Epictetus' claim that "we are disturbed not so much by events as by our beliefs about events".[18] The underlying claim is that what determines our actions and reactions in each and every situation is our belief-set, as stated in this passage of Epictetus:

> ... for all human beings there is one and the same origin [of action]. Just as for assent (*sunkatathesis*) the origin is the feeling that something is the case, and for rejection the origin is the feeling that it is not the case ... so too for motivation (*hormē*) towards something the origin is the feeling that it is beneficial to me (*sumpheron*). It is impossible to judge that something is beneficial but to desire something else, or to judge that something is appropriate (*kathēkon*), but to be motivated towards something else.[19]

Underlying these similarities is a shared cognitive view of emotions; emotions are not seen in either case as constituting a distinct sector of psychological experience, as they are in some other ancient and modern theories of emotion, but as shaped by beliefs or cognitions.[20] It might seem to be a difference between these two approaches that, for modern theory, cognitions are not necessarily conscious[21] whereas Stoic beliefs are – at least we may assume this to be so. However, the conscious/non-conscious distinction is not accentuated (or perhaps even recognized) in Stoic or other ancient psychologies; and if we do introduce it into Stoicism, the concept of "impressions" (*phantasiai*), which includes thoughts, emotions and

---

18 On this point of resemblance, see Robertson (2010) ch. 1, esp. 5–7, Herbert/Forman (2011) 268–269. See Epictetus, *Handbook* 5.
19 Epictetus, *Discourses* 1.18.1, trans. Brennan (2003) 268. The passage assumes the standard Stoic view that motivation to action or feeling depends on 'assent' to 'impressions' (i.e. the beliefs held at any one time); see Brennan (2003) 265–274.
20 On Stoicism see ref. in n. 19 and Graver (2007), chs. 1–2. On cognitive therapy, see Herbert/Forman (2011) 30–33.
21 See Herbert/Forman (2011) 269–271.

perceptions, spans both conscious and non-conscious processes.[22] Also, what is crucial for Stoicism, as for cognitive therapy, is not that the impressions are conscious but that they are causally effective in shaping action and emotion.[23] A second theme in Epictetus which brings it close to cognitive therapy (though also to ACT) is stress on the importance of "examining one's impressions", including thoughts and beliefs, to make sure they stand up to critical scrutiny as impressions one wants to endorse. Here is a typical passage:

> Practise, then, from the very beginning to say to every rough impression, 'You're an impression and not at all what you appear to be.' Then examine it and test it by the standards that you have, and first and foremost by this one, whether the impression relates to those things which are up to us (*eph' hēmin*) or those which aren't up to us; and if it relates to those things which aren't up to us, be ready to reply, 'That's nothing to me'.[24]

A key dimension of cognitive therapy is that the client is led to recognize and reject a whole series of cognitive errors, such as exaggerated or unjustified beliefs about herself or others' attitudes to her.[25] This procedure might be seen as comparable with the Stoic examination of impressions; however, as brought out shortly, the scope of this theme is more ambitious in Stoicism and embraces core ethical beliefs and commitments.

Although these similarities between cognitive and Stoic therapy are striking, and have been recognized, the points of contact with ACT are, arguably, still more suggestive. This might seem initially surprising, since ACT presupposes a psychological framework that is rather different from the Stoic one. For ACT, the causal agents in human psychology are not just cognitions but also a whole set of factors, including beliefs, emotions, and facts in one's situation, which form what is described as the 'functional context' for the psychological problem.[26] This approach, on the face of it, might seem closer to ancient psychological views opposed to the Stoic one, notably the Platonic-Aristotelian approach advocated by Plutarch and Galen, which subdivides the psyche between rational and non-rational parts, and which places beliefs and reasoning in one part and emotions in the other. However, I am not sure that ACT would want to endorse that kind of sharp division; and, certainly ACT, like CBT in general, presupposes

---

22 On 'impressions' (*phantasiai*) in Stoicism, see Long/Sedley (1987), sections 39 and 53. On impressions as not necessarily conscious, see Gill (1991) 188.
23 See text to nn. 19–20, and Herbert/Forman (2011) 15–17.
24 Epictetus, *Handbook* 1.5, trans. Hard (2014) 287, modified.
25 On this feature in cognitive therapy, see Herbert/Forman (2011) 30–33, 35–37; also refs. in n. 13.
26 See text to n. 15.

that the therapeutic process produces change that bears equally on beliefs and emotions and leads to modifications in both respects.[27] In spite of this difference, Epictetus' stress on the importance of "examining impressions", without necessarily endorsing them, is suggestively close to the critical exploration of influences on one's psychological state that constitutes the first stage of the ACT therapeutic process.[28] However, more striking still are similarities that arise in connection with key features of the second stage in ACT noted earlier.[29] The first is (in ACT) distinguishing between features of our situation – or mind-set – that we can or cannot change. This evokes a key theme in Epictetus, on recognising the difference between what is and is not "up to us" or "in our power" (*eph' hēmin*) as agents and shaping our actions and feelings accordingly.

> Some things are up to us, and others are not up to us. Up to us are opinion, motivation, desire, aversion, and in a word whatever is of our own doing; not up to us are our body, property, reputation, position of authority, and, in a word, whatever is not of our own doing.[30]

The second feature is closely linked with this. In Epictetus, the main point of "examining impressions" and of distinguishing what is and is not "up to us" is an ethical one. The aim is to make sure that the impressions shaping our actions and feelings are in line with our core ethical convictions – or at least with convictions whose force we can be led to recognize.[31] Similarly, in ACT, a crucial role is given to testing how far the shaping influences on our psychological state, including beliefs and emotions, are in line with our deepest ethical commitments – a process described as "values-clarification".[32] Thirdly, ACT lays great emphasis on the crucial importance of commitment to undertake change in the key respects affecting one's problem, and on recognising that we are in fact capable of forming and acting on this commitment.[33] This point evokes strongly the theme

---

[27] On the contrast between Plutarch or Galen and Stoic thinking on this point, see Gill (2006) ch. 4, esp. 219–266. On ACT, considered in relation to other CBT therapies, see Herbert/Forman (2011) ch. 10.

[28] On the two main stages in ACT see refs in n. 17.

[29] See n. 16.

[30] Epictetus, *Handbook* 1.1, trans. Hard (2014), modified. On this theme in ACT, see Hayes/Strosahl/Wilson (1999) 78–79.

[31] Relevant here is Epictetus' three-stage programme in practical ethics, designed for someone wanting to become 'virtuous and good' (*kalos kai agathos*) (*Discourses* 3.2.1–5). See Gill (2006) 372–382; also on Epictetus' use of discourse to promote effective reflection on core values, Long (2002) 52–86; on similar themes in Marcus Aurelius' *Meditations* (e.g. 3.6, 3.11), see Gill (2013a) xl–xlii.

[32] See Hayes/Strosahl/Wilson (1999) 221–228.

[33] See Hayes/Strosahl/Wilson (1999) 243–248.

in Epictetus that what is constitutive of adult humans is our capacity for decision or choice (*prohairesis*), a capacity which underlies the other two features shared by Stoicism and ACT. This passage in Epictetus sums up several of these themes:

> So where is progress to be found? If any of you turns away from external things to concentrate his efforts on his own power of choice (*prohairesis*), to cultivate it and perfect it, so as to bring it into harmony with nature, raising it up and rendering it free, unhindered, unobstructed, trustworthy, self-respecting ... if he bathes as a trustworthy person, and eats as a self-respecting person, putting his guiding principles (*proēgoumena*) into action in relation to anything he has to deal with ... this is the person who is really making progress ...[34]

So, despite some differences in psychological assumptions, I think these similarities go rather deeply into the nature of the two projects, those of ACT psychotherapy and Stoic ethical or therapeutic guidance.

These points of resemblance have certain further contemporary and in a sense practical implications. One implication is that, despite the general differences between ancient and modern psychotherapy noted earlier, there is scope for quite close convergence between Stoic and CBT methods of therapeutic guidance. CBT methods can be used, without inappropriateness, to enhance Stoic-style psychotherapeutic guidance under modern conditions and Stoic ideas can also be used to inform CBT-style psychotherapeutic guidance.

The scope for convergence underlies some recent activities of a public engagement project in which a number of people are involved, including myself, 'Stoicism Today'. The aim of this project is to present Stoic ethical ideas and practices in a form that makes them accessible to a broad public audience and potentially helpful to them in reflecting on their lives and managing them. This project represents a collaboration between scholars of Stoic ethics and CBT psychotherapists, together with a writer on practical philosophy.[35] The main focus of our collaborative work has been developing on-line courses for self-guidance: these have included week-long courses ('Live like a Stoic for a week'), and a four-week course, 'Stoic mindfulness and resilience training'. These courses represent an amalgam of key themes in Stoic ethics and modern psychotherapeutic or life-guidance approaches.[36] The production of these courses has involved a kind

---

[34] Epictetus, *Discourses*, 1.4.18, 20; see also 1.4.6–15, 1.17.13–18; Long (2002) 207–230.
[35] Those most closely involved: academics, Gabriele Galluzzo, Christopher Gill, and Patrick Ussher (Exeter), Massimo Pigliucci (New York) John Sellars (Royal Holloway, London); philosophical writer Jules Evans; psychotherapists Gill Garratt, Tim LeBon, Donald Robertson; also Gref Lopez and Greg Sadler.
[36] These courses have been posted on the blog:http://modernstoicism.com/stoicism-today-blog; and the courses, along with reports on their effectiveness, are often available on the blog.

of two-way dialogue: CBT methods, including meditative exercises, are used to enable people to embed Stoic attitudes into their daily lives, and Stoic ideas are used to inform modern psychotherapeutic guidance.

The combination of psychotherapeutic and Stoic themes emerges most clearly in the four-week 'Stoic mindfulness and resilience training' course devised by Donald Robertson. Thus, for instance, the theme of recognising the distinction between what is and is not 'up to us' (what does and does not fall within our agency or control) in week one is followed by a focus on 'value-clarification' in week two, including discussion of the Stoic distinction between virtues and 'indifferents', such as health or property. The linkage brings out the salient Stoic claim that progress towards developing the virtues is something that is 'up to us', as agents, whereas acquiring 'indifferents' such as health and property is not.[37] Analogously, week three introduces the idea of 'cognitive distancing' (in more Stoic terms, suspending value judgements or "examining your impressions"), as a key element in the preparation for 'resilience-building' in week four. Week four presents the Stoic exercise of mental "preparation for disaster" (*praeparatio malorum*).[38] It also shows how the distinctively Stoic response to disaster, or the prospect of disaster, depends on recognising the crucial distinction between what is and is not 'up to us', the importance of the contrast between virtue and 'indifferents', and the need to "examine our impressions" to ensure that our thoughts match our deepest moral convictions. In other words, the distinctively Stoic response to disaster depends on recognising that what matters, ultimately, is not the loss of 'indifferents' such as health or property, a loss which we normally treat as a disaster. What matters, ultimately, is something that is 'up to us', namely the scope for developing virtue, which external events cannot affect. As this summary indicates, the course uses modern psychotherapeutic language and meditative exercises, and aims to bring out the value of these exercises and advice for therapeutic purposes. However, the course also highlights the point that its effectiveness as advice depends on seeing the force of the Stoic ideas underlying the advice and on recognising the interconnections between these ideas, in a way that affects attitudes and behaviour as well as conceptual thinking. Hence, despite the broader differences between ancient and modern psychotherapy as practices, the collaborative courses show how they can be used to inform each other.[39]

---

[37] For these themes in Stoicism or CBT (esp. ACT) see the preceding discussion; on the distinction between virtue and 'indifferents', see Long/Sedley (1987) section 58.
[38] For this exercise (also used by other philosophical schools), see Cicero, *Tusculans* 3.3.52–54.
[39] This course is available from time to time on the 'Stoicism Today' blog. On the Stoic ideas presented in the course, see also Robertson (2013) chs. 8–9, which underlines the connections between these themes and their role in providing a basis for emotional resilience.

The 'Stoicism Today' collaboration has been very successful in engaging large numbers of non-specialists with Stoic ideas.[40] Obviously, the attempt to present Stoic ideas as life-guidance or psychotherapeutic advice raises a number of broader questions, some of which have been debated in public events organized by the group or in articles on the 'Stoicism Today' blog.[41] One of these questions is how far Stoic 'therapy' (which is fundamentally ethical in orientation) is compatible with the aims as well as the methods of CBT, though it should be stressed that we are not pretending to offer CBT psychotherapy as such but rather psychotherapeutic guidance informed by Stoicism. However, in considering these questions, it is worth bearing in mind the specific similarities highlighted here between Stoic therapy and CBT. The 'Stoicism Today' project, that is to say, is based on what are, arguably, substantive points of resemblance. How far these points of resemblance can reasonably be pressed, and how far they can be deployed effectively in the development of effective on-line courses and other resources, is a question still to be pursued, at both the theoretical and practical levels. But that these similarities exist is, I think, a matter of academic and potentially practical interest.

---

40 The on-line 'Live like a Stoic' course was followed by over 2,000 users in 2013 and over 2,500 users in 2014. The 'Stoic Mindfulness and Resilience Training' course was followed by over 500 users in 2014 and over 1000 in 2015. The Stoic public events in London have attracted participants of over 200 (in 2013), over 300 (in 2014). There are detailed reports by Tim LeBon on the questionnaire feedback on the 2013 and 2014 'Live Like a Stoic' courses, and Donald Robertson has received very positive feedback on the 'Stoic Mindfulness and Resilience Training' course. Patrick Ussher has prepared two volumes, *Stoicism Today*, based on posts on the 'Stoicism Today' blog, which have been down-loaded over 5,000 times and is being translated into several other languages. This information covers activities up till 2015; since then the numbers of those involved has continued to grow.
41 See the volumes, *Stoicism Today*, cited in n. 40.

Bibliography

Abraham (1911): K. Abraham, "Notes of Psychoanalytic Research and Therapy of Manic Depressive Disorders", in: *Selected Papers of Karl Abraham*, London, 136–156.
Abramiuk (2012): M.A. Abramiuk, *The Foundations of Cognitive Archaeology*, Cambridge, MA.
Adamson (2007): G. Adamson, *Thinking Through Craft*, London.
Adcock (1927): F.E. Adcock, "The Breakdown of the Thirty Years Peace, 445–431 BC", in: *The Cambridge Ancient History* 5, 165–192.
Adkins (1960): A.W.H. Adkins, *Merit and Responsibility: A Study in Greek Values*, Chicago.
Aeschylus (1972): Aeschyli *septem quae supersunt tragoedias*, ed. by D. Page, Oxford.
Albrecht (2003): M. von Albrecht, *Cicero's Style. A Synopsis*, Leiden.
Aldag/Fuller (1993): R.J. Aldag and S.R. Fuller, "Beyond Fiasco: A Reappraisal of the Groupthink Phenomenon and a New Model of Group Decision Processes", in: *Psychological Bulletin* 113, 533–552.
Alexander (1990): M. Alexander, *Trials in the Late Roman Republic. 149 BC to 50 BC*, Toronto.
Alford (1992): C.F. Alford, "Greek Tragedy and the Place of Death in Life: A Psychoanalytic Perspective", in: *Psychoanalysis and Contemporary Thought* 15, 129–159.
Alford (1996): C.F. Alford, "Greek Tragedy, Confusion, and Melanie Klein. Or is there an *Oresteia* Complex?", in: *American Imago* 50, 1–27.
Allen (1990): R. Allen, *Psychophysiology of the Human Stress Response*, College Park, MD.
Allan (2006): W. Allan, "Divine Justice and Cosmic Order in Early Greek Epic", in: *Journal of Hellenic Studies* 126, 1–35.
Andrews-Hanna/Smallwood/Spreng (2014): J.R. Andrews-Hanna, J. Smallwood, and R.N. Spreng, "The Default Network and Self-generated thought: Component Processes, Dynamic Control, and Clinical Relevance", in: *Annals of the New York Academy of Sciences* 1316, 29–52.
Arikha (2007): N. Arikha, *Passions and Tempers: A History of the Humours*, New York.
Aristotle (1995): *The Complete Works of Aristotle: The Revised Oxford Translation*, 2 vols., ed. by J. Barnes, Oxford.
Aristotle (2006): Aristotle, *On Rhetoric*, ed. by G. Kennedy, Oxford.
Armstrong (2005): R.H. Armstrong, *A Compulsion for Antiquity: Freud and the Ancient World*, Ithaca.
Arrindell et al. (1991): W. Arrindell et al., "Phobic Dimensions III. Factor Analytic Approaches to the Study of Common Phobic Fears: An Updated Review of Findings Obtained with Adult Subjects", in: *Advances in Behaviour Research and Therapy* 13, 73–130.
Arrow/McGrath/Berdahl (2000): H. Arrow, J.E. McGrath, J.R. Berdahl, *Small Groups as Complex Systems: Formation, Coordination, Development, and Adaptation*, Thousand Oaks, CA.
Arthur (1982): M.B. Arthur, "Cultural Strategies in Hesiod's *Theogony*: Law, Family, Society", in: *Arethusa* 15, 63–82.
Arthur (1983): M.B. Arthur, "The Dream of a World without Women: Poetics and the Circles of Order in the Theogony Prooemium", in: *Arethusa* 16, 97–112.
Atran (1993): S. Atran, *Cognitive Foundations of Natural History*, Cambridge.
Atwater (1992): P.M.H. Atwater, "Is There a Hell? Surprising Observations About the Near-Death Experience", in: *Journal of Near-Death Studies* 10.3, 149–160.
Austin (1969): N. Austin, "Telemachos Polymechanos", in: *California Studies in Classical Antiquity* 3, 45–63.

Austin (1975): N. Austin, *Archery at the Dark of the Moon: Poetic Problems in Homer's* Odyssey, California.
Aziz-Zadeh/Damasio (2008): L. Aziz-Zadeh and A. Damasio, "Embodied Semantics for Actions: Findings From Functional Brain Imaging", in: *Journal of Physiology* 102, 35–39.
Aziz-Zadeh/Wilson/Rizzolatti/Iacobini (2006); L. Aziz-Zadeh, S.M. Wilson, G. Rizzolatti and M. Iacoboni, "Congruent Embodied Representations for Visually Presented Actions and Linguistic Phrases Describing Actions", in: *Current Biology* 16, 1818–1823.
Badian (1985): E. Badian, "A Phantom Marriage Law", in: *Philologus* 129, 82–98.
Badian (1993): E. Badian, *From Plataea to Potidaea: Studies in the History and Historiography of the Pentecontaetia*, Baltimore, MD.
Bakhtin (1981): M. Bakhtin, *The Dialogic Imagination: Four Essays*, trans. C. Emerson and M. Holquist, Austin.
Bakhtin (1984): M. Bakhtin, *Problems of Dostoevsky's Poetics*, trans. C. Emerson, Minneapolis.
Bakhtin (1986): M. Bakhtin, *Speech Genres and Other Late Essays*, trans. V.W. McGee, Austin.
Bakker (1997): E.J. Bakker, *Poetry in Speech: Orality and Homeric Discourse*, Ithaca.
Bakker (2005): E.J. Bakker, *Pointing at the Past: From Formula to Performance in Homeric Poetics*, Cambridge, MA.
Bakker (2013): E.J. Bakker, *The Meaning of Meat and the Structure of the Odyssey*, Cambridge.
Ball (2002): H.K. Ball, "Subversive Materials: Quilts as Social Text", in: *The Alberta Journal of Educational Research* 48.3, 1–29.
Balot (2014): R.K. Balot, *Courage in the Democratic Polis: Ideology and Critique in Classical Athens*, New York.
Bamborough (1989–2000): J.B. Bamborough, "Introduction", in: Burton (1632/1989–2000), viii-xxxvi.
Barker/Christensen (2015): E.T.E. Barker and J.P. Christensen, "Odysseus' Nostos and the *Odyssey*'s Nostoi", in: G. Scafoglio (ed.), *Studies on the Greek Epic Cycle*, Pisa, 85–110.
Barkley-Brown (1989): E. Barkley-Brown, "African American Women's Quilting: A Framework for Conceptualizing and Teaching African American Women's History", in: *Signs: Journal of Women in Culture and Society* 14.4, 921–929.
Barnes (2011): T. Barnes, *Constantine*, Oxford.
Baron (2005): R.S. Baron, "So Right it's Wrong: Groupthink and the Ubiquitous Nature of Polarised Group Decision Making", in: *Advances in Experimental Social Psychology* 37, 219–253.
Barone/Eisner (2012): T. Barone and E. Eisner, *Arts Based Research*, Thousand Oaks.
Barrett (2011): L. Barrett, *Beyond the Brain: How Body and Environment Shape Animal and Human Minds*, New Jersey.
Barsalou (1983): L. Barsalou, "Ad hoc categories", in: *Memory & Cognition* 11, 211–227.
Batstone (2002): W.W. Batstone, "Catullus and Bakhtin: The Problems of a Dialogic Lyric", in: R.B. Branham (ed.), *Bakhtin and the Classics*, Evanston, 99–136.
Beard/Crawford (1999): M. Beard and M. Crawford, *Rome in the Late Republic: Problems and Interpretations*, London (2nd edition).
Beck/Alford (2009): A.T. Beck and B.A. Alford, *Depression: causes and treatment*, Philadelphia.
Begbie (1915): H. Begbie, *On the Side of Angels*, London.
Bekoff (2007): M. Bekoff, *The Emotional Lives of Animals*, Novato.
Bentley (1826): R. Bentley, *Q. Horatius Flaccus*, Leipzig (Originally published in Cambridge, 1711).
Benveniste (1971): E. Benveniste, *Problems in General Linguistics*, Miami.

Bergren (1983): A.L.T. Bergren, "Language and the Feminine in Early Greek Thought", in: *Arethusa* 16, 69–95.
Bergson (1971): L. Bergson, "Eiron und Eironeia", in: *Hermes* 99, 409–422.
Bettini (2009): M. Bettini, "Comparare i Romani. Per un'antropologia del mondo antico", in: *Studi italiani di filologia classica* 7.4, 1–47.
Bettini (2011): M. Bettini, *The Ears of Hermes*, trans. W.M. Short, Columbus, OH.
Bibring (1953): E. Bibring, "The Mechanisms of Depression", in P. Greenacre (ed.), *Affective Disorders*, New York, 13–48.
Biegler (2011): P. Biegler, *The Ethical Treatment of Depression: Autonomy Through Psychotherapy*, Cambridge, MA.
Bilu (2013): Y. Bilu, "'We Want to See our King': Apparitions in Messianic Habad", in: *Journal of the Society for Psychological Anthropology* 41, 98–126.
Bitzer (1968): L.F. Bitzer, "The Rhetorical Situation", in: *Philosophy & Rhetoric* 1.1, 1–14.
Blackburne et al. (2014): L.K. Blackburne, M. Eddy, P. Kalra, D. Yee, P. Sinha, and J.D.E. Gabrieli, "Neural Correlates of Letter Reversal in Children and Adults", in: *PLoS One* 3, 9.5, e98386.
Blair (2007): R. Blair, *The Actor, Image, and Action: Acting and Cognitive Neuroscience*, Oxford.
Blais et al. (2008): C. Blais, R.E. Jack, C. Scheepers, D. Fiset, and R. Caldara: "Culture Shapes How We Look at Faces", in: *PLoS One* 3, no. 8 e3022.
Blom (2010): J.D. Blom, *A Dictionary of Hallucinations*, The Hague.
Boddy (1915): A. Boddy, Interview in the *Sunderland Echo*, 16 August 1915.
Boden (2008): M. Boden, *Mind as Machine: A History of Cognitive Science*, Oxford.
Boegehold (1986): A.J. Boegehold, "Gestures and Interpretations of Greek Literature", in: *American Journal of Archaeology* 90, 181.
Boegehold (1999): A.J. Boegehold, *When a Gesture Was Expected: A Selection of Examples from Archaic and Classical Greek Literature*, New Jersey.
Bonifazi (2009): A. Bonifazi, "Inquiring into *Nostos* and its Cognates", in: *American Journal of Philology* 130, 481–510.
Borch-Jacobsen (1990): M. Borch-Jacobsen, "Analytic Speech: From Restricted to General Rhetoric", in: J. Bender and D. Wellbery (eds), *The Ends of Rhetoric: History, Theory, Practice*, Stanford, 128–139.
Botha (2007): M. Botha, *Metaphor and Its Moorings*, Bern.
Bowlby (2009): R. Bowlby, "Psychoanalysis", in: B. Graziosi, P. Vasunia, and G. Boys-Stones (eds), *The Oxford Handbook of Hellenic Studies*, Oxford, 802–810.
Boyd (2005): B. Boyd, "Literature and Evolution: A Bio-cultural Approach", in: *Philosophy and Literature* 29.1, 1–23.
Boyd (2009): B. Boyd, *On the Origin of Stories: Evolution, Cognition, and Fiction*, Cambridge, MA.
Boys-Stones/Haubold (2010): G.R. Boys-Stones and J.H. Haubold (eds), *Plato and Hesiod*, Oxford.
Bratich and Brush (2011): J.Z Bratich and H.M Brush, "Fabricating Activism: Craft-Work, Popular Culture, Gender", in: *Utopian Studies* 22.2, 233–260.
Braund/Gilbert (2003): S. Braund and G. Gilbert, "An ABC of Epic *ira*: Anger, Beasts, and Cannibalism", *Yale Classical Studies* 32, 250–285.
Bremmer (2002): J. Bremmer, *The Rise and Fall of the Afterlife*, London and New York.
Brennan (2003): T. Brennan, "Stoic Moral Psychology", in B. Inwood (ed.), *The Cambridge Companion to the Stoics*, Cambridge, 257–294.
Brown (1982): T.S. Brown, "Herodotus' Portrait of Cambyses", in: *Historia: Zeitschrift für alte Geschichte* 31.4, 387–403.

Brown (2000): W.S. Brown (ed.), *Understanding Wisdom: Sources, Science, and Society*, Philadelphia.
Brugman (1990): C. Brugman, "What is the INVARIANCE HYPOTHESIS?", in: *Cognitive Linguistics* 1.2, 257–266.
Bruner (1986): J. Bruner, *Actual Minds, Possible Worlds*, Cambridge.
Brunschwig (1996): J. Brunschwig, "Aristotle's Rhetoric as a 'Counterpart' to Dialectic", in: A. Rorty (ed.), *Essays on Aristotle's Rhetoric*, Berkeley and Los Angeles, 34–55.
Büchner (1941): W. Büchner, "Über den Begriff der Eironeia", in: *Hermes* 4, 339–358.
Buckner/Vincent (2007): R.L. Buckner and J. Vincent, "Unrest at Rest: Default Activity and Spontaneous Network Correlations", in: *Neuroimage* 37.4, 1091–1096.
Budelmann (2017): F. Budelmann, "Performance, Re-performance and Pre-performance in Pindaric Epinician", in: R. Hunter and A. Uhlig (eds), *Reperformance in Ancient Culture*, Oxford, 42–46.
Burgess (2014): J. Burgess, "Framing Odysseus: The Death of the Suitors", in: Christopoulos/Paizi-Apostolopoulou (2014), 337–354.
Burkert (1997): W. Burkert, "The Song of Ares and Aphrodite: On the Relationship between the Odyssey and the Iliad", in: G.M. Wright and P.V. Jones (eds and trans.), *Homer. German Scholarship in Translation*, Oxford, 249–262.
Burnett (1979): A.P. Burnett, "Desire and Memory; Sappho fr. 94", in: *Classical Philology* 74, 16–27.
Burnett (1983): A.P. Burnett, *Three Archaic Poets: Archilochus, Alcaeus, Sappho*, Cambridge, MA.
Burton (1632/1989–2000): R. Burton, *The Anatomy of Melancholy*, 6 vols., ed. by T. Faulkner, N. Kiessling, and R. Blair, Vols I-III: Text; vols IV-VI: Commentary by J.B. Bamborough and M. Dodsworth, Oxford.
Butrica (1984): J.L. Butrica, *The Manuscript Tradition of Propertius*, Toronto, Buffalo and London.
Butrica (1997): J.L. Butrica, "Editing Propertius", in: *The Classical Quarterly* 47, 176–208.
Cacioppo/Petty (1984): J.T. Cacioppo and R.E. Petty "The Efficient Assessment of Need for Cognition", in: *Journal of Personality Assessment* 48.3, 306–307.
Cairns (2005a): D.L. Cairns, "Bullish Looks and Sidelong Glances: Social Interaction and the Eyes in Early Greek Culture", in: Cairns (2005b), 123–155.
Cairns (2005b): D.L. Cairns (ed.), *Body Language in the Greek and Roman Worlds*, Swansea.
Cairns (2008): D. Cairns, "Look Both Ways: Studying Emotion in Ancient Greek", in: *Critical Quarterly* 50.4, 43–62.
Cairns (2009): D.L. Cairns, "Weeping and Veiling: Grief, Display, and Concealment in Ancient Greek Culture", in: T. Fögen (ed.), *Tears in the Greco-Roman World*, Berlin, 37–57.
Cairns (2012): D.L. Cairns, "Vêtu d'impudeur et enveloppé de chagrin. Le rôle des métaphores de 'l'habillement' dans les concepts d'émotion en Grèce ancienne", in: F. Gherchanoc and V. Huet (eds), *Le vêtement antique. S'habiller/se déshabiller dans le monde antique*, Paris, 175–187.
Cairns (2013): D. Cairns, "A Short History of Shudders", in: A. Chaniotis and P. Ducrey (eds), *Unveiling Emotions II – Emotions in Greece and Rome: Texts, Images, Material Culture*, Stuttgart, 85–107.
Cairns (2016): D.L. Cairns, "Mind, Body, and Metaphor in Ancient Greek Concepts of Emotion", in: *L'Atelier du centre de recherche historique* 16.
Cairns/Fulkerson (2015): D. Cairns and L. Fulkerson, *Emotions Between Greece and Rome* (BICS Supplement 125), Institute of Classical Studies, London.
Callahan (1989): W.A. Callahan, "Discourse and Perspective in Daoism: A Linguistic Interpretation of Ziran", in: *Philosophy East and West* 39, 171–189.

Campbell (1982): D.A. Campbell, *Greek Lyric Poetry, Vol. 1: Sappho and Alcaeus*, Cambridge, MA.
Campbell (1915): P. Campbell, *Back of the Front*, London.
Canevaro (2014): L.G. Canevaro, "Genre and Authority in Hesiod's *Works and Days*", in:
    C. Werner, B.B. Sebastiani and A. Dourado-Lopes (eds), *Gêneros Poéticos na Grécia Antiga: Confluências e Fronteiras*, São Paulo, 23–48.
Canevaro (2015): L.G. Canevaro, *Hesiod's* Works and Days: *How to Teach Self-Sufficiency*, Oxford.
Canevaro (2017): L.G. Canevaro, "Fraternal conflict in Hesiod's *Works and Days*", in:
    P. Bassino, L.G. Canevaro and B. Graziosi (eds), *Conflict and Consensus in Early Hexameter Poetry*, Cambridge, 173–189.
Cannon (1929): W.B. Cannon, *Bodily Changes in Pain, Hunger, Fear and Rage: An Account of Recent Researches into the Function of Emotional Excitement*, New York.
Cannon (1932): W. Cannon, *The Wisdom of the Body*, New York.
Cannon (1953): W. Cannon, *Bodily Changes in Pain, Hunger, Fear, and Rage*, Boston.
Canter (1936): H. Canter, "Irony in the orations of Cicero", in: *American Journal of Philology* 57.4, 457–464.
Carr (1961): E.H. Carr, *What is History?*, Harmondsworth.
Cartwright/Zander (1968): D. Cartwright and D. Zander, *Group Dynamics: Research and Theory*, New York.
Case and Dalley (1992): C. Case and T. Dalley, *The Handbook of Art Therapy*, London.
Caswell (1990): C. Caswell, *A Study of Thumos in Early Greek Poetry*, Leiden.
Cawkwell (1997): G. Cawkwell, *Thucydides and Peloponnesian War*, New York.
Chafe (1994): W.L. Chafe, *Discourse, Consciousness, and Time*, Chicago.
Chaitin (1996): G.D. Chaitin, *Rhetoric and Culture in Lacan*, Cambridge.
Chaston (2010): C. Chaston, *Tragic Props and Cognitive Function: Aspects of the Function of Images in Thinking* (Mnemosyne Supplements 317), Leiden.
Christopoulos/Paizi-Apostolopoulou (2014): M. Christopoulos and M. Paizi-Apostolopoulou (eds), *Crime and Punishment in Homeric and Archaic Epic*, Ithaca.
Cialdini/Goldstein (2004): R.B. Cialdini and N.J. Goldstein, "Social Influence: Compliance and Conformity", in: *Annual Review of Psychology* 55, 591–621.
Cixous (2000): H. Cixous, "The Laugh of the Medusa", in: K. Oliver (ed.), *French Feminisms*, Lanham, 257–275.
Clark (2008): A. Clark, *Supersizing the Mind: Embodiment, Action, and Cognitive Extension*, Oxford.
Clark/Chalmers (1998): A. Clark and D. Chalmers, "The Extended Mind", *Analysis*, 7–19.
Clark/Gerrig (1984): H. Clark and R. Gerrig, "On the Pretense Theory of Irony", in: *Journal of Experimental Psychology* 113.1, 121–126.
Clarke (2002): D. Clarke, "Rumours of Angels: a Legend of the First World War", in: *Folklore*, October.
Clarke (2004): D. Clarke, *The Angel of Mons*, Chichester.
Clarke (1967): H. Clarke, *The Art of the* Odyssey, Englewood Cliffs.
Clarke (1999): M. Clarke, *Flesh and Spirit in the Songs of Homer*, Oxford.
Clarke (2005): M. Clarke, "The Semantics of Ancient Greek Smiles", in: Cairns (2005b), 37–53.
Clay (1983): J.S. Clay, *The Wrath of Athena: Gods and Men in the* Odyssey, Princeton.
Clay (1993): J.S. Clay, "The Education of Perses: Fom 'Mega Nepios' to 'Dion Genos' and Back", in: *Materiali e discussioni per l'analisi dei testi classici* 31, 23–33.
Clay (2003): J.S. Clay, *Hesiod's Cosmos*, Cambridge.

Clay (2011): J.S. Clay, *Homer's Trojan Theater: Space, Vision, and Memory in the* Iliad, Cambridge.
Clements (2000): R.E. Clements, "The Sources of Wisdom", in: Brown (2000), 15–34.
Clifton (1963): G. Clifton, "The Mood of the Persai of Aeschylus", in: *Greece and Rome* 10.2, 111–117.
Clinton (1992): K. Clinton, *Myth and Cult: the Iconography of the Eleusinian Mysteries*, Stockholm.
Clinton (2004): K. Clinton, "Epiphany in the Eleusinian Mysteries", in: *Illinois Classical Studies* 29, 85–109.
Colombetti (2014): G. Colombetti, *The Feeling Body: The Affective Sciences Meet the Enactive Mind*, Cambridge.
Connerton (1989): P. Connerton, *How Societies Remember*, Cambridge.
Connor (1984): W.R. Connor, *Thucydides*, Princeton, NJ.
Conte (1986): G.B. Conte, *The Rhetoric of Imitation. Genre and Poetic Memory in Virgil and Other Latin Poets*, Ithaca, NY.
Cook (1995): E. Cook, *The* Odyssey *in Athens: Myths of Cultural Origins*, Ithaca.
Cook (2014): E. Cook, "Structure as Interpretation in the Homeric *Odyssey*", in: R. Scodel and D. Cairns (eds), *Defining Greek Narrative*, Edinburgh, 76–100.
Corbeill (2002): A. Corbeill, "Ciceronian Invective", in: J. May (ed.), *Brill's Companion to Cicero: Oratory and Rhetoric*, 197–217.
Corbett and Housley (2011): S. Corbett and S. Housley, "The Craftivist Collective Guide to Craftivism", in: *Utopian Studies* 22.2, 344–351.
Cramer/Borsboom/Aggen/Kendler (2011): A.O.J. Cramer, D. Borsboom, S.H. Aggen, and K.S. Kendler, "The Pathoplasticity of Dysphoric Episodes: Differential Impact of Stressful Life Events on the Pattern of Depressive Symptom Inter-correlations", in: *Psychological Medicine* 42, 957–965.
Critchley (1979): M. Critchley, "The Idea of Presence", in: *The Divine Banquet of the Brain and Other Essays*, New York, pp. 1–12.
Crowley (2012): J. Crowley, *The Psychology of the Athenian Hoplite: The Culture of Combat in Classical Athens*, Cambridge.
Crowley (2014): J. Crowley, "Beyond the Universal Soldier: Combat Trauma in Classical Antiquity", in: Meineck/Konstan (2014), 105–130.
Cvetkovich (2012): A. Cvetkovich, *Depression: A Public Feeling*, London.
Dalley (1984): T. Dalley (ed.), *Art as Therapy: An Introduction to the Use of Art as a Therapeutic Technique*, London.
Damasio (1999): A. Damasio, *The Feeling of What Happens: Body and Emotion in the Making of Consciousness*, New York.
Damasio (2008): A. Damasio, *Descartes' error: Emotion, reason and the human brain*, London.
Damasio (2010): A. Damasio, *Self Comes to Mind: Constructing the Conscious Brain*, New York.
Damasio (2012): A. Damasio, *Self Comes to Mind: Constructing the Conscious Brain*, New York.
Damasio/Carvalho (2013): A. Damasio and G.B. Carvalho "The Nature of Feelings: Evolutionary and Neurobiological Origins", in: *Nature Reviews Neuroscience* 14.2, 143–152.
Damasio/Damasio (2006): A. Damasio and H. Damasio, "Minding the body", in: *Daedalus* 135.3, 15–22.
Danek (1988): G. Danek, *Epos und Zitat: Studien zur Quellen der* Odyssee, Vienna.
Danesi/Perron (1999): M. Danesi and P. Perron, *Analyzing Culture*, Bloomington, IN.
Darwin (2009): C. Darwin, *The Expression of the Emotions in Man and Animals* [1872], ed. by P. Ekman, London and New York.

Davie (2007): J. Davie, *Seneca: Dialogues and Essays*, trans. J. Davie with introduction and notes by T. Reinhardt, Oxford.
Dehaene (2013): S. Dehaene, "Inside the Letterbox: How Literacy Transforms the Human Brain", in: *Cerebrum*, June 7.
De Jong (2001): I. de Jong, *A Narratological Commentary on the Odyssey*, Cambridge.
Deignan (2003): A. Deignan, "Metaphoric Expressions and Culture", in: *Metaphor and Symbol*, 18.1, 255–271.
de Lauretis (1987): T. de Lauretis, *Technologies of Gender: Essays on Theory, Film, and Fiction*, Bloomington.
Deleuze (1983): G. Deleuze, *Nietzsche and Philosophy*, trans. H. Tomlinson, New York and London.
Deleuze (1990): G. Deleuze, *The Logic of Sense*, trans. M. Lester, London.
Deleuze (1994): G. Deleuze, *Difference and Repetition*, trans. P. Patton, New York.
Deleuze (2004): G. Deleuze, *Desert Islands and Other Texts: 1953–1974*, ed. by D. Lapoujade, trans. M. Taormina, New York.
Deleuze/Guattari (1983): G. Deleuze and F. Guattari, *Anti-Oedipus: Capitalism and Schizophrenia*, trans. R. Hurley, M. Seem, and H.R. Lane, Minneapolis.
Deleuze/Guattari (1987): G. Deleuze and F. Guattari, *A Thousand Plateaus: Capitalism and Schizophrenia*, trans. B. Massumi, Minneapolis and London.
Denzin and Lincoln (1994): N.K. Denzin and Y.S. Lincoln (eds), *Handbook of Qualitative Research* (2nd edition), London.
de Romilly (1963): J. de Romilly, *Thucydides and Athenian Imperialism*, trans. P. Thody, Oxford.
Desai et al. (2011): R. Desai, J. Binder, L. Conant, Q. Mano, and M. Seidenberg, "The Neural Career of Sensory-Motor Metaphors", in: *Journal of Cognitive Neuroscience* 23, 2376–2386.
Desai et al. (2013): R. Desai, L. Conant, J. Binder, H. Park, and M. Seidenberg, "A Piece of the Action: Modulation of Sensory Motor Regions by Action Idioms and Metaphors", in: *NeuroImage* 83, 862–869.
Desai et al. (2011): R.H. Desai, J.R. Binder, L.L. Conant, Q.R. Mano, and M.S. Seidenberg, "The neural Career of Sensory-motor Metaphors", in: *Journal of Cognitive Neuroscience* 23.9, 2376–2386.
Detienne (2000): M. Detienne, *Comparer l'incomparable*, Paris.
Detienne (2005): M. Detienne, *Les Grecs et nous*, Paris.
Devereaux (forthcoming): J.J. Devereaux, "Embodied Historiography: Models for Reasoning in Tacitus' *Annales*", in: W. Short (ed.), *Embodiment in Latin Semantics*, Amsterdam.
Dietrich (1965): B.C. Dietrich, *Death, Fate and the Gods: The Development of a Religious Idea in Greek Popular Belief and Homer*, London.
Dilthey (1976): W. Dilthey, "The Development of Hermeneutics", in: H.P. Rickman (ed.), *Selected Writings*, Cambridge, 247–263.
Dobos/Tao (2011): G. Dobos and I. Tao, "The Model of Western Integrative Medicine: The Role of Chinese Medicine", in: *Chinese Journal of Integrative Medicine* 17, 11–20.
Dobson (2010): K.S. Dobson (ed.), *Handbook of Cognitive Behavioural Therapies*, New York.
Dodds (1951): E.R. Dodds, *The Greeks and the Irrational*, Berkeley.
Doherty (1995): L. Doherty, *Siren Songs: Gender, Audiences and Narrators in the Odyssey*, Ann Arbor.
Dosse (2010): F. Dosse, *Gilles Deleuze and Félix Guattari: Intersecting Lives*, trans. D. Glassman, New York.
Dougherty (2001): C. Dougherty, *The Raft of Odysseus: The Ethnographic Imagination of Homer's Odyssey*, New York.

Duffy (2005): A. Duffy, "Someone Told Me to Get Up", in: *National Post*, June 6.
Dunbar-Soule (1976): M. Dunbar-Soule Dobson, "Oracular Language: Its Style and Intent in the Delphic Oracles and Aeschylus' *Oresteia* and the Delphic Oracle", in: *Harvard University Archives HU* 90.10932.20.
Eardley/Bishop/Prescott (2012): S. Eardley, F.L. Bishop, and P. Prescott, "A Systematic Literature Review of Complementary and Alternative Medicine Prevalence in EU", in: *Research in Complementary Medicine* 19, Suppl. 2, 1661–4119.
Edelman (2006): G.M. Edelman, "The Embodiment of Mind", *Daedalus* 135.3, 23–32.
Ehninger (1968): D.W. Ehninger, "On Systems of Rhetoric", in: *Philosophy and Rhetoric* 1, 131–144.
Eisner (1981): E.W. Eisner, "On the Differences between Scientific and Artistic Approaches to Qualitative Research", in: *Educational Researcher* 10.4, 5–9.
Ekman/Friesen (2003): P. Ekman and W.V. Friesen, *Unmasking the Face: a Guide to Recognizing Emotions in the human face,* Los Altos, CA.
Ekman/Levenson/Friesen (1983): P. Ekman, R. Levenson, and W. Friesen, "Autonomic Nervous System Activity Distinguishes Among Emotions", in: *Science* 221, 1208–1210.
Elbert/Schauer (2014): T. Elbert and M. Schauer, "18 Epigenetic, Neural and Cognitive Memories of Traumatic Stress and Violence", in: *Psychology Serving Humanity: Proceedings of the 30th International Congress of Psychology: Volume 2: Western Psychology*, Oxford, 215–227.
Embry (2011): D.D. Embry, "Behavioral Vaccines and Evidence-Based Kernels: Nonpharmaceutical Approaches for the Prevention of Mental, Emotional, and Behavioural Disorders", in: *Psychiatric Clinics of North America* 34,1–24.
Epictetus (1964): Epictetus, *Moral Discourses*. Ed. with an Introduction by T. Gould, New York.
Euripides (1904/1962): Euripidis *fabulae*, tomus II, ed. by G. Murray, Oxford.
Evans (1977): J.D.G. Evans, *Aristotle's Concept of Dialectic,* Cambridge.
Evans (1997): R.J. Evans, *In Defence of History*, London.
Everly/Lating (2012): G. Everly and J. Lating, *A Clinical Guide to the Treatment of the Human Stress Response,* New York.
Eysenck (1952): H.J. Eysenck, "The Effects of Psychotherapy: An Evaluation", in: *Journal of Consulting Psychology* 16, 319–324.
Fagan (2011): G.G. Fagan, *The Lure of the Arena: Social Psychology and the Crowd at the Roman Games Social Psychology and the Crowd at the Roman Games,* Cambridge.
Farrell (2003): J. Farrell, "Classical Genre in Theory and Practice", in: *New Literary History* 34, 383–408.
Feather (1982): N.T. Feather, "Actions in Relation to Expected Consequences", in: *Expectations and Actions*, Hillsdale, 53–95.
Feeney (1998): D. Feeney, *Literature and Religion at Rome: Cultures, Contexts, and Beliefs*, Cambridge.
Feldherr (1998): A. Feldherr, *Spectacle and Society in Livy's History*, Los Angeles.
Feldman (2006): J. Feldman, *From Molecule to Metaphor: A Neural Theory of Language*, Cambridge, MA.
Felson-Rubin (1994): N. Felson-Rubin, *Regarding Penelope: From Character to Poetics*, Princeton.
Felson/Slatkin (2014): N. Felson and L. Slatkin, "*Nostos, Tisis,* and Two Forms of Dialogism in Homer's *Odyssey*", in: Christopoulos/Paizi-Apostolopoulou (2014), 211–222.

Fenik (1974): B. Fenik, *Studies in the Odyssey*, Wiesbaden.
Fernyhough (2012): C. Fernyhough, *Pieces of Light*, New York.
Fillmore (1985): C. Fillmore, "Frames and the Semantics of Understanding", in: *Quaderni di semantica* 6.2, 222–254.
Fink (1999): B. Fink, *A Clinical Introduction to Lacanian Psychoanalysis: Theory and Practice* (2nd edition), Cambridge, MA.
Finkelberg (1995): M. Finkelberg, "Patterns of Human Error in Homer", in: *Journal of Hellenic Studies* 115, 15–28.
Finley (1942): J.H. Finley, *Thucydides*, Cambridge, MA.
Finley (2003): S. Finlay, "Arts-based Inquiry in QI: Seven Years from Crisis to Guerrilla Warfare", in: *Qualitative Inquiry* 9.2, 281–296.
Finley/Knowles (1995): S. Finley and J.G. Knowles, "Researcher as Artist/Artist as Researcher", in: *Qualitative Inquiry* 1.1, 110–142.
Flannery (2001): M.C. Flannery, "Quilting: A Feminist Metaphor for Science", in: *Qualitative Inquiry* 7.5, 628–645.
Fogel (2013): A. Fogel, *Body Sense: The Science and Practice of Embodied Self-Awareness*, New York.
Foley (1985): H.P. Foley, *Ritual Irony. Poetry and Sacrifice in Euripides*, Ithaca.
Forbes (1950): P.B.R. Forbes, "Hesiod versus Perses", in: *The Classical Review* 64.3/4, 82–87.
Forde (1989): S. Forde, *The Ambition to Rule: Alcibiades and the Politics of Imperialism in Thucydides*, Ithaca, NY.
Forsyth (2009) D.R. Forsyth, *Group Dynamics*, Belmont.
Foster (2010): E. Foster, *Thucydides, Pericles, and Periclean Imperialism*, New York.
Foucault (1988): M. Foucault, *The History of Sexuality*, Volume 3, *The Care of the Self*, New York.
Frame (1978): D. Frame, *The Myth of Return in Early Greek Epic*, New Haven.
Frass/Strassl/Friehs (2012): M. Frass, R.P. Strassl, H. Friehs *et.al.*, "Use and Acceptance of Complementary and Alternative Medicine Among the General Population and Medical Personnel: A Systematic Review", in: *The Ochsner Journal* 12, 45–56.
Freud (1953): S. Freud, *The Standard Edition of the Complete Psychological Works of Sigmund Freud, Volume VII (1901–1905): A Case of Hysteria, Three Essays on Sexuality and Other Works*, trans. J. Strachey, London.
Freud (1954–74): S. Freud, *The Standard Edition of the Complete Psychological Works of Sigmund Freud* (24 vols.; trans. and ed. by J. Strachey with A. Freud, A.Strachey, and A. Tyson), London.
Freud (1955): S. Freud, *The Standard Edition of the Complete Psychological Works of Sigmund Freud, Volume XVIII (1920–1922): Beyond the Pleasure Principle, Group Psychology and Other Works*, trans. J. Strachey, London.
Galen (1976): Galen, *On the Affected Parts.* trans. and ed. by R.E. Seigel, Basel.
Galinksy (1981): K. Galinsky, "Augustus' Legislation on Morals and Marriage", in: *Philologus* 125, 126–144.
Gallagher (2005): S. Gallagher, *How the Body Shapes the Mind*, Oxford.
Garvie (1986): A.F. Garvie, *Aeschylus' Choephori*, Oxford.
Gaskin (1990): R. Gaskin, "Do Homeric Heroes Make Real Decisions?", in: *The Classical Quarterly* 40, 1–15.
Geertz (1973): C. Geertz, *The Interpretation of Cultures*, New York.
Geertz (1983): C. Geertz, *Local Knowledge: Further Essays in Interpretive Anthropology*, New York.
Geiger (2009): J. Geiger, *The Third Man Factor*, New York.
Geiger (2013): J. Geiger, *The Angel Effect*, Philadelphia.

Gibbs (1992): R. Gibbs, "Why Idioms Mean What They Do", in: *Journal of Memory and Language* 31, 485–506.

Gibbs (1994): R. Gibbs, *The Poetics of Mind: Figurative Thought, Language, and Understanding*, Cambridge.

Gibbs (2005): R. Gibbs, "Embodiment in Metaphorical Imagination", in: D. Pecher and R. Zwann (eds), *Grounding Cognition: The Role of Perception and Action in Memory, Language and Thinking*, Cambridge, 65–92.

Gibbs (2006a): R.W. Gibbs, "Metaphor Interpretation as Embodied Simulation", in: *Mind and Language* 21, 434–458.

Gibbs (2006b): R.W. Gibbs, *Embodiment and Cognitive Science*, Cambridge.

Gibbs/Colston (1995): R. Gibbs and H. Colston, "The Cognitive Psychological Reality of Image Schemas and Their Transformations", in: *Cognitive Linguistics* 6, 347–378.

Gill (1985): C. Gill, "Ancient Psychotherapy", in: *Journal of the History of Ideas* 46, 307–325.

Gill (1991): C. Gill, "Is There a Concept of Person in Greek Philosophy?", in S. Everson (ed.), *Companions to Ancient Thought 2: Psychology*, Cambridge, 166–193.

Gill (1996): C. Gill, *Personality in Greek Epic, Tragedy and Philosophy: The Self in Dialogue*, Oxford.

Gill (2006): C. Gill, *The Structured Self in Hellenistic and Roman Thought*, Oxford.

Gill (2009): C. Gill, "Seneca and Selfhood", in: S.Bartsch and D. Wray (eds), *Seneca and the Self*, Cambridge, 65–83.

Gill (2010): C. Gill, *Naturalistic Psychology in Galen and Stoicism*, Oxford.

Gill (2011): C. Gill, "Self", in: M. Finkelberg (ed.), *The Homeric Encyclopedia: Volume II*, Oxford.

Gill (2013a): C. Gill, *Marcus Aurelius' Meditations Book 1–6, Translated with an Introduction and Commentary*, Oxford.

Gill (2013b): C. Gill, "Philosophical Therapy as Preventive Psychological Medicine", in: W. Harris (ed.), *Mental Disorders in the Classical World*, Leiden, 339–360.

Gilroy (2006): A. Gilroy, *Art Therapy, Research and Evidence-Based Practise*, London.

Glenberg/Sato/Cattaneo/Riggio/Palumbo/Buccino (2008): A. Glenberg, M. Sato, L. Cattaneo, L. Riggio, D. Palumbo, and G. Buccino, "Processing Abstract Language Modulates Motor System Activity", in: *Quarterly Journal of Experimental Psychology* 61.6, 905–919.

Goette (2007): H.R. Goette, "An Archaeological Appendix", in: P. Wilson (ed.), *The Greek Theatre and Festivals: Documentary Studies*, Oxford, 116–121.

Goffman (1967): E. Goffman, *Interaction Ritual: Essays on Face-to-face Behaviour*, New York.

Goldhill (1984): S. Goldhill, *Language, Sexuality, Narrative: The* Oresteia, Cambridge.

Goldie (2010): P. Goldie (ed.), *The Oxford Handbook of Philosophy of Emotion*, Oxford.

Goldstein (2013): D. Goldstein, "Wackernagel's Law and the Fall of the Lydian Empire", in: *Transactions of the American Philological Association* 143, 325–347.

Gomme/Andrewes/Dover (1959): A.W. Gomme, A. Andrewes, and, K.J. Dover, *A Historical Commentary of Thucydides*, Vol. 1, Oxford.

Gowland (2006): A. Gowland, "The Problem of Early Modern Melancholy", in: *Oxford: Past and Present* 191, 77–120.

Gowland (2007): A. Gowland, *The Worlds of Renaissance Melancholy: Robert Burton in Context*, Cambridge.

Grady (1997): J. Grady, *Foundations of Meaning: Primary Metaphors and Primary Scenes*, Ph.D. dissertation, University of California, Berkeley.

Grady (1999): J. Grady, "A Typology of Motivation for Conceptual Metaphor", in: R. Gibbs and G. Steen (eds), *Metaphor in Cognitive Linguistics*, Amsterdam, 79–100.

Graf (1984): F. Graf, *Eleusis und die orphische Dichtung Athens in vorhellenistischer Zeit*, Berlin and New York.
Grant (1995): M. Grant, *Greek and Roman Historians: Information and Misinformation*, New York.
Graver (2007): M. Graver, *Stoicism and Emotion*, Chicago.
Graziosi/Haubold (2010): B. Graziosi and J.H. Haubold, *Homer. Iliad, Book VI*, Cambridge.
Green (1975): A. Green, "Orestes and Oedipus", in: *International Review of Psychoanalysis* 2, 355–364.
Green/McCreery (1975): C. Green and C. McCreery, *Apparitions*, Oxford.
Greene (1996): E. Greene, "Apostrophe and Women's Erotics in the Poetry of Sappho", in: *Reading Sappho: Contemporary Approaches*, Berkeley, 233–247.
Greene (2005): E. Greene, *Women Poets in Ancient Greece and Rome*, Norman.
Greene (1963): W.C. Greene, *Moira, Fate and Evil in Greek Thought*, New York.
Greer (2014): B. Greer, *Craftivism: The Art of Craft and Activism*, Vancouver.
Greetham (2010): D.C. Greetham, *The Pleasures of Contamination: Evidence, Text, and Voice in Textual Studies*, Bloomington and Indianapolis.
Gregory (2004): R.L. Gregory, *The Oxford Companion to the Mind*, Oxford.
Greyson (2014a): B. Greyson, "Near-Death Experiences", in: E. Cardeña, S.J. Lynn, and S. Krippner (eds), *Varieties of Anomalous Experience: Examining the Scientific Evidence*, 2nd edition, Washington, DC, 333–368.
Greyson (2014b): B. Greyson, Interview with Bruce Greyson at https://www.youtube.com/watch?v=IawBPkZCi3U.
Grice (1975): H.P. Grice, "Logic and Conversation", in: P. Cole and J. Morgan (eds), *Syntax and Semantics. Vol. 3: Speech Acts*, New York, 41–58.
Grice (1978): H.P. Grice, "Further Notes on Logic and Conversation", in: P. Cole (ed.), *Syntax and Semantics. Vol. 9*, New York, 113–128.
Griffin (1976): M. Griffin, *Seneca: A Philosopher in Politics*, Oxford.
Griffin (1980): J. Griffin, *Homer on Life and Death*, Oxford.
Griffith (1983): M. Griffith, "Personality in Hesiod", in: *Classical Antiquity* 2, 37–65.
Grillo (2014): L. Grillo, "A Double *sermocinatio* and a Resolved Dilemma in Cicero's *Pro Plancio*", in: *The Classical Quarterly* 64.1, 214–225.
Grillo (2015): L. Grillo, *Cicero's De Provinciis Consularibus. Introduction and Commentary*, Oxford.
Gruen (1974): E. Gruen, *The Last Generation of the Roman Republic*, Berkeley.
Guattari (1995): F. Guattari, *Chaosmosis: An Ethico-Aesthetic Paradigm*, trans. P. Bains and J. Pefanis, Bloomington and Indianapolis.
Gutiérrez Pérez (2008): R. Gutiérrez Pérez, "A Cross-Cultural Analysis of Heart Metaphors", in: *Revista Alicantina de Estudios Ingleses* 21, 25–56.
Haberlandt/Berian/Sandson (1980): K. Haberlandt, C. Berian, and J. Sandson, "The Episode Schema in Story Processing", in: *Journal of Verbal Learning and Verbal Behavior* 19, 635–650.
Habinek (2005a): T. Habinek, *Ancient Rhetoric and Oratory*, Malden, MA, and Oxford.
Habinek (2005b): T. Habinek, *The World of Roman Song: From Ritualized Speech to Social Order*, Baltimore.
Habinek (2011): T. Habinek, "The Tentacular Mind: Stoicism, Neuroscience, and the Configurations of Physical Reality", in: B.M. Stafford (ed.), *A Field Guide to a New Meta-Field: Bridging the Humanities-Neuroscience Divide*, Chicago, 64–83.
Haddad (2002): G. Haddad, *Le jour où Lacan m'a adopté. Mon analyse avec Lacan*, Paris.
Hadot (1969), I. Hadot, *Seneca und die griechische-römische Tradition der Seelenleitung*, Berlin.

Hallett (1973): J.P. Hallett, "The Role of Women in Roman Elegy: Counter–Cultural Feminism", in: *Arethusa* 6, 103–124.
Hallett/Van Nortwick (1996): J.P. Hallett and T. Van Nortwick (eds), *Compromising Traditions: Personal Voice in Classical Scholarship*, London.
Halliwell (1990): S. Halliwell, "Traditional Greek Conceptions of Character", in: C. Pelling (ed.), *Characterization and Individuality in Greek Literature*, Oxford, 32–59.
Halperin (1990): D.M. Halperin, "Why is Diotima a Woman?", in: J.J. Winkler and F.I. Zeitlin (eds), *Before Sexuality: The Construction of Erotic Experience in the Ancient Greek World*, Princeton, 257–308.
Hamberg (1945): P.G. Hamberg, "The Columns of Trajan and Marcus Aurelius and their Narrative Treatment", in: *Studies in Roman Imperial Art*, Copenhagen, 104–161.
Hampe/Grady (2005): B. Hampe and J. Grady (eds), *From Perception to Meaning: Image Schemas in Cognitive Linguistics*, Berlin.
Han/Ma (2014): S. Han and Y. Ma, "Cultural differences in Human Brain Activity: A Quantitative Meta-analysis", in: *NeuroImage* 99, 293–300.
Hansen (1991): M.H. Hansen, *Democracy in the Age of Demosthenes: Structure, Principles, and Ideology*, Oxford.
Harrington (2001): A. Harrington, "Dilthey, Empathy, and Verstehen: A Contemporary Reappraisal", in: *European Journal of Social Theory* 4, 311–329.
Harris (2006): W.V. Harris, "A Revisionist View of Roman Money", in: *Journal of Roman Studies* 96, 1–24.
Harris (2015): W.V. Harris, "Republican Riches", in: *Times Literary Supplement*, 9 January 2015.
Harrison (1960): E.L. Harrison, "Notes on Homeric Psychology", in: *Phoenix* 14, 63–80.
Harrison (1927/1962): J. Harrison, *Themis: A Study of the Social Origins of Greek Religion*, Ohio.
Hass-Cohen/Carr (2008): N. Hass-Cohen and R. Carr, *Art Therapy and Clinical Neuroscience*, London.
Hatfield/Rapson/Le (2011): E. Hatfield, R.L. Rapson, and Yen-Chi L. Le, "Emotional Contagion and Empathy", in: J. Decety and W. Ickes (eds), *The Social Neuroscience of Empathy*, Cambridge, MA, 19.
Haubold (2010): J.H. Haubold, "Shepherd, Farmer, Poet, Sophist: Hesiod on his own Reception", in Boys-Stones/Haubold (2010), 11–30.
Haugeland (1985): J. Haugeland, *Artificial Intelligence: The Very Idea*, Cambridge, MA.
Haury (1955): A. Haury, *L'ironie et l'humour chez Cicéron*, Leiden.
Hawthorn (2014): G. Hawthorn, *Thucydides on Politics: Back to the Present*, Cambridge.
Hawton/Salovskis/Kirk/Clark (1989): K. Hawton, P. Salovskis, J. Kirk, and D. Clark (eds), *Cognitive Behaviour Therapy for Psychiatric Problems: A Practical Guide*, Oxford.
Hayes/Strosahl/Wilson (1999): S. Hayes, K. Strosahl, and K. Wilson (eds), *Acceptance and Commitment Therapy: An Experiential Approach to Behavior Change*, New York.
Heckhausen (1977): H. Heckhausen, "Achievement Motivation and its Constructs: A Cognitive Model", in: *Motivation and Emotion* 1, 283–330.
Herbert/Forman (2011): J. Herbert and E. Forman (eds), *Acceptance and Mindfulness in Cognitive Behavior Therapy: Understanding and Applying the New Therapies*, Hoboken.
Herman (2010): J.L. Herman, *Trauma and Recovery: From Domestic Abuse to Political Terror*, London.
Herman (2011): G. Herman, "Greek Epiphanies and the Sensed Presence", *Historia* 60, 127–157.
Heubeck/West/Hainsworth (1988): A. Heubeck, S. West, and J.B. Hainsworth, *A Commentary on Homer's* Odyssey, *Volume 1*, Oxford.

Heyworth (2007): S.J. Heyworth, *Cynthia: A Companion to the Text of Propertius*, Oxford and New York.
Hill (1945): A. Hill, *Art Versus Illness: A Story of Art Therapy*, London.
Hinds (1998): S. Hinds, *Allusion and Intertext: Dynamics of Appropriation in Roman Poetry*, Cambridge.
Hogan (2001): S. Hogan, *Healing Arts: The History of Art Therapy*, London.
Holland (1999): E. Holland, *Deleuze and Guattari's Anti-Oedipus: Introduction to Schizoanalysis*, London and New York.
Holland (2012): E. Holland, "Deleuze and psychoanalysis", in: D.W. Smith and H. Somers-Hall (eds), *The Cambridge Companion to Deleuze*, Cambridge, 307–336.
Hollandare/Johnsson/Randestad/Tilfors (2011): F. Hollandare, S. Johnsson, M. Randestad, M. Tilfors *et. al.*, " Randomized Trial of Internet-Based Relapse Prevention for Partially Remitted Depression", in: *Acta Psychiatrica Scandinavica* 124, 285–294.
Honeck (1997): R.P. Honeck, *A Proverb in Mind: The Cognitive Science of Proverbial Wit and Wisdom*, New York.
Horn/Masunaga (2000): J.L. Horn and H. Masunaga, "On the Emergence of Wisdom: Expertise Development", in: Brown (2000), 245–276.
Hornblower (1991): S. Hornblower, *A Commentary on Thucydides*, Vol. 1, Oxford.
Hornblower (1994): S. Hornblower, "Narratology and Narrative Technique in Thucydides", in: *Greek Historiography*, Oxford, 131–166.
Hornblower (2008): S. Hornblower, *A Commentary on Thucydides,* Vol. 3, Oxford.
Huffziger/Kuehner (2009): S. Huffziger and C. Kuehner, "Rumination, Distraction, and Mindful Self-Focus in Depressed Patients", in: *Behaviour Research and Therapy* 47.3, 224–230.
Hughes (2008): J. Hughes, "Fragmentation as Metaphor in the Classical Healing Sanctuary", in: *Social History of Medicine*, 21.2, 217–236.
Hunter (2014): R. Hunter, *Hesiodic Voices: Studies in the Ancient Reception of Hesiod's* Works and Days, Cambridge.
Hutcheon (1994): L. Hutcheon, *Irony's Edge: The Theory and Politics of Irony,* London.
Irigaray (1985): L. Irigaray, *This Sex which is not One*, trans. C. Porter and C. Burke, Ithaca.
Isager/Skydsgaard (1992): S. Isager and J.E. Skydsgaard, *Ancient Greek Agriculture: An Introduction*, New York.
Jack (2013): R.E. Jack, "Culture and Facial Expressions of Emotion", in: *Visual Cognition* 21.9–10, 1248–1286.
Jackson (1986): S. Jackson, *Melancholia and Depression: From Hippocratic Times to Modern Times*, London.
Jaeger (1926): W. Jaeger, "Solons Eunomia", in: *Sitzungsberichte der Preussischen Akademie der Wissenschaften* 11, 69–85.
Jahn (1987): T. Jahn, *Zum Wortfeld 'Seele-Geist' in der Sprache Homers*, Munich.
Jakobson (1956): R. Jakobson, "Two Aspects of Language and Two Types of Aphasic Disturbances", in R. Jakobson and M. Halle, *Fundamentals of Language,* The Hague, 53–82.
James (2003): S.L. James, *Learned Girls and Male Persuasion: Gender and Reading in Roman Love Elegy*, Berkeley, Los Angeles and London.
Janan (2001): M. Janan, *The Politics of Desire: Propertius IV*, Berkeley, Los Angeles and London.
Janan (2012) "Lacanian Psychoanalytic Theory and Roman Love Elegy", in: B.K. Gold (ed.), *A Companion to Roman Love Elegy*, Malden and Oxford, 375–89.
Janis (1972): I. Janis, *Victims of Groupthink*, Boston.
Janis (1982): I. Janis, *Groupthink: Psychological Studies of Policy Decisions and Fiascoes*, Boston.

Jansen et al. (1995): A.S. Jansen et al., "Central Command Neurons of the Sympathetic Nervous System: Basis of the Fight-or-Flight Response", in: *Science* 270, 644–646.

Johnson (1987): M. Johnson, *The Body in Mind*, Chicago.

Johnston (1990): S. Iles Johnston, *Hekate Soteira: a Study of Hekate's Roles in the Chaldean Oracles and Related Literature*, Oxford.

Jones (1953): E. Jones, *Sigmund Freud: Life and Work, The Young Freud, 1856–1900*, London.

Jorgensen/Miller/Sperber (1984); J. Jorgensen, G. Miller, and D. Sperber, "Test of the Mention Theory of Irony", in: *Journal of Experimental Psychology: General* 113.1, 112–120.

Joshua/Markman (2012): I. Joshua and A.B. Markman, "Embodied Cognition as a Practical Paradigm: Introduction to the Topic, the Future of Embodied Cognition", in: *Topics in Cognitive Science* 4.4 685–691.

Jouanna (2000): J. Jouanna, "Hippocrates", in: J. Brunschwig and G.E.R. Lloyd (eds), *Greek Thought: A Guide to Classical Knowledge*, Cambridge.

Kallet (2001): L. Kallet, *Money and the Corrosion of Power in Thucydides: The Sicilian Expedition and its Aftermath*, Berkeley, CA.

Kam/Handy (2013): J.W.Y. Kam and T.C. Handy, "The Neurocognitive Consequences of the Wandering Mind: A Mechanistic Account of Sensory-Motor Decoupling", in: *Frontiers in Psychology* 4.

Kaschak/Jones/Coyle/Sell (2009): M. Kaschak, J. Jones, M. Coyle and A. Sell, "Language and Body", in: R. Wagner, C. Schatschneider, and C. Phythian-Sense (eds), *Beyond Decoding: The Behavioral and Biological Foundations of Reading Comprehension*, Guilford, 3–26.

Kaster (2005): R.A. Kaster, *Emotion, Restraint, and Community in Ancient Rome*, New York.

Kaster (2006): R. Kaster, *Cicero: Speech on behalf of Publius Sestius*, Oxford.

Katz (1991): M. Katz, *Penelope's Renown*, Princeton.

Kay (2014): P. Kay, *Rome's Economic Revolution*, Oxford.

Kearns (2004): E. Kearns, "The Gods in the Homeric Epics", in: R. Fowler (ed.), *The Cambridge Companion to Homer*, Cambridge, 59–73.

Kelley (1992): E. Kelley, *The Metaphorical Basis of Language: A Study in Cross-Cultural Linguistics*, New York.

Kendler/Zachar/Craver (2011): K.S. Kendler, P. Zachar, and C. Craver, "What Kinds of Things are Psychiatric Disorders?", in: *Psychological Medicine* 41, 1143–1150.

Kennedy (1993): D.F. Kennedy, *The Arts of Love: Five Studies in the Discourse of Roman Love Elegy*, Cambridge.

Killingsworth/Gilbert (2010): M.A. Killingsworth and D.T. Gilbert, "A Wandering Mind is an Unhappy Mind", in: *Science* 330.6006, 932.

King (1975–76): J.K. King, "Propertius' Programmatic Poetry and the Unity of the *Monobiblos*", in: *Classical Journal* 71, 108–124.

Klein/Segal (1997): M. Klein and H. Segal, *Envy and Gratitude, and Other Works 1946–1963*, London.

Klinger (1975): E. Klinger, "Consequences of Commitment to and Disengagement from Incentives", in: *Psychological Review* 82, 1–25.

Knoblich (2006): G. Knoblich, *Human Body Perception from the Inside Out*, Oxford.

Knowles/Cole (2008): J.G. Knowles and A.L. Cole (eds), *Handbook of the Arts in Qualitative Research: Perspectives, Methodologies, Examples, and Issues*, Los Angeles.

Knowles/Moon (2006): M. Knowles and R. Moon, *Introducing Metaphor*, London.

Koch (2012): C. Koch, *Consciousness: Confessions of a Romantic Reductionist*, Cambridge, MA.

Koning (2010): H. Koning, *Hesiod: the Other Poet*, Leiden.

Konstan (2006): D. Konstan, *The Emotions of the Ancient Greeks* (Studies in Aristotle and Classical Literature 5), Toronto.
Konstan (2010): D. Konstan, "Ridiculing a Popular War: Old Comedy and Militarism in Classical Athens", in: D.M. Pritchard (ed.), *War, Democracy, and Culture in Classical Athens*, Cambridge, 184–200.
Konstan (2011): D. Konstan, *Pity Transformed*, London.
Kopytin/Lebedev (2015): A. Kopytin and A. Lebedev, "Therapeutic Functions of Humour in Group Art Therapy with War Veterans", in: *International Journal of Art Therapy: Inscape* 20.2, 40–53.
Kövecses (1986): Z. Kövecses, *Metaphors of Anger, Pride, and Love: A Lexical Approach to the Structure of Concepts*, Amsterdam.
Kövecses (1995): Z. Kövecses, "Anger: Its Language, Conceptualization, and Physiology in the Light of Cross-Cultural Evidence", in: J. Taylor and R. MacLaury (eds), *Language and the Cognitive Construal of the World*, Berlin, 181–196.
Kövecses (2000): Z. Kövecses, *Metaphor and Emotion: Language, Culture, and the Body in Human Feeling*, Cambridge.
Kövecses (2005): Z. Kövecses, *Metaphor in Culture: Universality and Variation*, Cambridge.
Kövecses (2006): Z. Kövecses, *Language, Mind and Culture*, Oxford.
Kowert (2002): P.A. Kowert, *Groupthink or Deadlock: When do Leaders Learn from their Advisors*, Albany.
Kroll (1978): B.M. Kroll, "Cognitive Egocentrism and the Problem of Audience Awareness in Written Discourse", in: *Research in the Teaching of English* 12.3, 269–281.
Kubiak (1981): D.P. Kubiak, "The Orion Episode of Cicero's Aratea", in: *Classical Journal* 77.1, 12–22.
Kuhl (1981): J. Kuhl, "Motivational and Functional Helplessness: The Moderating Effect of State Versus Action Orientation", in: *Journal of Personality and Social Psychology* 40, 155–170.
Kullman (1985): W. Kullman, "Gods and Men in the *Iliad* and the *Odyssey*", in: *Harvard Studies in Classical Philology* 89, 1–23.
Kuzmičová (2013): A. Kuzmičová, "The Words and Worlds of Literary Narrative", in L. Bernaerts et al. (eds), *Stories and Minds: Cognitive Approaches to Literary Narrative*, Lincoln, 107–128.
La Bua (1998): G. La Bua, "Elementi innici nelle orazioni ciceroniane", in: *Res Publica Litterarum* 21, 134–154.
Lacan (1991): J. Lacan, "The Topic of the Imaginary", in: J.-A. Miller (ed.), *The Seminar of Jacques Lacan: Book 1: Freud's Papers on Technique, 1953–1954*, trans. J. Forrester, New York and London, 73–88.
Lacan (2006): J. Lacan, "The Mirror Stage as Formative of the *I* Function as Revealed in Psychoanalytic Experience", in: B.Fink (ed.), *Écrits: The First Complete Edition in English*, New York, 75–81.
Lacan (2006): J. Lacan, *Écrits. The First Complete Edition in English*, trans. Bruce Fink, New York and London.
Lacey/Stilla/Sathian (2012): S. Lacy, R. Stilla, and K. Sathian, "Metaphorically Feeling: Comprehending Textural Metaphors Activates Somatosensory Cortex", in: *Brain and Language* 120.3, 416–421.
Lakoff/Turner (1989): G. Lakoff and M. Turner, *More Than Cool Reason*, Chicago.
Lakoff (1990): G. Lakoff, "The Invariance Hypothesis: Is Abstract Reason Based on Image-Schemas?", in: *Cognitive Linguistics* 1.1, 39–74.
Lakoff (1993): G. Lakoff, "The Contemporary Theory of Metaphor", in: A. Ortony (ed.), *Metaphor and Thought*, Cambridge, 202–251.

Lakoff (2008): G. Lakoff, "The Neural Theory of Metaphor", in: R. Gibbs (ed.), *The Cambridge Handbook of Metaphor and Thought,* Cambridge, 17–39.

Lakoff/Johnson (1980a): G. Lakoff and M. Johnson, "The Metaphorical Structure of the Human Conceptual System", in: *Cognitive Science* 4, 195–208.

Lakoff/Johnson (1980b): G. Lakoff and M. Johnson, *Metaphors We Live By,* Chicago.

Lakoff/Johnson (1999): G. Lakoff and M. Johnson, *Philosophy in the Flesh: The Embodied Mind and its Challenge to Western Thought,* New York.

Lakoff/Turner (1989): G. Lakoff and M. Turner, *More Than Cool Reason: A Field Guide to Poetic Metaphor,* Chicago.

Lamberton (1988): R. Lamberton, *Hesiod,* Newhaven.

Laplanche/Pontalis (1988): J. Laplanche and J.B. Pontalis, *The Language of Psychoanalysis,* London.

Lardinois (2005): A. Lardinois, "The Wisdom and Wit of Many: The Orality of Greek Proverbial Expressions", in: J. Watson (ed.), *Speaking Volumes: Orality and Literacy in the Greek and Roman Worlds,* Leiden, 93–108.

Lardinois/McClure (2001): A. Lardinois and L. McClure, *Making Silence Speak: Women's Voices in Greek Literature and Society,* Princeton.

Larson (2010): S. Larson, "Τεθνάκην δ' ἀδόλως θέλω: Reading Sappho's 'Confession' (fr. 94) through Penelope", in: *Mnemosyne* 63, 175–202.

Lateiner (1995): D. Lateiner, *Sardonic Smile: Nonverbal Behavior in Homeric Epic,* Ann Arbor.

Latimer (1930): J.F. Latimer, "Hesiod versus Perses", in: *Transactions and Proceedings of the American Philological Association* 61, 70–79.

Lazarus/Folkman (1991): R. Lazarus and S. Folkman, *Stress, Appraisal and Coping,* New York.

Le Rider (2002): J. Le Rider, *Freud, de l'Acropole au Sinaï. Le retour à l'Antique des modernes viennois,* Paris.

Lebeck (1971): A. Lebeck, *The Oresteia: A Study in Language and Structure,* Cambridge.

Lebow (2003): R.N. Lebow, *The Tragic Vision of Politics,* Cambridge.

Leclerc (1994): M.C. Leclerc, "L'attelage d'Hésiode: les difficultés d'une reconstitution", in: *Dialogues d'histoire ancienne* 20.2, 53–84.

LeDoux (1996): J. LeDoux, *The Emotional Brain,* New York.

LeDoux (1998): J. LeDoux, *The Emotional Brain: The Mysterious Underpinnings of Emotional Life,* London.

LeDoux (2000): J. LeDoux, "Emotion Circuits in the Brain", in: *Annual Review of Neuroscience* 23, 155–184.

Lee (1990): J.S. Lee, *Jacques Lacan,* Boston.

Lesky (2004): A. Lesky, "Divine and Human Causation in Homeric Epic", trans. L. Holford-Strevens, in: D.L. Cairns (ed.), *Oxford Readings in Homer's Iliad,* Oxford, 170–202.

Levenson et al. (1991): R. Levenson, L. Carstensen, W. Friesen, and P. Ekman, "Emotion, Physiology, and Expression in Old Age", in: *Psychology and Aging* 6, 28–35.

Levenson/Ekman/Friesen (1990): R. Levenson, P. Ekman, and W. Friesen, "Voluntary Facial Action Generates Emotion-specific Autonomic Nervous System Activity", in: *Psychophysiology* 27, 363–384.

Levine (1984): D.B. Levine, "Odysseus' Smiles", in: *Transactions of the American Philological Association* 114, 1–9.

Lewis/Fraser (1996): J. Lewis and M. Fraser, "Patches of Grief and Rage: Visitor Responses to the NAMES Project AIDS Memorial Quilt", in: *Qualitative Sociology* 19.4, 433–451.

Liamputtong/Rumbold (2008): P. Liamputtong and J. Rumbold (eds), *Knowing Differently: Arts-Based and Collaborative Research Methods*, New York.
Liebeschuetz (2003): W. Liebeschuetz, "The Structure and Function of the Melian Dialogue", in: *The Journal of Hellenic Studies* 88, 73–77.
Liu et al. (2013): Z. Liu et al., "Culture Influence on Aesthetic Perception of Chinese and Western Paintings: Evidence from Eye Movement Patterns", in: *Proceedings of the 6th International Symposium on Visual Information Communication and Interaction*, ACM, 72–78.
Lloyd (1979): G.E.R. Lloyd, *Magic, Reason, and Experience: Studies in the Origin and Development of Greek Science*, Cambridge.
Lloyd (2004): M. Lloyd, "The Politeness of Achilles: Off-Record Conversation Strategies in Homer and the Meaning of *kertomia*", in: *Journal of Hellenic Studies* 124, 75–89.
Lloyd (2007): G. Lloyd, *Cognitive Variations: Reflections on the Unity And Diversity Of The Human Mind*, Oxford.
Lloyd-Jones (1971): H. Lloyd-Jones, *The Justice of Zeus*, Berkeley.
Long (1986): A.A. Long, *Hellenistic Philosophy: Stoics, Epicureans, Sceptics*, Second Edition, Berkeley and Los Angeles.
Long (2002): A.A. Long, *Epictetus: A Stoic and Socratic Guide to Life*, Oxford.
Long/Sedley (1987): A.A. Long and D.N. Sedley, *The Hellenistic Philosophers*, Cambridge.
Longley/Pruitt (1980): J. Longley and D. Pruitt, "Groupthink: A Critique of Janis' Theory", in: L. Wheeler (ed.), *Review of Personality and Social Psychology*, Beverley Hills, CA, 153–186.
Lonsdale (1990): S.H. Lonsdale, *Creatures of Speech: Lion, Herding, and Hunting Similes in the Iliad*, Stuttgart.
Lund (2010): M. Lund, *Melancholy, Medicine and Religion in Early Modern England: Reading The Anatomy of Melancholy*, Cambridge.
Lundberg (2012): C. Lundberg, *Lacan in Public: Psychoanalysis and the Science of Rhetoric*, Tuscaloosa.
Lutterbie (2011): J. Lutterbie, *Toward a General Theory of Acting: Cognitive Science and Performance*, New York.
Machen (1915): A. Machen, *The Bowmen and Other Legends of the War*, London.
Macintosh (2010): F. Macintosh (ed.), *The Ancient Dancer in the Modern World: Responses to Greek and Roman Dance*, Oxford.
MacLachlan (2004): M. MacLachlan, *Embodiment: Clinical, Critical and Cultural Perspectives on Health and Illness*, McGraw-Hill.
Macleod (1983): C. Macleod, *Collected Essays*, Oxford.
Mahony (1974): P. Mahony, "Freud in the Light of Classical Rhetoric", in: *Journal of the History of the Behavioral Sciences* 10.4, 413–425.
Makara/Palkovits/Szentagothal (1983): G. Makara, M. Palkovits, and J. Szentagothal, "The Endocrine Hypothalamus and Hormonal Response to Stress", in: H. Selye (ed.), *Selye's Guide to Stress Research*, New York, 280–337.
Makari (2008): G. Makari, *Revolution in Mind: The Early Years of Psychoanalysis*, London.
Malabou (2012): C. Malabou, *The New Wounded: From Neurosis to Brain Damage*, New York.
Malafouris/Renfrew (2010): L. Malafouris and C. Renfrew, "The Cognitive Life of Things: Archaeology, Material Engagement and the Extended Mind", in: *The Cognitive Life of Things: Recasting the Boundaries of the Mind*, Oakville, CT, 1–12.
Marincola (2001): J. Marincola, *Greek Historians*, Oxford.
Marinone (2004): N. Marinone, *Cronologia ciceroniana*, Bologna.

Marks (2008): J. Marks, *Zeus in the* Odyssey, Washington D.C.
Marshall (1975): M.H.B. Marshall, "Urban Settlement in the Second Chapter of Thucydides", in: *The Classical Quarterly* 25, 26–40.
Martin (1984): R. Martin, "Hesiod, Odysseus, and the Instruction of Princes", in: *Transactions and Proceedings of the American Philological Association* 114, 29–48.
Martin (1993): R. Martin, "Telemachus and the Last Hero Song", in: *Colby Quarterly* 29, 222–240.
Martin (2012): L.H. Martin, "The Future of the Past: The History of Religions and Cognitive Historiography", in: *Future* 20, 155–171.
Masuda/Nisbett (2001): T. Masuda and R.E. Nisbett, "Attending Holistically Versus Analytically: Comparing The Context Sensitivity of Japanese and Americans", in: *Journal of Personality and Social Psychology* 81.5, 922–934.
Matchar (2013): E. Matchar, *Homeward Bound: Why Women Are Embracing the New Domesticity*, New York.
Maturana/Varela (1980): H. Maturana and F. Varela, *Autopoiesis and Cognition*, Dordrecht.
Maturana/Varela (1987): H. Maturana and F. Varela, *The Tree of Knowledge*, Berkeley, CA.
McConachie (2008): B.A. McConachie, *Engaging Audiences: A Cognitive Approach to Spectating in the Theatre*, New York.
McConachie/Blair (2013): B.A. McConachie and R. Blair, in: N. Shaugnessy (ed.), *Affective Performance and Cognitive Science: Body, Brain, and Being*, London.
McConachie/Hart (2006): B.A. McConachie and F.E. Hart (eds), *Performance and Cognition: Theatre Studies and the Cognitive Turn*, London and New York.
McDonnell (2006): M. McDonnell, *Roman Manliness: Virtus and the Roman Republic*, Cambridge.
McGann (1991): J.J. McGann, *The Textual Condition*, Princeton.
McGann (2001): J.J. McGann, *Radiant Textuality: Literature after the World Wide Web*, New York and Basingstoke.
McLaughlin (2011): K.A. McLaughlin, "The Public Health Impact of Major Depression: A Call for Interdisciplinary Prevention Efforts", in: *Prevention Science* 12, 361–371.
McNiff (1998): S. McNiff, *Arts-Based Research*, London.
McNiff (2008): S. McNiff, "Arts-Based Research", in: Knowles/Cole (2008), 29–40.
Meineck (2012): P. Meineck, "The Embodied Space: Performance and Visual Cognition in the Fifth Century Athenian Theatre", in: *New England Classical Journal* 39, 3–46.
Meineck (2011): P. Meineck, "The Neuroscience of the Tragic mask", in: *Arion*, 113–158.
Meineck/Konstan (2014): P. Meineck and D. Konstan (eds), *Combat Trauma and the Ancient Greeks*, New York.
Melucci (1995): A. Melucci, "The Process of Collective Identity", in: H. Johnson and B. Klandermans (eds), *Social Movements and Culture*, London, 41–63.
Mikulincer (1994): M. Mikulincer, *Human Learned Helplessness: A Coping Perspective*, New York.
Miller (2009a): F.W. Miller, "Homer's Challenge to Philosophical Psychology", in: W. Wians (ed.), *Logos and Muthos: Philosophical Essays in Greek Literature*, Albany, 29–50.
Miller (2012): G. Miller, *Rendez-vous chez Lacan*, Paris.
Miller (2009b): J.F. Miller, *Apollo, Augustus, and the Poets*, Cambridge.
Miller (2001): P.A. Miller, "Why Propertius is a Woman: French Feminism and Augustan Elegy", in: *Classical Philology* 96, 127–146.
Miller (2004): P.A. Miller, *Subjecting Verses: Latin Love Elegy and the Emergence of the Real*, Princeton.
Miller (2011): P.A. Miller, "What is a Propertian Poem?", in: *Arethusa* 44, 329–352.

Mills (1997): S. Mills, *Theseus, Tragedy, and the Athenian Empire*, New York.
Minchin (2001a): E. Minchin, "Similes in Homer: Image, Mind's Eye, and Memory", in: J. Watson (ed.), *Speaking Volumes: Orality and Literacy in the Greek and Roman World*, Leiden, 25–52.
Minchin (2001b): E. Minchin, *Homer and the Resources of Memory. Some Applications of Cognitive Theory to the Iliad and the Odyssey*, Oxford.
Minchin (2007): E. Minchin, "Describing and Narrating in Homer's *Iliad*", in: E.A. Mackay (ed.), *Signs of Orality: The Oral Tradition and Its Influence in the Greek and Roman World*, Leiden, 9–34.
Minchin (2008): E. Minchin, "Communication Without Words: Body Language, 'Pictureability', and Memorability in the *Iliad*", in: *Ordia prima* 7, 17–38.
Mitchell/Eclsteom (2009): D.H. Mitchell and D. Eckstein, "Jury Dynamics and Decision-Making: A Prescription for Groupthink", in: *International Journal for Academic Research* 1, 163–169.
Modell (2009): A. Modell, "Metaphor: The Bridge between Feelings and Knowledge", in: *Psychoanalytic Inquiry* 29.1, 6–11.
Mommsen/Krueger/Watson (1985): T. Mommsen, P. Krueger, and A. Watson (eds), *The Digest of Justinian*, Vol. 4. Philadelphia.
Montefusco (2005): L.C. Montefusco, "ἐναργεία et ἐνεργεία: l'evidence d'une démonstration qui signifie les choses en acte", in: M. Armisen Marchetti (ed.), *Demonstrare. Voir et faire voir: forme de la demonstration à Rome, Actes du colloque international des 18, 19 et 20 novembre 2004, Université de Toulouse-le-Mirail*, Toulouse, 43–58.
Morson/Emerson (1990): G.S. Morson and C. Emerson, *Mikhail Bakhtin: Creation of a Prosaics*, Stanford.
Most (2002): G.W. Most, "Freuds Narziβ: Reflexionen über einen Selbstbezug", in: A.-B. Renger (ed.), *Narcissus: Ein Mythos von der Antike bis zum Cyberspace*, Stuttgard and Weimar, 117–131.
Most (2007): G.W. Most, "Il narciso di Freud: Reflessioni su un caso di autoreflessività", trans. M. Telò, in: *Studi italiani di filologia classica*, 4.5, 201–221.
Moulthrop (1994): S. Moulthrop, "Rhizome and Resistance: Hypertext and the Dreams of a New Culture", in: G.P. Landow (ed.), *Hyper/Text/Theory*, Baltimore and London, 299–319.
Mrazek/Haggerty (1994): P.J. Mrazek and R.J. Haggerty (eds), *Reducing Risks for Mental Disorders: Frontiers for Preventive Intervention Research*, Washington, DC.
Murnaghan (1987): S. Murnaghan, *Disguise and Recognition in the Odyssey*, Princeton.
Murnaghan (2002): S. Murnaghan, "The Trials of Telemachus: Who was the *Odyssey* Meant for?", in: *Arethusa* 35, 233–253.
Nagler (1978): M.N. Nagler, *Spontaneity and Tradition: A Study in the Oral Art of Homer*, Berkeley.
Nelson (1996): S. Nelson, "The Drama of Hesiod's Farm", in: *Classical Philology* 91.1, 45–53.
Nelson (1998): S. Nelson, *God and the Land: The Metaphysics of Farming in Hesiod and Vergil*, New York and Oxford.
Nicholson (1992): J. Nicholson, *Cicero's Return from Exile*, New York.
Nisbet (1961): R. Nisbet, *M. Tulli Ciceronis in Calpurnium Pisonem oratio*, Oxford.
Nisbet (2004): G. Nisbet, "Hesiod 'Works and Days': A Didaxis of Deconstruction?", in: *Greece and Rome* 51.2, 147–163.
Nisbett (2004): R. Nisbett, *The Geography of Thought: How Asians and Westerners Think Differently... and Why*, New York.
Noë (2009): A. Noë, *Out of Our Heads: Why You Are Not Your Brain, and Other Lessons from the Biology of Consciousness*, New York.

Nolen-Hoeksema (2000): S. Nolen-Hoeksema, "The Role of Rumination in Depressive Disorders and Mixed Anxiety/Depressive Symptoms", in: *Journal of Abnormal Psychology* 109.3, 504.

Nolen-Hoeksema/Wisco/Lyubomirsky (2008): S. Nolen-Hoeksema, B.E. Wisco, and S. Lyubomirsky, "Rethinking Rumination", in: *Perspectives on Psychological Science* 3.5, 400–424.

Nowak (2011): M. Nowak, "The Complicated History of Einfühlung", in: *Argument* 1, 301–326.

Nünlist (2000): R. Nünlist, "Rhetorische Ironie – Dramatische Ironie: Definitions- und Interpretationsprobleme", in J.P. Schwindt (ed.), *Zwischen Tradition und Innovation: poetische Verfahren im Spannungsfeld klassischer und neuerer Literatur und Literaturwissenschaft*, Munich, 67–87.

Nussbaum (1994): M.C. Nussbaum, *The Therapy of Desire: Theory and Practice in Hellenistic Ethics*, Princeton.

O'Connell/Boat/Warner (2009): M.E. O'Connell, T. Boat, and K.E. Warner (eds), *Preventing Mental, Emotional and Behavioral Disorders Among Young People: Progress and Possibilities*, National Research Council (US) and Institute of Medicine (US) Committee on the Prevention of Mental Disorders and Substance Abuse Among Children, Youth, and Young Adults: Research Advances and Promising Intervention, Washington DC.

Oatley (1992): K. Oatley, *Best Laid Schemes: The Psychology of Emotions*, New York.

Oatley (1999): K. Oatley, " Why Fiction May Be Twice as True as Fact: Fiction as Cognitive and Emotional Simulation", in: *Review of General Psychology* 3.2, 101–117.

Oatley (2011): K. Oatley, *Such Stuff as Dreams: The Psychology of Fiction*, Malden and Oxford.

Oatley (2012): K. Oatley, *The Passionate Muse: Exploring Emotion in Stories*, New York.

Ober (1998): J. Ober, *Political Dissent in Democratic Athens*, Princeton, NJ.

Öhman (2008): A, Öhman, "Fear and Anxiety: Evolutionary, Cognitive, and Clinical Perspectives", in: M. Lewis, Jeannette Haviland-Jones, and Lisa Feldman Barrett (eds), *Handbook of Emotions*, Third Edition, New York, 709–729.

Ohry (2003): A. Ohry, "Extracampine Hallucinations", in: *The Lancet* 361, 161.

Oliensis (1997): E. Oliensis, "The Erotics of *Amicitia*: Readings in Tibullus, Propertius, and Horace". in: J.P. Hallett and M.B. Skinner (eds), *Roman Sexualities*, Princeton, 151–71.

Oliensis (2009): E. Oliensis, *Freud's Rome: Psychoanalysis and Latin Poetry*, Cambridge.

Olson (1995): D. Olson, *Blood and Iron: Stories and Storytelling in Homer's* Odyssey, Leiden.

Ong (1975): W. Ong, "The Writer's Audience is Always a Fiction", in: *Publications of the Modern Language Association of America* 90.1, 9–21.

Onians (1954): R. Onians, *The Origins of European Thought about the Body, the Mind, the Soul, the World, Time and Fate*, Cambridge.

Opsomer (1998): J. Opsomer, "The Rhetoric and Pragmatics of Irony/εἰρωνεία", in: *Orbis* 40.1, 1–34.

Opsomer (2000): J. Opsomer, "Εἰρωνεία and the Corpus Plutarcheum (with an Appendix on Plutarch's Irony)", in: L. Van der Stockt (ed.), *Rhetorical Theory and Practice in Plutarch*, Leuven, 309–329.

Orwin (1994): C. Orwin, *The Humanity of Thucydides*, Princeton, NJ.

Osborne (2004): R. Osborne, "Hoards, Votives, Offerings: The Archaeology of the Dedicated Object", in: *World Archaeology* 36.1, 1–10.

Overmier/Seligman (1967): J.B. Overmier and M.E.P. Seligman. "Effects of Inescapable Shock on Subsequent Escape and Avoidance Responding", in: *Journal of Comparative and Physiological Psychology* 63, 28–33.

Paas/Tuovinen/Tabbers/Van Gerven (2003): F. Paas, J.E. Tuovinen, H. Tabbers, and P.W.M. Van Gerven, "Cognitive Load Measurement as a Means to Advance Cognitive Load Theory", in: *Educational Psychologist* 38.1, 63–71.
Page (1944): D. Page, *The Homeric Odyssey*, Oxford.
Palmer (1992): M. Palmer, *Love of Glory and the Common Good. Aspects of the Political Thought of Thucydides*, Lanham, Md.
Palmer (1996): G. Palmer, *Toward a Theory of Cultural Linguistics*, Austin, TX.
Paloma et al. (2013): P.G. Paloma et al., "Embodiment Cognitive Science in Educational Field", in: *Procedia – Social and Behavioral Sciences* 106, 1054–1062.
Pampallona/Bollini/Tibaldi/Kupelnick/Munizza (2004): S. Pampallona, S. Bollini, G., Tibaldi, B. Kupelnick, C. Munizza, "Combined Pharmacotherapy and Psychological Treatment for Depression: A Systematic Review", in: *Archives of General Psychiatry* 61, 714–719.
Papastamati-von Moock (2014): C. Papastamati-von Mooc, "The Theatre of Dionysus Eleuthereus in Athens: New Data and Observations on its 'Lycurgan' Phase", in: Eric Csapo et al. (eds), *Greek Theatre in the Fourth Century B.C.*, Berlin and Boston, 15–76.
Pappas (2011): A. Pappas, "The Aesthetics of Ancient Greek Writing", in M. Dalbello and M. Lewis Shaw (eds), *Visible writings: Cultures, Forms, Readings*, New Brunswick, 37–54.
Parhon-Stefanescu/Procopiu-Constantinescu (1967): C. Parhon-Stefanescu and T. Procopiu-Constantinescu, "Considérations sur l'impression de présence", in: *Annales médico-psychologiques* 125, 253–260.
Park (2000): W. Park, "A Comprehensive Empirical Investigation of the Relationships among Variables of the Groupthink Model", in: *Journal of Organisational Behaviour* 21, 873–887.
Parry (1981): A. Parry, *Logos and Ergon in Thucydides*, Salem, NH.
Parvizi et al. (2012): J. Parvizi, J. Corentin, B.L. Foster, N. Withoft, V. Rangarajan, K.S. Weiner, and K. Grill-Spector, "Electrical Stimulation of Human Fusiform Face-Selective Regions Distorts Face Perception", in: *The Journal of Neuroscience* 32, no. 43, 14915–14920.
Paul (1982): G. Paul, "*Urbs Capta*: Sketch of an Ancient Literary Motif", in: *Phoenix* 36, 144–155.
Peirano (2013): I. Peirano, "*Ille ego qui quondam*: On Authorial (An)onymity", in: A. Marmodoro and J. Hill (eds), *The Author's Voice in Classical and Late Antiquity*, Oxford, 251–285.
Peirano (2014): I. Peirano, "Sealing the Book: the *Sphragis* as Paratext", in: L. Jansen (ed.), *The Roman Paratext: Frame, Texts, Readers*, Cambridge, 224–242.
Pelliccia (1995): H. Pelliccia, *Mind, Body, and Speech in Homer and Pindar*, Göttingen.
Pelling (2000): C. Pelling, *Literary Texts and the Greek Historian*, London.
Peradotto (1990): J. Peradotto, *Man in the Middle Voice: Name and Narration in the* Odyssey, Princeton.
Perelman/Olbrechts-Tyteca (1991): C. Perelman and L. Olbrechts-Tyteca, *The New Rhetoric: A Treatise on Argumentation*, Notre Dame.
Peterson (1985): C. Peterson, "Learned Helplessness: Fundamental Issues in Theory and Research", in: *Journal of Social and Clinical Psychology* 3, 248–254.
Peterson/Seligman (1983): C. Peterson and M.E.P. Seligman, "Learned Helplessness and Victimization", in: *Journal of Social Issues* 39, 103–116.
Petropoulos (2011): J.C.B. Petropoulos, *Kleos in a Minor Key: The Homeric Education of a Little Prince*, Washington D.C.
Phillimore (1901): J. Swinnerton Phillimore, *Sexti Properti Carmina*, Oxford.
Porges (2011): S. Porges, *The Polyvagal Theory*, New York.
Porter (2006): R. Porter (ed.), *The Cambridge History of Medicine*, Cambridge.

Postgate (1881): J.P. Postgate, *Select Elegies of Propertius*, London.
Powell (1988): A. Powell, *Athens and Sparta: Constructing Greek Political and Social History from 478 BC*, London.
Powers (2014): M. Powers, *Athenian Tragedy in Performance: A Guide to Contemporary Studies and Historical Debates*, Iowa City.
Prinz (2008): J. Prinz, "Is Consciousness Embodied?", in: P. Robbins and M. Aydede (eds), *The Cambridge Handbook of Situated Cognition*, Cambridge, 419–436.
Prinz (2012): J. Prinz, *Beyond Human Nature: How Culture and Experience Shape Our Lives*, London and New York.
Pritchard (2004): D. Pritchard, "Kleisthenes, Participation, and the Dithyrambic Contests of Late Archaic and Classical Athens", *Phoenix* 58.3/4, 208–228.
Pucci (1987): P. Pucci, *Odysseus Polutropos: Intertextual Readings in the* Iliad *and the* Odyssey, Ithaca.
Pucci (1998): P. Pucci, *The Song of the Sirens: Essays on Homer*, Lanham.
Race (2014): W.H. Race, "Phaeacian Therapy in Homer's *Odyssey*", in: Meineck/Konstan (2014), 47–66.
Radden (2003): J. Radden, "Is this Dame Melancholy? Equating Depression and Melancholia", in: *Psychiatry, Philosophy & Psychology* 10.1, 37–52.
Ravetz et al. (2013): A. Ravetz, A. Kettle, and H. Felcey (eds), *Collaboration Through Craft*, London.
Rawlings (1981): H.R. Rawlings, *The Structure of Thucydides' History*, Princeton, NJ.
Rayor (1991): D.J. Rayor, *Sappho's Lyre: Archaic Lyric and Women Poets in Ancient Greece*, Berkeley.
Rayor (1993): D.J. Rayor, "Korinna: Gender and the Narrative Tradition", in: *Arethusa* 26, 219–231.
Reason/Bradbury (2006): P. Reason and H. Bradbury (eds), *Handbook of Action Research: Concise Paperback Edition*, London.
Redican (1982): W.K. Redican, "Evolutionary Perspective on Human Facial Display", in P. Ekman (ed.), *Emotions in the Human Face*, 2nd edition, Cambridge, 212–280.
Reich (1946): W. Reich, *The Mass Psychology of Fascism*, trans. T.P. Wolfe, New York.
Reich (2012): W. Reich and L. Baxandall (eds), *Sex-Pol: Essays, 1929–1934*, London and New York.
Rein (1954): D.M. Rein, "Orestes and Electra in Greek Literature", in: *American Imago* 11, 1–10.
Reinhardt (1996): K. Reinhardt, "The Adventures in the *Odyssey*", trans. H. Flower, in: S. Schein (ed.), *Readings in the* Odyssey, Princeton, 63–132.
Rengakos (2006b): A. Rengakos, "Thucydides' Narrative: The Epic and Herodotean Heritage", in: Rengakos/Tsakmakis (2006a), 279–300.
Rengakos/Tsakmakis (2006a): A. Rengakos and A. Tsakmakis, *Brill's Companion to Thucydides*, Leiden.
Rhead (2014): J.D. Rhead, "The Deeper Significance of Integrative Medicine", in: *Journal of Alternative and Complementary Medicine* 20, 329–329.
Rhodes (1988): P.J. Rhodes, *Thucydides History II*, Warminster.
Ribbeck (1876): O. Ribbeck, "Ueber den Begriff des εἴρων", in: *Rheinisches Museum* 31, 381–400.
Rich (1972): A. Rich, "When We Dead Awaken: Writing as Re-Vision", in: *College English* 34.1, 18–30.
Richardson (2000): L. Richardson, "Writing: A Method of Inquiry" (Revised and Expanded), in: Denzin and Lincoln (eds), *Handbook of Qualitative Research* (2nd Edition), 923–949.

Richardson/Piggott (1982): N.J. Richardson and S. Piggott, "Hesiod's Wagon, Text and Technology", in: *Journal of Hellenic Studies* 102, 225–229.
Richmond (1928): O.L. Richmond, *Sexti Properti quae supersunt opera*, Cambridge.
Riedweg (1987): C. Riedweg, *Mysterienterminologie bei Platon, Philon, und Klemens von Alexandrien*, Berlin and New York.
Riggsby (2015): A.M. Riggsby, "Tyrants, Fire, and Dangerous Things", in: G. Williams and K. Volk (eds), *Roman Reflections: Studies in Latin Philosophy*, Oxford, 111–28.
Rimé (2007): B. Rimé, "The Social Sharing of Emotion as an Interface Between Individual and Collective Processes in the Construction of Emotional Climates", in: *Journal of social issues* 63.2, 307–322.
Rivolta (2014): D. Rivolta, "Cognitive and Neural Aspects of Face Processing", in: *Prosopagnosia*, Berlin and Heidelberg, 19–40.
Robbins (1990): E. Robbins, "Who's Dying in Sappho Fr. 94?", in: *Phoenix* 44, 111–121.
Robertson (2010): D. Robertson, *The Philosophy of Cognitive-Behavioral Therapy (CBT): Stoic Philosophy as Rational and Cognitive Psychotherapy*, London.
Robertson (2013): D. Robertson, *Stoicism and the Art of Happiness*, London.
Rokotnitz (2011): N. Rokotnitz, *Trusting Performance: A Cognitive Approach to Embodiment in Drama*, New York.
Rood (1998): T. Rood, *Thucydides: Narrative and Explanation*, Oxford.
Rosch (1973): E. Rosch, "Natural Categories", in: *Cognitive Psychology* 4, 328–350.
Rosch (1978): E. Rosch, "Principles of Categorization", in: E. Rosch and B. Lloyd (eds), *Cognition and Categorization*, Hillsdale, NJ, 27–48.
Rose (1979): G.P. Rose, "Odysseus' Barking Heart", in: *Transactions of the American Philological Association* 109, 215–230.
Rose (1997): P.W. Rose, "Ideology in the *Iliad*: Polis, Basileus, Theoi", in: *Arethusa* 30, 151–199.
Rose (2012): P.W. Rose, *Class in Archaic Greece*, Cambridge.
Roselli (2011): D.K. Roselli, *Theater of the People: Spectators and Society in Ancient Athens*, Austin.
Rosen (1990): R. Rosen, "Poetry and Sailing in Hesiod's *Works and Days*", in: *Classical Antiquity* 9, 99–113.
Rosenwein (2010): B.H. Rosenwein, "Problems and Methods in the History of Emotions", in: *Passions in Context* 1, 1–32.
Roth (2014): T.L. Roth, "How Traumatic Experiences Leave Their Signature on the Genome: An Overview of Epigenetic Pathways in PTSD", in: *Frontiers in Psychiatry* 5, 93, PMC4116797, retrieved 16 July 2015.
Roudinesco (1999): E. Roudinesco, *Jacques Lacan: An Outline of a Life and a History of a System of Thought*, trans. B. Bray, Cambridge.
Rowlands (2010): M. Rowlands, *The New Science of the Mind: From Extended Mind to Embodied Phenomenology*, Cambridge, MA.
Rubin (1995): D.C. Rubin, *Memory in Oral Traditions: The Cognitive Psychology of Epic, Ballads, and Counting-Out Rhymes*, Oxford and New York.
Russo (2012): J. Russo, "Re-thinking Homeric Psychology: Snell, Dodds and their Critics", in: *Quaderni Urbinati di cultura classica* 101, 11–28.
Russo/Simon (1968): J. Russo and B. Simon, "Homeric Psychology and the Oral Epic Tradition", in: *Journal of the History of Ideas* 28, 483–498.
Rüter (1969): K. Rüter, *Odysseeinterpretationen: Untersuchungen zum ersten Buch und zur Phaiakis*, Göttingen.

Rutherford (1992): R.B. Rutherford, *Homer: Odyssey. Books XIX and XX*, Cambridge.
Sacks (2012): O.Sacks, *Hallucinations*, New York and Toronto.
Saïd (2011): S. Saïd, *Homer and the* Odyssey, Oxford.
Sansò (2014): A. Sansò, "Cognitive Linguistics and Greek", in: G. Giannakis (ed.), *Encyclopedia of Ancient Greek Language and Linguistics*, Vol. 2, Leiden, 308–311.
Saxonhouse (2006): A.W. Saxonhouse, *Free Speech and Democracy in Ancient Athens*, Cambridge.
Schacter (2012): D.L. Schacter et al., "The Future of Memory: Remembering, Imagining, and the Brain", in: *Neuron* 76.4, 677–694.
Schadewaldt (1936): W. Schadewaldt, "Zu Sappho", in: *Hermes* 71, 363–373.
Schadewaldt (1950): W.Schadewaldt, *Sappho: Welt und Dichtung: Dasein in der Liebe*, Potsdam.
Schadewaldt (1958): W. Schadewaldt, "Der Prolog der Odyssee", in: *Harvard Studies in Classical Philology* 63, 15–32.
Schmidt (2007): J. Schmidt, *Melancholy and the Care of the Soul: Religious, Moral Philosophy and Madness in Early Modern England*, Aldershot.
Schnapp-Gourbeillon (1981): A. Schnapp-Gourbeillon, *Lions, héros, masques: les représentations de l'animal chez Homère*, Paris.
Schubart (1902): W. Schubart, "Neue Bruchstücke der Sappho und des Alkaios", in: *Sitzungsberichte der königlich Preussischen Akademie der Wissenschaften zu Berlin*, 195–209.
Schubart (1907): W. Schubart, *Berliner Klassikertexte* 5.2, Berlin.
Schubert/Waldzus/Seibt (2008): T. Schubert, S. Waldzus, and B. Seibt, "The Embodiment of Power and Communalism in Space and Bodily Contact", in G. Semin and E. Smith (eds), *Embodied Grounding: Social, Cognitive, Affective, and Neuroscientific Approaches*, Cambridge, 160–183.
Schwartz/Power (2000): A.J. Schwartz and F.C. Power, "Maxims to Live by: The Art and Science of Teaching Wise Sayings", in: Brown (2000), 393–412.
Scodel (2008): R. Scodel, *Epic Facework: Self-presentation and Social Interaction in Homer*, Swansea.
Scodel (2014): R. Scodel, "Narrative Focus and Elusive Thought in Homer", in: D.L. Cairns and R. Scodel (eds), *Defining Greek Narrative*, Edinburgh, 55–74.
Scully (1986): S. Scully, "Studies of Narrative and Speech in the *Iliad*", in: *Arethusa* 19, 135–153.
Seaford (1994): R. Seaford, *Reciprocity and Ritual*, Oxford.
Seaford (1996): R. Seaford, *Euripides Bacchae*, Warminster.
Seaford (1997): R. Seaford, "Thunder, Lightning and Earthquake in the *Bacchae* and the *Acts of the Apostles*", in: A.B. Lloyd (ed.), *What is a God?*, London, 139–151.
Seaford (2005): R. Seaford, "Mystic Light in Aeschylus' *Bassarai*", in: *The Classical Quarterly* 55, 602–606.
Seaford (2010): R. Seaford, "Mystic Light and Near-Death Experience", in: M. Christopoulos et al. (eds), *Light and Darkness in Ancient Greek Religion*, Lanham, 201–206.
Seaford (2012): R. Seaford, *The Social Construction of Space and Time in the Tragedies of Aeschylus*, Cambridge.
Seaford (2013): R. Seaford, "The Politics of the Mystic Chorus", in: J. Billings, F. Budelmann and F. Macintosh (eds), *Choruses Ancient and Modern*, Oxford, 261–279.
Segal (1994): C. Segal, *Singers, Heroes and Gods in the* Odyssey, Ithaca.
Seligman/Maier (1967): M.E.P. Seligman, and S.F. Maier, "Failure to Escape Traumatic Shock", in: *Journal of Experimental Psychology* 74, 256–262.

Sennett (2008): R. Sennett, *The Craftsman*, London.
Settis (1988): S. Settis, "La Colonna: strategie di composizione, strategie di lettura", in: S. Settis et al. (eds), *La colonna traiana*, Turin, 60–129.
Shanske (2006): D. Shanske, *Thucydides and the Philosophical Origins of History*, Cambridge.
Sharrock (2000): A.R. Sharrock, "Constructing Characters in Propertius", in: *Arethusa* 33, 263–284.
Shay (2003): J. Shay, *Odysseus in America: Combat Trauma and the Trials of Homecoming*, London.
Shay (2010): J. Shay, *Achilles in Vietnam: Combat Trauma and the Undoing of Character*, London.
Sheets-Johnstone (1999): M. Sheets-Johnstone, "Emotion and Movement: A Beginning Empirical-phenomenological Analysis of their Relationship", in: *Journal of Consciousness Studies* 6, 259–277.
Sherif/Sherif (1956): M. Sherif and C.W. Sherif, *An Outline of Social Psychology*, New York.
Sherman et al. (1989): R. Sherman, J. Arena, C. Sherman, and J. Ernst, "The Mystery of Phantom Pain: Growing Evidence for Psychophysiological Mechanisms", in: *Biofeedback and Self-Regulation* 14.4, 267–280.
Shore (1996): B. Shore, *Culture in Mind*, Oxford.
Short (2012): W.M. Short, "A Roman Folk Model of the Mind", in: *Arethusa* 45.1, 109–147.
Short (2013): W.M. Short, "'Transmission' Accomplished? Latin's Alimentary Metaphors of Communication", in: *American Journal of Philology* 134.2, 247–275.
Shorter (2011): A. Shorter, *How Everyone Became Depressed: The Rise and Fall of the Nervous Breakdown*, Oxford and New York.
Simon (1978): B. Simon, *Mind and Madness in Ancient Greece: The Classical Roots of Modern Psychiatry*, Ithaca and London.
Singer (2013): P.N. Singer (ed.), *Galen: Psychological Writings*, Cambridge.
Skinner (1985): E.A. Skinner, "Action, Control Judgments, and the Structure of Control Experience", in: *Psychological Review* 92, 39–58.
Skinner (1996): M.B. Skinner, "Woman and Language in Archaic Greece, or, Why is Sappho a Woman?", in: E. Greene (ed.), *Reading Sappho: Contemporary Approaches*, Berkeley, 175–192.
Sluiter (2011): I. Sluiter, "Deliberation, Free Speech, and the Marketplace of Ideas", in: T. van Haaften, H. Jansen, J. de Jong, and W. Koetsenruijter (eds), *Bending Opinion*, Leiden, 25–49.
Smith (1999): R. Smith, "Logic", in: J. Barnes (ed.), *The Cambridge Companion to Aristotle*, Cambridge, 27–65.
Snell (1960): B. Snell, *The Discovery of the Mind*, trans. T.G. Rosenmeyer, Oxford.
Snyder (1997): J. McIntosh Snyder, *Lesbian Desire in the Lyrics of Sappho*, New York.
Solms/Turnbul (2011): M. Solms and O.H. Turnbull, "What Is Neuropsychoanalysis?", in: *Neuropsychoanalysis* 13.2, 133–145.
Sommerstein (1989): A. Sommerstein, *Aeschylus*: Eumenides, Cambridge.
Sommerstein (2010): A. Sommerstein, *Aeschylean Tragedy*, Bristol.
Sorabji (2000): R. Sorabji, *Emotion and Peace of Mind: From Stoic Agitation to Christian Temptation*, Oxford.
Spengel (1953): L. Spengel, *Rhetores Graeci. Vol 3*, Leipzig.
Sperber/Wilson (1981): D. Sperber and D. Wilson, "Irony and the Use-Mention Distinction", in: P. Cole (ed.), *Radical pragmatics*, New York, 295–318.
Stadter (1993): P.A. Stadter, "The Form and Content of Thucydides' Pentekontaetia", in: *Greek, Roman, and Byzantine Studies* 34, 35–72.

Stahl (1973): H.-P. Stahl, "Speeches and Course of Events in Books Six and Seven of Thucydides", in: P.A. Stadter (ed.), *The Speeches in Thucydides: A Collection of Original Studies with a Bibliography*, Chapel Hill, NC, 60–77.

Stahl (1985): H.-P. Stahl, *Propertius: "Love" and "War": Individual and State under Augustus*, Berkeley, Los Angeles and London.

Stahl (2006): H.-P. Stahl, "Narrative Unity and Consistency of Thought: Composition of Event Sequences in Thucydides", in: Rengakos/Tsakmakis (2006a), 301–334.

Stanford (1983): W.B. Stanford, *Greek Tragedy and the Emotions: An Introductory Study*, London.

Stehle (1996): E. Stehle, "Sappho's Gaze: Fantasies of a Goddess and Young Man", in: E. Greene (ed.), *Reading Sappho: Contemporary Approaches*, Berkeley, 193–225.

Stehle (1997): E. Stehle, *Performance and Gender in Ancient Greece: Nondramatic Poetry in Its Setting*, Princeton.

Stoklosa (2012): A. Stoklosa, "Chasing the Bear: William James on Sensations, Emotions and Instincts", in: *William James Studies* 9, 72.

Storr (1979): A. Storr, *The Art of Psychotherapy*, London.

Strauss (1964): L. Strauss, *The City and Man*, Chicago.

Suedfeld/Geiger (2008): P. Suedfeld and J. Geiger, "The Sensed Presence as a Coping Resource in Extreme Environments", in: J. Harold Ellens (ed.), *Miracles: God, Science, and Psychology in the Paranormal*, vol. III, Westport, 1–15.

Suedfeld/Mocellin (1987): P. Suedfeld and J.S.P. Mocellin, "The 'Sensed Presence' in Unusual Environments", in: *Environment and Behaviour* 19.1, 33–35.

Sullivan (1988): S.D. Sullivan, *Psychological Activity in Homer: A Study of Phrên*, Ottawa.

Sulloway (1979): F. Sulloway, *Freud: Biologist of the Mind*, Cambridge, MA.

Sunstein (2006): C. Sunstein, *Infotopia: How Many Minds Produce Knowledge*, Oxford and New York.

Sutton/Williamson (2014): J. Sutton and K. Williamson, "Embodied remembering", in: L. Shapiro (ed.), *The Routledge Handbook of Embodied Cognition*, Abingdon-on-Thames.

Syme (1939): R. Syme, *The Roman Revolution*, Oxford.

Tandy/Neale (1996): D. Tandy and W.C. Neale, *Hesiod's Works and Days: A Translation and Commentary for the Social Sciences*, Berkeley/London.

Tarlow (2012): S. Tarlow, "The Archaeology of Emotion and Affect", in: *Annual Review of Anthropology* 41, 170.

Tarrant (2006): R. Tarrant, "Propertian Textual Criticism and Editing", in: H.C. Günther (ed.), *Brill's Companion to Propertius*, Leiden and Boston, 45–65.

Taylor (1989): J. Taylor, *Linguistic Categorization: Prototypes in Linguistic Theory*, Oxford.

Taylor (1964): L.R. Taylor, "Magistrates of 55 in Cicero's *Pro Plancio* and Catullus 52", in: *Athenaeum* 42, 12–28.

Teffeteller (2003): A. Teffeteller, "Homeric Excuses", in: *The Classical Quarterly* 53, 15–31.

Thagard (1999): P. Thagard, *How Scientists Explain Disease*, Princeton.

Thalmann (1988): W.G. Thalmann, "Thersites: Comedy, Scapegoats and Heroic Ideology in the *Iliad*", in: *Transactions of the American Philological Association* 118, 1–28.

Thalmann (1998): W.G. Thalmann, *The Swineherd and the Bow*, Ithaca.

't Hart (1990): P. 't Hart, *Groupthink in Government: A Study of Small Groups and Policy Failure*, Amsterdam.

Thelen et al. (2001): E. Thelen, G. Schoner, C. Scheier, and L. Smith, "The Dynamics of Embodiment: A Field Theory of Infant Preservative Reaching", in: *Behavioral and Brain Sciences* 24, 1–86.

Theodorou (1993): Z. Theodorou, "Subject to Emotion: Exploring Madness in Orestes", in: *The Classical Quarterly* 43, 32–46.
Thibodeau/Boroditsky (2011): P. Thibodeau and L. Boroditsky, "Metaphors We Think With: The Role of Metaphor in Reasoning", in: *PLoS ONE* 6.2, e16782, doi:10.1371/journal.pone.0016782.
Thibodeau/Boroditsky (2013): P. Thibodeau and L. Boroditsky, "Natural Language Metaphors Covertly Influence Reasoning", in: *PLoS ONE* 8.1, e52961, doi:10.1371/journal.pone.0052961.
Thomas (1995): R. Thomas, "Written in Stone? Liberty, Equality, Orality and the Codification of Law", in: *Bulletin of the Institute of Classical Studies* 40.1, 59–74.
Thomas (2012): L. Thomas, *Building Student Engagement and Belonging at a Time of Change in Higher Education*, London.
Thomson (1941/1980): G. Thomson, *Aeschylus and Athens: A Study in the Social Origins of Drama*, London.
Tieleman (2003): T. Tieleman, *Chrysippus' On Affections: Reconstruction and Interpretation*, Leiden.
Tilmouth (2005): C. Tilmouth, "Burton's 'Turning Picture': Argument and Anxiety in the *Anatomy of Melancholy*", in: *The Review of English Studies*, New Series 56, 524–549.
Timpanaro (2005): S. Timpanaro, *The Genesis of Lachmann's Method*, trans. G.W. Most, Chicago and London.
Todorov (1982): T. Todorov, *Theories of the Symbol*, Ithaca.
Tomkins (1962): S.S. Tomkins, *Affect Imagery Consciousness: The Positive Affects (Vol. 1, ch. 9)*, New York.
Torrance (2013): I. Torrance, *Metapoetry in Euripides*, Oxford.
Tribble (2011): E.B. Tribble, *Cognition in the Globe: Attention and Memory in Shakespeare's Theatre*, New York.
Tribble/Sutton (2011): E.B. Tribble and J. Sutton, "Cognitive Ecology as a Framework for Shakespearean Studies", in: *Shakespeare Studies* 39, 94–103.
Tritle (2002): L. Tritle, *From Melos to My Lai: A Study in Violence, Culture and Social Survival*, London.
Tritle (2014): L. Tritle, "Ravished Minds in the Ancient World", in: Meineck/Konstan (2014), 87–104.
Tsakmakis (1995): A. Tsakmakis, *Thukydides über die Vergangenheit*, Tubingen.
Tsouna (2007): V. Tsouna, *The Ethics of Philodemus*, Oxford.
Tudebodis (1866): P. Tudebodis, "Historia de Hierosolymitano Itinere", in: *Recueil des Historiens des Croisades. Historiens Occidentaux* III, Paris [original publication: c. 1100].
Turner (1990): M. Turner, "Aspects of the Invariance Hypothesis", in: *Cognitive Linguistics* 1.2, 247–255.
Turner (1996): M. Turner, *The Literary Mind: The Origins of Thought and Language*, Oxford.
Twesten (1815): A. Twesten, *Commentatio critica de Hesiodi carmine quod inscribitur Opera et Dies*, Kiel.
Usdin (1976): E. Usdin, *Catecholamines and Stress*, Oxford.
Ustinova (2013): Y. Ustinova, "To Live in Joy and Die with Hope: Experiential Aspects of Ancient Greek Mystery Rites", in: *Bulletin of the Institute of Classical Studies* 56.2, 110–123.
Vallée-Tourangeau/Anthony/Austin (1998): F. Vallée-Tourangeau, S. Anthony, and N. Austin, "Strategies for Generating Multiple Instances of Common and Ad-Hoc Categories", in: *Memory* 6, 555–592.

Van den Zwaal (1988): P. Van den Zwaal, "Psychoanalysis as a Rediscovery of Classical Rhetoric", in: F. Ackerman and A.J. Vanderjagt (eds), *Rodolphus Agricola Phrisius, 1444–1485*, Leiden, New York, Kobenhavn, and Köln, 302–311.

Van der Valk (1949): M. van Der Valk, *Textual Criticism of the Odyssey*, Leiden.

Van Noorden (2014): H. Van Noorden, *Playing Hesiod: The 'Myth of the Races' in Classical Antiquity*, Cambridge.

Van Nortwick (2009): T. Van Nortwick, *The Unknown Odysseus: Alternate Worlds in Homer's Odyssey*, Ann Arbor.

Van Straten/Cuijpers/Smits (2008): A. Van Straten, P. Cuijpers, and N. Smits, "Effectiveness of a Web-Based Self-help Intervention for the Symptoms of Depression, Anxiety, and Stress: Randomized Controlled Trial", in: *Journal of Medical Internet Research* 10, e7.

Van Voorhees (2011): Benjamin W. Van Voorhees *et al.*, "Internet-Based Depression Prevention over the Life Course: a Call for Behavioral Vaccines", in: *Psychiatric Clinics of North America* 34.1, 167–183.

Varela/Rosch/Thompson (1992): F.J. Varela, E. Rosch, and E. Thompson, *The Embodied Mind: Cognitive Science and Human Experience*, Cambridge, MA.

Vargados (forthcoming): A. Vargados, *Hesiod's Verbal Craft: Studies in Hesiod's Conception of Language and its Ancient Reception*, Oxford.

Ventura/Fernandes/Cohen/Morais/Kolinsky/Dehaene (2013): P. Ventura, T. Fernandes, L. Cohen, J. Morais, R. Kolinsky, and S. Dehaene, "Literacy Acquisition Reduces the Influence of Automatic Holistic Processing of Faces and Houses", in: *Neuroscience Letters* 554, 105–109.

Verdenius (1985): W.J. Verdenius, *A Commentary on Hesiod Works and Days vv.1-382*, Leiden.

Vernant (1990): J.-P. Vernant, "Intimations of the Will in Greek Tragedy", in: *Myth and Tragedy in Ancient Greece*, trans. J. Lloyd, New York.

Voigt (1971): E.-M. Voigt, *Sappho et Alcaeus. Fragmenta*, Amsterdam.

Volk (2002): K. Volk, *The Poetics of Latin Didactic: Lucretius, Vergil, Ovid, Manilius*, Oxford.

Walsh (2011): R. Walsh, "Lifestyle and Mental Health", in: *American Psychologist* 66, 579–592.

Ward/Stapleton (2012): D. Ward and M. Stapleton, "Es are good: Cognition as Enacted, Embodied, Embedded, Affective and Extended", in: F. Paglieri (ed.), *Consciousness in Interaction: The Role of the Natural and Social Environment in Shaping Consciousness*, Amsterdam, 89–104.

Watters (2010): E. Watters, *Crazy Like Us: The Globalization of the American Psyche*, London.

Wear (1985): A. Wear, "Explorations in Renaissance writings on the Practice of Medicine", in: A. Wear, R.K. French, and I.M. Lonie (eds), *The Medical Renaissance of the Sixteenth Century*, Cambridge, 118–145.

Webb (1997): R. Webb, "Imagination and the Arousal of the Emotions in Greco-Roman Rhetoric", in: S. Braund and C. Gill (eds), *The Passions in Roman Thought and Literature*, Cambridge, 112–127.

Webb (2009): R. Webb, *Ekphrasis, Imagination and Persuasion in Ancient Rhetorical Theory and Practice*. Burlington.

Weiss (1993): P. Weiss, "Die Vision Constantins", in: J. Bleicken (ed.), *Colloquium aus Anlass des 80. Geburstages von Alfred Heuss* (Frankfurter althistorische Studien 13), Kallmünz, 143–169 [trans. into English by A.R. Birley, with revisions and additions by the author as "The Vision of Constantine", *Journal of Roman Archaeology* 2003, 16, 237–259].

Wertheimer (1923): M. Wertheimer, "Untersuchungen zur Lehre von der Gestalt, II", in: *Psychologische Forschung* 4, 301–350.

West (1965): M.L. West, "Tryphon *De Tropis*", in: *The Classical Quarterly* 15.2, 230–248.
West (1978): M.L. West, *Hesiod Works and Days*, Oxford.
Whalley (2014): K. Whalley, "Epigenetics: Early Trauma Alters Sperm RNA", in: *Nature Reviews Neuroscience* 15.6, 349–349.
Wheeldon (1989): M. Wheeldon, "True Stories: The Reception of Historiography in Antiquity", in: A. Cameron (ed.), *History as Text: The Writing of Ancient History*, London, 33–63.
White (2007): M. White, *Maps of Narrative Practice*, New York.
White (2011): M. White, *Narrative Practice: Continuing the Conversations*, New York.
Wichers (2014): M. Wichers, "The Dynamic Nature of Depression: a New Micro-Level Perspective of Mental Disorder that Meets Current Challenges", in: *Psychological Medicine* 44, 1349–1360.
Wieland (1996): C. Wieland, "Matricide and Destructiveness: Infantile Anxieties and Technological Culture", in: *British Journal of Psychotherapy* 12, 300–313.
Wilcox (2010): C. Wilcox, *Groupthink: An Impediment to Success*, Bloomsfield.
Wilkowski et al. (2009): B. Wilkowski, B. Meier, M. Robinson, M. Carter, and R. Feltman, "'Hot-headed' is More than an Expression: The Embodied Representation of Anger in Terms of Heat", in: *Emotion* 9, 464–477.
Williams (1993): B. Williams, *Shame and Necessity*, Berkeley.
Williams/Bargh (2008): L. Williams and J. Bargh, "Experiencing Physical Warmth Promotes Interpersonal Warmth", in: *Science* 322, 606–607.
Williamson (1996): M. Williamson, "Sappho and the Other Woman", in: E. Greene (ed.), *Reading Sappho: Contemporary Approaches*, Berkeley, 248–264.
Wilson (2002): M. Wilson, "Six Views of Embodied Cognition", in: *Psychonomic Bulletin and Review* 9, 625–636.
Wilson/Gibbs (2007): N.L. Wilson and R.W. Gibbs, "Real and Imagined Body Movement Primes Metaphor Comprehension", in: *Cognitive Science* 31, 721–731.
Wilson/Sperber (2012): D. Wilson and D. Sperber, *Meaning and Relevance*, Cambridge.
Winkler (1996): J.J. Winkler, "Gardens of Nymphs: Public and Private in Sappho's Lyrics", in: E. Greene (ed.), *Reading Sappho: Contemporary Approaches*, Berkeley, 89–109.
Winkler/Zeitlin (1992): J.J. Winkler and F.I. Zeitlin, *Nothing to do with Dionysos? Athenian Drama in its Social Context*, Princeton.
Winnington-Ingram (1983): R.P. Winnington-Ingram, *Studies in Aeschylus*, Cambridge.
Wiseman (1993): T. Wiseman, "Lying Historians: Seven Types of Mendacity", in: C. Gill and T. Wiseman (eds), *Lies and Fiction in the Ancient World,* Exeter, 122–146.
Woodman (1988): A. Woodman, *Rhetoric in Classical Historiography,* Portland.
Wyatt (1909): W.F. Wyatt, "The Intermezzo of *Odyssey* 11, and the Poets Homer and Odysseus", in: *Studi Micenei ed Egeo-Anatolici* 27, 235–253.
Wyke (1987): M. Wyke, "Written Women: Propertius' *Scripta Puella*", in: *Journal of Roman Studies* 77, 47–61.
Wyke (1989): M. Wyke, "Mistress and Metaphor in Augustan Elegy", in: *Helios* 16, 25–47.
Yarbus (1967): A.L. Yarbus, *Eye Movements During Perception of Complex Objects*, New York.
Yu (2003): N. Yu, "Metaphor, Body and Culture: The Chinese Understanding of Gallbladder and Courage", in: *Metaphor and Symbol* 18.1, 13–31.
Yu (2008): N. Yu, "Metaphor from Body and Culture", in: R. Gibbs (ed.), *The Cambridge Handbook of Metaphor and Thought,* Cambridge, 247–261.
Yunis (1996): H. Yunis, *Taming Democracy: Models of Political Rhetoric in Classical Athens*, Ithaca, NY.

Zaborowski (2003): R. Zaborowski. "Tadeusz Zieliński and the Homeric Psychology", in: *Eos* 90, 291–300.
Zachar (2014): P. Zachar, *A Metaphysics of Psychopathology*, Cambridge, MA.
Zajko/O'Gorman (2013): V. Zajko and E. O'Gorman (eds), *Classical Myth and Psychoanalysis: Ancient and Modern Stories of the Self*, Oxford.
Zeitlin (1965): F.I. Zeitlin, "The Motif of Corrupted Sacrifice in Aeschylus' Oresteia", in: *Transactions of the American Philological Association* 96, 463–508.
Zieliński (2002): T. Zieliński, "Homeric Psychology", in: *Organon* 31, 15–45.
Zlatev (2007): J. Zlatev, "Spatial Semantics", in: H. Cuyckens and D. Geeraerts (eds), *The Oxford Handbook of Cognitive Linguistics*, Oxford, 318–350.
Zoccola (2007): V. Zoccola, "L'ironia nell'*Hecyra di Terenzio*", in: *Orpheus* 28.1–2, 265–301.
Zunshine (2006): L. Zunshine, *Why We Read Fiction: Theory of Mind and the Novel*, Columbus.
Zunshine (2015): L. Zunshine, *The Oxford Handbook of Cognitive Literary Studies*, London.
Zwann/Madden (2005): R. Zwann and C. Madden, "Embodied Sentence Comprehension", in: D. Pecher and R. Zwann (eds), *Grounding Cognition: The Role of Perception and Action in Memory, Language, and Thinking*, Cambridge, 224–245.

Index

πικρός 71, 72, 73, 74, 75

acceptance and commitment therapy (ACT) 285
a cognitive historiography 84
Acts of the Apostles 257
Aeschylus 8, 65, 67, 68, 69, 71, 72, 75, 91, 110, 158, 160, 161, 163, 165, 166, 167, 168
Aeschylus' trilogy 8, 165
Affect(ive)/cultural neuroscience/neuroscientist 77
afterlife 172
anger 17, 36, 38, 39, 41, 42, 55, 56, 67, 68, 69, 71, 72, 73, 236, 243, 269, 280
animal sacrifice 258
animation 53
animus 28
anticipated audience response 150
anxiety 36, 38, 39, 40, 41, 65, 66, 85, 115, 116, 132, 184, 231, 237, 258
apparition (*phasma*) 96
archaic 22, 142, 191, 204
Aristophanes Frogs 256
Aristotelianism 264, 270
Aristotle 9, 53, 67, 68, 77, 78, 80, 226, 227, 228, 229, 230, 231, 232, 233, 266, 270
Art therapy 109, 112, 113, 114, 117
assemblage 184
Athens 8, 85, 91, 92, 160, 165, 236, 239, 242, 246, 248, 250, 251, 252, 253
Attic theater 63
audience 4, 6, 7, 38, 41, 43, 45, 47, 56, 57, 62, 64, 65, 67, 68, 69, 71, 73, 77, 78, 79, 80, 83, 85, 86, 88, 89, 91, 92, 93, 111, 115, 129, 130, 131, 133, 134, 137, 142, 143, 144, 145, 147, 151, 152, 153, 154, 156, 157, 160, 162, 166, 167, 189, 190, 197, 201, 210, 212, 217, 218, 219, 220, 221, 223, 232, 236, 258, 289
audience empathic responses 62, 63
authenticity 108
authority 49, 50, 65, 147, 149, 156, 160, 169, 182, 183, 185, 231, 288

Bacchae 255, 256, 257, 258, 259
Bakhtin 194
behaviourism 284
beliefs 42, 83, 94, 100, 169, 202, 229, 247, 248, 269, 270, 271, 279, 280, 284, 285, 286, 287, 288
belief schema 284
bio-cultural approach 82, 83, 85
biology 82, 83, 90, 226
blood imagery 76
Buddhism 285
Burton, R. 9, 277

catharsis 78, 162, 166
choice (prohairesis) 289
Christianity 105, 106, 107, 255, 268, 269
Cicero 8, 21, 24, 46, 48, 49, 50, 53, 54, 55, 56, 60, 222, 234
Cixous 190, 191, 196, 203
clinical perspective 131
Clytemnestra 159, 160, 162, 163, 166, 167
cognition 2, 13, 14, 15, 16, 45, 47, 78, 79, 81, 82, 83, 84, 85, 86, 87, 88, 152, 157, 274, 284, 285, 286, 287
cognitive 7, 9, 10, 28, 45, 47, 49, 62, 63, 65, 67, 68, 70, 71, 76, 93, 142, 143, 144, 145, 146, 151, 156, 157, 266, 269, 270, 271, 272, 273, 274, 275, 276, 284, 285, 286, 287
cognitive and behavioural psychotherapy (CBT) 276, 278, 279, 280, 281, 283, 284, 285, 286, 287, 289, 290, 291
cognitive distancing 290
cognitive embodiment 78, 79
cognitive neuroscience 273
cognitive psychiatry 273
cognitive psychology 6, 13, 15, 130, 143, 284
cognitivism 262, 274
collaboration/collective 1, 58, 87, 110, 117, 118, 119, 121, 164, 168, 172, 179, 188, 248, 250, 289, 291
collective psyche 250
communication 9, 111, 210, 278, 281, 282

community 7, 62, 65, 74, 109, 110, 120, 121, 163
comparative cognitive approach 86
conceptual metaphor 13, 16, 43, 49, 50
conformism 106, 152, 240, 245, 249, 250, 274
conjunctions 21, 76, 96, 184
Constantine 105, 106, 107
constructionist 81, 82
'container' metaphor 68
continuity 148, 169
cooperative principle 210, 211, 221
counter-transference 232
Cynthia 174, 175, 176, 177, 180, 183, 184

damnatio memoriae 50
Darwin 41, 42, 80
decision-making 38, 136, 139, 239, 240, 241, 242, 243, 244, 245, 250, 252
declarative memory 154
defense mechanism 260
Deleuze, Gilles 8, 172, 174, 178, 180, 181, 183, 186
dēmos 243, 245, 248, 249, 250, 252
De Oratore 46, 54, 57, 60, 208
depersonalization 260
depression 122, 132, 262, 275, 276
derealization 260
desire 2, 3, 8, 35, 38, 66, 68, 69, 120, 165, 171, 172, 173, 174, 175, 176, 180, 181, 183, 184, 185, 187, 188, 193, 196, 198, 199, 200, 203, 215, 224, 226, 239, 246, 250, 260, 288
developmental psychology 8
dialectical 225, 226, 227, 228, 229, 230, 231, 238
dialogism 196, 197
didactic poetry 144
Dionysos 91, 255, 258, 259
discours and parole 232
discoveries/anagnōriseis 78
disgust 6, 56, 67, 72, 73, 74
disposition 58, 64, 67, 70, 148, 224, 265, 272, 277
dissociation 80, 260
distaste 73, 75, 76
distributed cognition 78, 79, 83, 84

dream 164, 185, 224, 229, 233
Du Laurens, A. 268

echoic irony 213
education 110, 125, 136, 148, 157
Ekman, Paul 80
elegy 8, 172, 173, 182, 186
Eleusinian mysteries 255, 256, 258
ellipsis 223, 225
embellishment 105
embodied 5, 6, 7, 13, 14, 15, 16, 26, 36, 47, 51, 53, 54, 57, 58, 59, 60, 62, 77, 78, 79, 80, 81, 82, 122, 189, 262
embodied cognition 5, 6, 47, 62, 72
embodied emotion 78, 80
embodied framework 47, 54
embodied metaphor 6, 62, 67, 76
embodiment theory 81
emotion 9, 32, 38, 39, 41, 42, 47, 53, 55, 56, 57, 58, 59, 60, 62, 63, 64, 66, 67, 70, 72, 73, 76, 78, 80, 86, 87, 112, 114, 116, 117, 130, 146, 230, 236, 237, 243, 269, 274, 275, 278, 280, 282, 284, 285, 286, 287, 288
emotional communities 7, 76, 81
emotional contagion 54, 56, 80, 86
emotionological framework 49, 53
enactivist couplings 16
enargeia 6, 53
Eos 201
ephebe 159
epic 21, 32, 78, 129, 130, 131, 137, 138, 140, 146, 155, 189, 200, 202, 217
epigenetics 82
ethics 278, 279, 289
ethos 9, 66, 70, 223, 225, 230, 231, 232, 235, 237
eudaimonia 270, 279
Euripides 78, 90, 91, 92, 161, 167, 169, 255, 256, 257, 259
Eusebius of Caesarea 105
exercise 9, 197, 266, 268, 270, 271, 272, 290
expectancy model 260
experientialist 6, 14, 15

faculty psychology 262, 264
fear 7, 39, 40, 41, 57, 58, 59, 64, 66, 67, 70, 72, 78, 81, 111, 114, 117, 241, 242, 243, 244, 245, 247, 248, 249, 250, 251, 255, 257, 264, 267, 269, 271, 272, 275, 284
feminine voice 8, 190, 191, 203
feminist criticism 8, 190
"fight-or-flight" response 26
figurative 15, 17, 23, 24, 35, 49, 213
folk psychology 6, 7, 131, 133
fragment 178 256
free associations 224, 225, 227, 234, 235
functional contextualism 285
functionalism 14, 273
funeral 243, 258

Galen 263, 267, 279, 287
gestalt 15, 16
Gestalt 155
gestalt structures 15
greed (pleonexia) 239, 245
Grice, P 208, 210, 211, 213, 217
Groupthink 9, 253
Guattari, Félix 8, 172, 173, 174, 178, 180, 181, 183, 186
gustatory metaphors 6, 67, 69, 71, 74, 76

habit 14, 71, 122, 266, 268, 270, 272, 273, 275, 277
habituation 272, 277
hallucination/hallucinatory 168, 169, 260
happiness 279, 280
Harrison, Jane Ellen 159, 162
healing (remedy) 7, 122, 266, 272, 276
Herodotus 51, 54, 58, 77, 101, 208
Hesiod 7, 142, 143, 144, 145, 146, 147, 148, 149, 150, 151, 152, 153, 154, 155, 156, 157, 160
historiography 6, 61, 84, 85
history 1, 2, 46, 47, 60, 78, 80, 82, 95, 102, 105, 107, 110, 112, 151, 173, 188, 239, 244, 266, 278, 279, 280, 284
Homer 6, 7, 32, 35, 42, 43, 45, 53, 129, 201, 217
Homeric psychology 130, 131
homogeneity 95

honour 102, 244, 247
hypertext 186

imagery 42, 44, 56, 76, 100, 107, 112, 158, 165, 201
image schema 6, 7, 28
imagination 63, 111, 255, 264, 265, 266, 268, 269, 270, 271, 274, 275
impression (phantasia) 286
initiation ritual 257
intertextuality 217
inventio 47
Irigaray, Luce 189, 190, 191, 195, 202, 203
irony (*eironeia*) 236
Isocrates 78
iteration 49, 54, 55, 56, 58, 172
iterative 54

Jones, Ernest 223
Jorgensen, J. 213

kinetic memory 146
Klein, Melanie 168, 175
krasis 270

language 6, 13, 15, 16, 17, 26, 35, 37, 47, 49, 59, 60, 63, 64, 67, 68, 69, 71, 72, 76, 82, 89, 90, 138, 139, 158, 160, 163, 170, 190, 200, 213, 215, 224, 228, 229, 232, 249, 290
Learned helplessness 129
Learned Helplessness 7
LeMeSurier 70, 71
Livy 20, 21, 25, 49, 50, 56, 57, 59
logos 9, 223, 224, 230
lust (*erōs*) 25, 72, 239, 245
lyric poetry 8, 189
lyric self or selves 193, 194, 196

madness 68, 78, 158, 161, 163, 164, 165, 167, 168, 169, 170, 267
male (symbolic) discourse 200
mask 7, 63, 77, 78, 85, 89, 92, 93
mask perception 77
matricide 164, 166, 168, 170
medicine 262, 264, 269, 273, 276

326 —— Index

melancholy 262, 263, 264, 265, 266, 267, 268, 269, 271, 272, 273, 275, 276, 277
memory 44, 46, 48, 51, 53, 56, 59, 63, 91, 104, 105, 117, 146, 152, 154, 156, 194, 195, 196, 198, 229, 264, 265, 274
mention theory of irony 213
metaphor 6, 7, 13, 18, 32, 34, 35, 36, 38, 41, 42, 43, 46, 62, 82, 163, 164, 173, 200, 201, 211, 212, 232, 267
method 4, 9, 58, 80, 108, 109, 113, 118, 120, 122, 154, 224, 228, 229, 231, 235, 262, 270, 280, 281, 283, 284, 289, 290, 291
metonymy 49, 53, 225
Mikkel Borch-Jacobsen 230
Miller, G. 213
mind-body 38, 274
mindfulness 276, 284, 285, 289, 290
mirror-stage 175
mnemonic 83, 152
Monobiblos 171
morality 246, 247, 249
moral processing 73, 76
motus animi 60, 282
mystic initiation 255, 257, 258
myth 2, 3, 69, 78, 115, 151, 152, 153, 160, 161, 164, 223, 257, 258, 259, 261

Nachträglichkeit 229
narrative strategy 151
nature 14, 15, 20, 60, 61, 64, 65, 69, 75, 80, 87, 98, 116, 117, 120, 131, 152, 162, 163, 181, 183, 226, 227, 233, 237, 241, 242, 244, 247, 251, 253, 257, 289
near death experience 9, 255
need for cognition 145, 152, 157
neurobiology 227, 275
neurotransmitter 27

Odysseus 6, 32, 35, 36, 37, 38, 39, 40, 41, 42, 43, 44, 45, 129, 200, 201
Odyssey 6, 7, 45, 129, 132, 133, 200
oracle 51, 101, 158, 160, 161, 163, 166
orality 144
Orestes 8, 158

paralipsis 235
paranoia 174

passions 262, 264, 265, 266, 268, 273, 274, 275, 276, 280
paternalism 158
pathos 9, 60, 223, 225, 230, 232, 235, 237
performance 62, 63, 66, 71, 72, 77, 78, 79, 80, 85, 116, 131, 132, 145, 152, 155, 196, 197, 200, 203, 225
periphrasis 225
persuasion 54, 74, 143, 163, 165, 210, 225, 229, 230, 231, 233, 234, 235, 236, 238
phantasy 270
philology 2, 8, 10, 171, 187, 188
physiology 17, 274
Plater, F. 268
Plato 63, 64, 78, 80, 92, 189, 228, 229, 236, 256, 257, 259
Plato Phaedo 259
Plato Phaedrus 256, 257
Plautus 21
Plutarch 62, 77, 92, 96, 101, 202, 255, 256, 257, 258, 279, 287
pollution 65, 74, 76
polyphonic poetry 190
pretence theory of irony 217
prevention 272, 273, 276, 277
Prinz, Jesse 15, 64, 79, 81
procedural memory 154
procession 164, 165, 170, 258
Propertius 8, 21, 188
proprioceptive 27
Prudentia 60
psychoanalysis 1, 2, 3, 5, 113, 114, 172, 223, 224, 225, 226, 227, 229, 230, 231, 233, 234, 235, 238, 278, 279, 280, 283

Quintilian 6, 53, 188, 209, 210, 211, 213, 217, 219, 220, 234

rationalization 248
reception 3, 4, 8, 10, 81, 143, 145, 156, 157, 187
remembering 58, 61, 70, 118, 143, 145, 146, 152, 158, 170, 192, 193, 194, 198, 199, 265
reputation 102, 148, 231, 288
responsibility 129, 163, 167, 169, 170

reversals/peripeteiai 78
rhetoric 1, 6, 9, 47, 50, 53, 54, 55, 56, 58, 60, 74, 142, 208, 210, 211, 218, 220, 224, 225, 226, 229, 230, 231, 232, 233, 234, 235, 236, 243
Rhetorica ad Herennium 208, 209, 210, 211
rhetorical 6, 8, 47, 48, 55, 60, 144, 147, 152, 158, 201, 210, 238, 244, 245
ritual/ritualism 9, 62, 65, 71, 76, 83, 86, 161, 166, 169, 255, 257, 258, 259, 261
role-playing 144, 146
rumination 134, 138, 275

Sallust 58, 59
Sappho 8, 189, 191, 192, 193, 194, 195, 196, 197, 198, 199, 200, 201, 203
schizoanalysis 184, 185, 186
Scipio 22, 25, 50
self care 268, 269, 277
self-interest 244, 245, 247, 252
self-knowledge 274
"semnai theai" 166
Sensed Presence 108
Sensed Presence and non-Sensed Presence 7
sensorimotor interaction 15
Seven Against Thebes 6, 62, 65, 69
social production 180
soul-moving/psychagôgia 78
Sperber, D. 213
sphragis 179, 187
stemmatics 171
stereotype 27, 121, 248, 249
Stoicism 9, 269, 286, 287, 289, 291
Stoicism Today project 123
Stoics 264, 269, 270
supplication 212, 213, 258
synesthesia 67

teaching 47, 92, 113, 125, 144, 148, 149, 152, 153, 154, 156, 157
technology 112

Telemachy 131, 136, 137
testimony/nies 100, 101, 234
theology 262, 263
therapy 7, 9, 85, 109, 110, 112, 113, 114, 117, 223, 224, 225, 226, 227, 229, 231, 276, 278, 279, 280, 281, 282, 283, 284, 285, 286, 287, 291
The Votives Project 111
Thucydides 9, 49, 60, 85, 253
transference 56, 224, 225, 230, 231, 232, 235, 237, 238
trauma 7, 85, 95, 100, 113, 230, 278
trope 189, 209, 210, 217, 219, 220, 233, 234, 235, 236
truth 4, 8, 46, 47, 52, 60, 148, 149, 150, 151, 152, 211, 225, 227, 228, 229, 232, 233, 236

universal 4, 7, 17, 56, 65, 81, 82, 83, 87, 95, 156, 164, 180, 227, 244, 260
universalist 81
up-to-us (*eph' hēmin*) 288

values 6, 8, 64, 65, 66, 74, 82, 105, 120, 121, 142, 152, 156, 189, 195, 216, 220, 222, 235, 236, 241, 268, 269, 290
Vergil 20
violation 65
virtual votives 111
virtue 53, 54, 98, 220, 279, 280, 290
voice 8, 94, 97, 98, 100, 114, 155, 172, 174, 176, 177, 178, 186, 187, 188, 189, 190, 191, 195, 196, 199, 203, 213

wedding 199, 258
Weyer, J. 268
Wilson, D. 36, 213
Winnicott, Donald 114

Xenophon 77, 80